Praise for
League of Denial

"Meticulously documented and endlessly chilling."

—*New York Times*

"*League of Denial* may turn out to be the most influential sports-related book of our time."

—*Boston Globe*, **Best Sports Books of 2013**

"The book should come with a warning label for football fans: Watching a game will never be the same after you read it . . . [Fainaru-Wada and Fainaru] ask tough questions of the NFL without taking their conclusions too far."

—**NPR, Best Books of 2013**

"It is meticulously researched, artfully structured, engaging, and well written. . . . This is an informative, intriguing, and sobering book about power and control. I recommend it strongly."

—**Nate Jackson,** *Washington Post*

"Journalistically bruising."

—**Peter King**

"Clear-eyed and devastating."

—*San Francisco Chronicle*

"Mark Fainaru-Wada and Steve Fainaru's book *League of Denial* should be required reading in secondary schools for all athletes. Those of us outside the lines will be wiser as well for having invested just a few hours to read it."

—**Tim Cowlishaw,** *Dallas Morning News*

LEAGUE OF DENIAL

THE NFL, CONCUSSIONS,

AND THE

BATTLE FOR TRUTH

MARK FAINARU-WADA
AND STEVE FAINARU

THREE RIVERS PRESS

NEW YORK

Originally published in hardcover in the United States by Crown Archetype,
an imprint of the Crown Publishing Group, a division of Random House LLC,
New York, in 2013.

Library of Congress Cataloging-in-Publication Data is available upon request.

ISBN 978-0-7704-3756-5
eBook ISBN 978-0-7704-3755-8

Printed in the United States of America

Cover design by Michael Nagin
Cover photograph: Nick Veasey/Getty Images

10 9 8 7 6 5 4 3 2 1

First Paperback Edition

To the three remarkable women in our lives—

Nicole,

Maureen,

and our mother, Ellen Gilbert

CONTENTS

Authors' Note   ix

Principal Characters   xi

Prologue: Bird Brains   1

PART ONE   DISCOVERY

1. The Nutcracker   13
2. Psych 101   31
3. "Dad Is in Ohio"   47
4. Fuck You, Jerry Maguire   63
5. The Mike Webster Health Care System   83
6. The Vanilla Guy   106

PART TWO   DENIAL

7. Galen of Pergamon   125
8. Onyemalukwube   148
9. The Dissenters   166
10. "The Lady Doth Protest Too Much"   188
11. A Man of Science   207
12. The Brain Hunters   229

PART THREE   RECKONING

13. The Art of Disease   249
14. Big Football   266
15. "Please, See That My Brain Is Given to the NFL's
    Brain Bank"   286
16. Concussion, Inc.   306
17. Buzzards   324

Epilogue: Scars of the Gladiators   341

Afterword   353
Acknowledgments   363
Source Notes   367
Bibliography   391
Photo Insert Credits   397
Index   399

AUTHORS' NOTE

This book benefited greatly from the work of people who joined us at different stages of the research. Sabrina Shankman, a reporter for *Frontline,* the PBS investigative news program, spent nearly a year on the project, conducting numerous interviews and gathering information on everything from the biomechanics of helmet testing to the NFL's courtship of mommy bloggers. She is a tireless, smart, and resourceful reporter and a wonderful colleague. Her work can be found throughout the book. Kevin Fixler, a recent graduate of the UC Berkeley Graduate School of Journalism and a freelance sportswriter based in Denver, and Maureen Fan, the former Beijing correspondent for the *Washington Post,* also contributed essential research. We were fortunate to have such outstanding collaborators, each of whom strengthened the book in ways that are visible and others that are not.

PRINCIPAL CHARACTERS

THE NATIONAL FOOTBALL LEAGUE

Paul J. Tagliabue, *Commissioner, 1989–2006*
Roger S. Goodell, *Commissioner, 2006–*
Jeff Pash, *Executive Vice President and General Counsel*
Greg Aiello, *Director of Communications*

THE NFL MILD TRAUMATIC BRAIN INJURY COMMITTEE

Elliot J. Pellman, M.D., *Chairperson, 1994–2007*
Ira R. Casson, M.D., *Cochairman, 2007–2009*
David C. Viano, Ph.D., *Cochairman, 2007–2009*
Henry Feuer, M.D.
Mark R. Lovell, Ph.D.
Joseph F. Waeckerle, M.D.
Joseph C. Maroon, M.D.

THE DISSENTERS

Kevin M. Guskiewicz, Ph.D., ATC, *University of North Carolina, Chapel Hill*
Robert C. Cantu, M.D., *Emerson Hospital, Concord, Massachusetts*
Julian E. Bailes Jr., M.D., *NorthShore Neurological Institute, Evanston, Illinois*
William B. Barr, Ph.D., *New York University Medical Center, New York, New York*
Leigh Steinberg, *Sports Agent, Newport Beach, California*

THE OMALU GROUP

Bennet I. Omalu, M.D., *Chief Medical Examiner, San Joaquin County, Lodi, California*

Julian E. Bailes Jr., M.D., *NorthShore Neurological Institute, Evanston, Illinois*

Robert P. Fitzsimmons, *Attorney, Wheeling, West Virginia*

Garrett Webster, *son of Mike Webster, Moon Township, Pennsylvania*

THE BU GROUP

Christopher Nowinski, *Sports Legacy Institute, Boston University Center for the Study of Traumatic Encephalopathy, Boston, Massachusetts*

Ann C. McKee, M.D., *Edith Nourse Rogers Memorial Veterans Hospital*

Robert C. Cantu, M.D., *Emerson Hospital, Concord, Massachusetts*

Robert A. Stern, Ph.D., *Boston University School of Medicine, Boston, Massachusetts*

KEY NFL PLAYERS

Troy Aikman, *Quarterback, Dallas Cowboys, 1989–2000*

Harry Carson, *Linebacker, New York Giants, 1976–1988*

Dave Duerson (deceased), *Defensive Back, Chicago Bears, 1983–1989; New York Giants, 1990; Phoenix Cardinals, 1991–1993*

John Grimsley (deceased), *Linebacker, Houston Oilers, 1984–1990; Miami Dolphins, 1992–1993*

Merril Hoge, *Running Back, Pittsburgh Steelers, 1987–1993; Chicago Bears, 1994*

Ted Johnson, *Linebacker, New England Patriots, 1995–2004*

Terry Long (deceased), *Guard, Pittsburgh Steelers, 1984–1991*

John Mackey (deceased), *Tight End, Baltimore Colts, 1963–1971; San Diego Chargers, 1972*

Tom McHale (deceased), *Guard, Tampa Bay Buccaneers, 1987–1992; Philadelphia Eagles, 1993–1994; Miami Dolphins, 1995*

Gary Plummer, *Linebacker, San Diego Chargers, 1986–1993; San Francisco 49ers, 1994–1997*

Junior Seau (deceased), *Linebacker, San Diego Chargers, 1990–2002;
 Miami Dolphins, 2003–2005; New England Patriots, 2006–2009*
Justin Strzelczyk (deceased), *Guard-Tackle, Pittsburgh Steelers,
 1990–1998*
Al Toon, *Wide Receiver, New York Jets, 1985–1992*
Andre Waters (deceased), *Safety, Philadelphia Eagles, 1984–1993;
 Arizona Cardinals, 1994–1995*
Mike Webster (deceased), *Center, Pittsburgh Steelers, 1974–1988;
 Kansas City Chiefs, 1989–1990*
Steve Young, *Quarterback, Los Angeles Express (USFL), 1984–1985;
 Tampa Bay Buccaneers, 1985–1986; San Francisco 49ers,
 1987–1999*

LEAGUE OF DENIAL

BIRD BRAINS

Behold the mighty woodpecker.

On average, it weighs about 2 ounces and can generate up to 1,000 g forces while pecking at tree limbs 12,000 times a day. Yet the woodpecker's brain remains pristine and unscathed, a fact that has intrigued researchers for decades. Nature essentially has turned the woodpecker into a shock absorber from beak to foot. The bird's uneven bill deflects much of the impact of its incessant head banging. A third interior eyelid prevents its eyeballs from popping out. The woodpecker's tongue is one of the most unusual features in nature. It extends from the back of the bird's mouth and through its right nostril, finally wrapping itself snugly around the entire crown of the head. Chinese researchers who subjected the great spotted woodpecker and the Eurasian hoopoe to super-slow-motion replay and CT scans concluded that the tongue serves as a kind of safety belt for the brain.

In the late 2000s, Julian Bailes displayed a woodpecker skull in a jar on top of his desk in Morgantown, West Virginia. Bailes was a top neurosurgeon and a former team doctor for the Pittsburgh Steelers. He incurred the wrath of the NFL when he joined a small group of researchers who concluded that football was causing brain damage in an alarming number of former players. During a closed-door meeting in 2007 that was attended by the NFL commissioner, Roger Goodell, and

200 team doctors, trainers, and players, a neurologist affiliated with the league had mocked Bailes, rolling his eyes as Bailes showed slides of diseased brain tissue collected from dead players. "I'm a man of science!" the NFL's neurologist had bellowed, implying that Bailes was not. It was an ugly scene, one of many that took place during those strange years when the National Football League went to war against science.

Every once in a while, someone would ask Bailes about the curious object on his desk. Bailes loved football—he had been an all-state linebacker in Louisiana—and even though the NFL was attacking him, he surrounded himself with artifacts of the sport: a shelf filled with old helmets of the Steelers, Cardinals, Chiefs, and Rams; deflated footballs; a panoramic photo of Pittsburgh's Three Rivers Stadium, where he once had worked; and a signed photo of the legendary Steelers linebacker Jack Lambert, snarling and toothless. "My whole life was football," Bailes would say. He would pick up the tiny bird brain from his desk and explain that if only NFL players were built like woodpeckers, none of this would have happened.

September 28, 2002, is one of the most significant dates in the history of American sports. You won't find it in the record books.

That morning, on a stainless steel autopsy table inside the Allegheny County coroner's office in Pittsburgh, Pennsylvania, lay the body of Mike Webster, the legendary center of the Pittsburgh Steelers. He had been stripped to his blue jeans, and his stomach had been injected with embalming fluid. Even in death, Webster looked formidable, with a muscular thickness from head to foot, a body that seemed designed to absorb and mete out punishment. But on closer inspection, it was a body that showed horrific signs of wear. Late in Webster's life, his personal physician had noticed that the skin on his forehead had become "fixed to his scalp," a shelf of scar tissue built up over 17 years of pro football. Odd bulges protruded from his back, varicose veins spidered down his legs, and deep cracks ran along the bottoms of his feet. His fingers were thick and crooked like splayed branches. Webster's ex-wife, peering into his casket, had noticed that his fingers remained curled so that "it looked like he was still holding a football." Webster was 50 years old when he died, but a lot of people thought he looked 70.

Five years earlier, when Webster was inducted into the Hall of Fame, his old quarterback, Terry Bradshaw, introduced him as "the best center that's ever played the game, the best to ever put his hands down on a football." Bradshaw, bald except for a fringe of blond hair, looking like a TV evangelist in his gold Hall of Fame sport coat, gazed up to the gray skies and cried: "One more time, let me put my hands under Mike Webster's butt!" Webster, looking sheepish and befuddled, bent over in his khakis and hiked the ball to Bradshaw as the crowd roared. That was in 1997. Webster was already a very sick man. How sick, only a few people knew. Steelers fans had heard some of the stories: that Webster was broke and jobless and living in his truck, that his body was falling apart, that he was seeing a psychiatrist. The reality was far worse: Webster, a kind, thoughtful man during his playing days—many imagined he would go on to a successful career in coaching or perhaps broadcasting, like Bradshaw—had been transformed into a completely different person.

Webster had accumulated an arsenal of weapons that included a Sig Sauer P226 semiautomatic pistol, an AR-15 semiautomatic assault rifle, and a .357 Magnum revolver. He talked frequently about killing NFL officials, including Steelers executives and members of the league's disability board, whom he blamed for his financial troubles. Webster had become addicted to Ritalin, a stimulant normally prescribed to children with attention-deficit disorder, finding that it was the only thing that got him through the day.

Webster, more than anyone, knew how sick he was, and he believed his illness was connected to the game to which he had given his life. Webster once went six seasons without missing a single offensive play; later, when asked by a doctor if he had ever been involved in a car crash, he replied: "Oh, probably about 25,000 times or so." He read constantly, even during the worst of his illness, and he would pore over literature on head trauma and brain disease, putting exclamation points in the margins and circling terms that he thought applied to him, such as "ice pick headache" and "disinhibition" and "dysfluency." He wrapped duct tape around his crooked fingers so that he could grasp a pen to write thousands of letters—some ranting and paranoid, some desperate, some incomprehensible—on any scrap of paper he could find. One read:

What Do I do, I am over fucking overwhelmed . . . what to Do . . . Have NO way Be able to Help my Kids Everyone other Family Dependents and Keep Them Healthy Safe. . . . Maybe me worthless piece of crap but can NOT Let That Get to me have to Keep Trying Keep Work at all this but How Do I Do anything Now?

As Webster lay dead inside the coroner's office that September morning, a silver Mercedes-Benz turned into the back parking lot. A small, dapper forensic pathologist named Bennet Omalu climbed out. It was a mild fall day in Pittsburgh, not yet cold, the start of another football season. Outside the building, TV trucks and reporters had gathered with the news that "Iron Mike" Webster, the indestructible force of four Super Bowl champions, the center of gravity of the Steeler dynasty— "our *strength*," Bradshaw had called him—was inside on a slab.

Omalu was on call to perform autopsies that Saturday because he was the most junior pathologist in the office. He had been out clubbing the night before.

"What's going on?" he asked his colleagues.

"It's Mike Webster. His body is in there," one of them whispered.

"Who is Mike Webster?" asked Omalu.

Over the last year or so, people sometimes have asked us: Is ESPN really going to let you write this book?

It is an interesting question. We are employees of the company once known as the Entertainment and Sports Programming Network but now commonly identified by its initials—a media empire that operates seven 24-hour sports channels, a website that attracts more than 37 million unique visitors every month, a radio network of more than 400 stations, and numerous other sports-related enterprises. The centerpiece of ESPN's empire is its lucrative relationship with the National Football League. The network pays the NFL—and, by extension, its 32 franchises—$1.9 billion per year to broadcast *Monday Night Football*. That's $112 million per game, nearly the average budget for the Harry Potter films.

ESPN's bet on the NFL is based on its own market research, which distinguishes the average sports fan from what the network likes to call "avids"—people who follow their sports regularly and crave information about them the way they crave food. According to ESPN's internal data, by 2012 there were 85 million NFL avids—more than a quarter of the nation. The network has been able to pinpoint almost the exact moment when pro football permanently surpassed baseball as America's pastime: the fall of 1994, when, not coincidentally, a seven-month strike wiped out the World Series. In some major cities today, having a pro football team is a higher priority than providing basic services. The city of Oakland and Alameda County, for example, shell out over $30 million each year to support the Raiders; by 2012, Oakland, with one of the worst crime rates in the nation, had cut 200 police officers to save money.

The national obsession with football, which blew right through the recession, has turned the NFL into the richest and most powerful sports league in the nation and a ubiquitous presence in our lives. ESPN's research has discovered that for the first time, more people prefer watching games on television to attending them. The NFL is broadcast over five networks—including its own—and brings in annual rights fees of $5 billion. In the fall of 2012, 23 of the 25 top-rated shows on TV were NFL games. Once, when the league moved a game from Sunday to Tuesday because of a blizzard, a spokesman predicted that the ratings would be unaffected because the NFL is the "ultimate reality show" and impervious even to acts of God.

The players—the larger-than-life men on whom this $10 billion industry was built—participate in what the historian and former Kansas City Chiefs offensive lineman Michael Oriard has described as "contact ballet." The violence, of course, has always been a big part of football's appeal, but it's cinematic and filtered, almost like a war movie. The destructive force behind the sport was seldom considered. In 2004, a football-loving physicist at the University of Nebraska named Tim Gay set out to calculate the magnitude of a Dick Butkus hit. Applying Newton's second law of motion, he calculated that Butkus, who played at 245 pounds (about 30 pounds lighter than many linebackers today), generated 1,150 pounds of force when slamming into a running back of approximately the same size. "That's the weight of a small adult killer whale!" Gay added helpfully. But rarely did fans dwell on the implications for the men on either side of that transaction.

And then, one Saturday morning in 2002, an obscure forensic pathologist cut open Mike Webster's skull.

That decision—and its consequences, growing by the day—is the subject of this book. There has never been anything like it in the history of sports: a public health crisis that emerged from the playing fields of our twenty-first-century pastime. A small group of research scientists put football under a microscope—literally. What they found was not the obvious, as many people later would claim. We all knew that football was violent and dangerous, that one hit could break your neck or even kill you. No, what the researchers were saying was that the essence of football—the unavoidable head banging that occurs on every play, like a woodpecker jackhammering at a tree—can unleash a cascading series of neurological events that in the end strangles your brain, leaving you unrecognizable.

The researchers who made this discovery—you could count them on one hand—thought NFL executives would embrace their findings, if only to make their product safer. That is not what happened. Instead, the league used its economic, political, and media power to attack pioneering research and try to replace it with its own. Its resources, of course, were considerable. For years, the NFL would co-opt an influential medical journal whose editor in chief was a consultant to the New York Giants. The league used that journal, which some researchers would come to ridicule as "the Journal of No NFL Concussions," to publish an unprecedented series of papers, several of which were rejected by peer reviewers and editors and later disavowed even by some of their own authors. The papers portrayed NFL players as superhuman and impervious to brain damage. They included such eye-popping assertions as "Professional football players do not sustain frequent repetitive blows to the brain on a regular basis." The NFL's flawed research was shaped by a web of conflicting interests. Riddell, the league's official helmet maker, used the research to create and successfully market a helmet it claimed significantly reduced concussions in children—a claim that triggered an investigation by the Federal Trade Commission, which concluded it was false.

The NFL's strategy seemed not unlike that of another powerful industry, the tobacco industry, which had responded to its own existential threat by underwriting questionable science through the creation of its own scientific research council and trying to silence anyone who contradicted it. There are many differences, as we shall see, but one is that football's health crisis featured not millions of anonymous victims but very public figures whose grotesque demises seemed almost impossible to reconcile with their personas. One eight-year NFL veteran would kill himself by drinking antifreeze. Another prominent player would crash his Ford pickup into a tanker truck while leading police on a high-speed chase. Two players, Dave Duerson and Junior Seau, would fire handguns into their chests; Seau, one of the finest linebackers to play the game, used a .357 Magnum that his family didn't know he owned to shoot himself in a guest room of his beach house filled with the memorabilia of a 20-year career. As the crisis grew, the brains of those famous players became valuable scientific commodities. A macabre race ensued among researchers to harvest and study them—even while the bodies were still warm. Minutes after Seau's body was carted out of his house, his oldest son, Tyler, began getting calls seeking his father's brain.

The story is far from over. As this book was being written, nearly 6,000 retired players and their families were suing the league and Riddell for negligence and fraud. Their argument was that the NFL had "propagated its own industry-funded and falsified research" to conceal the link between football and brain damage. One week before the start of the 2013 season, the NFL settled the case—agreeing to pay the players $765 million, plus an expected $200 million in legal fees. The NFL did not admit wrongdoing, but the settlement hardly resolved the question at the core of the league's concussion crisis: How dangerous is football to one's brain? Unlike smoking, there was no scientific consensus about the risks of playing football. One neurosurgeon connected to the NFL said children were more likely to sustain a brain injury riding a bike or falling down. Another neurosurgeon, also connected to the league, called for abolishing tackle football entirely for children younger than 14.

The prevalence of chronic traumatic encephalopathy (CTE)—the name for the insidious disease found in the brains of Seau, Duerson, and the others—is also unknown. The leading expert on the subject is a blond Green Bay Packers fan named Ann McKee, who works out of a redbrick building at the Department of Veterans Affairs outside Boston in an office cluttered with football helmets, bobblehead dolls, and a Packers cheesehead resting atop a plastic heart. In a nearby building, the largest collection of NFL brains is stored in a freezer at −80 degrees Celsius.

By the fall of 2012, McKee had examined the brains of 34 former NFL players. Thirty-three had CTE. We asked her what percentage of NFL players probably had it.

The following exchange ensued:

McKee: I don't think everybody has it, but I think it's going to be a shockingly high percentage.

Question: If you believe that there is a shockingly high number of football players who are bound to suffer from it, how can we even justify having people play professional football?

McKee: Well, I think, you know . . . how come I just don't say, "Let's ban football immediately"?

Question: Yeah.

McKee: I think I would lose my audience.

That brings us back to the question: What's in it for ESPN to support this book? Why would the network that stages the rough equivalent of a Harry Potter movie every week let us dig into a subject that examines the darkest underside of the network's biggest product.

ESPN—itself worth an estimated $40 billion—subsists on sports information, any sports information, much the way the *Wall Street Journal* and CNBC subsist on financial information. "The value of the NFL to us is the ubiquity of the sport across all our platforms all the time," John Skipper, now ESPN's president, explained to the *New York Times* when asked about the staggering contract in 2011. "It's just stupendous for us. It's daily product—we don't have a day without the NFL."

From its modest beginnings, journalism has been part of ESPN's DNA. We work out of a cubbyhole of the empire, an investigative reporting unit with the unusual mandate to investigate the very products that ESPN is selling. It is, in many respects, a journalistic minefield. But for a network that traffics in sports information, one piece of sports information is in particularly high demand these days: Is football killing its players?

Do we really want to know?

- - -

"You mean that guy who was on TV?" Bennet Omalu asked his colleagues as he arrived at the coroner's office.

Omalu had seen the reports of Webster's death, the stories about his life unraveling over the final few years. Omalu didn't think much about it. He had never attended a football game. He found the sport brutal and strange, "extraterrestrials running around a large field and tackling one another, sometimes in a ferocious manner."

Omalu himself was something of an alien. At that moment, his visa had lapsed, and he was in the process of renewing it to stay in the United States. He was a small man, about 5-feet-6 and black, with a voice that went up several octaves when he was excited, which was often, and a perfectly round head, like a 16-inch softball. Omalu had been born in the middle of Nigeria's civil war in the short-lived secessionist nation of Biafra. He came to the United States in 1994 and immediately began collecting degrees. He obtained his medical license in Indiana and Pennsylvania (later he would add California and Hawaii); an MBA; a master's degree in public health; and board certifications in anatomic pathology, clinical pathology, forensic pathology, neuropathology, and medical management.

Omalu's specialty was the science of death.

A deeply spiritual man, he believed, in fact, that he could talk to the dead. Before dissecting his subjects—murder victims, people who had died of unknown or suspicious causes—he carried on internal conversations with the people laid out before him, imploring the dead to help him figure out what had caused their demise.

Now he talked to Webster.

"Mike, you need to help me. I know there's something wrong, but you need to help me tell the world what happened to you."

Omalu used a scalpel to make a Y-shaped incision along the length of Webster's torso. He peeled back Webster's abdomen, which was thick and taut from the embalming fluid. He removed Webster's rib cage with a small oscillating saw. He inspected the internal organs in situ and then removed them one by one. He weighed the organs—the liver, the pancreas, the heart—on a scale and then sliced them into pieces on a plastic cutting board before placing them in jars.

The assistant then propped up the back of Webster's head on a rubber tee. She made incisions across the scalp and over the ears. She pushed the rough skin of Webster's forehead over his eyes and pulled back his scalp to reveal the top of his head. To see the skull exposed is to understand the preciousness of its contents, the brain's utter indispensability to who we are. The brain sits inside a quarter-inch-thick vault of bony plates, in a bath of cerebrospinal fluid. It is not easy to remove. The autopsy suite filled with the high-pitched whine of the circular saw as bone dust rose from Webster's head.

For all the punishment Webster's body had absorbed, his brain looked normal. It had no visible bruises or aneurysms within its soft gray folds. In its natural state, the brain is almost gelatinous; to examine it further would require soaking it for weeks in a tub of formaldehyde and water, a process known as fixing. The process stiffens the brain until it can be sliced like pound cake and then shaved into slivers to be viewed under a microscope.

But that wouldn't be necessary here. The official cause of Webster's death was "acute myocardial infarction"—a heart attack. The assistant began to gather Webster's brain with his other organs, to be placed back inside his body.

Omalu paused. The death certificate had noted somewhat mysteriously that Webster suffered from "depression secondary to postconcussion syndrome." Omalu thought about the reports he had seen on television that morning about Webster's erratic behavior. He thought about a previous patient, a battered woman whose autopsy had shown signs of brain disease. "It was a decision that you just make in the spur of the moment," he later would say.

"Fix the brain," he ordered.

The assistant balked. Webster's brain was normal, wasn't it? He had died of a heart attack.

"*Fix* the brain," Omalu said, this time more firmly.

PART ONE

DISCOVERY

1

THE NUTCRACKER

On Monday morning, July 15, 1974, Mike Webster took the field for the first time as a Pittsburgh Steeler. It was the opening day of training camp. Not the official opening—that had taken place the day before, with routine meetings, room assignments, and the distribution of playbooks and equipment. This was the real opening of camp, when Chuck Noll and his coaching staff would toss out "the raw meat to find who's hungriest." Thousands of fans made the pilgrimage out to Saint Vincent College in Latrobe, Pennsylvania, about an hour east of Pittsburgh. The cars snaked down Route 30 and parked in a cornfield, the faithful walking the last mile to the tiny Benedictine school.

They had turned out not only for practice but for one particular drill, a bloody annual rite so notorious that it had two names. Noll, always bland and officious, used its more decorous name: the Oklahoma drill, said to derive from its origins at the University of Oklahoma under Bud Wilkinson. But others had a more descriptive name that seemed closer to its essence: the Nutcracker. Its champions included Vince Lombardi, who viewed it as nothing less than a test of manhood. The players dreaded it. Future generations would look back and cringe at the ritual, almost a form of human cockfighting, thinking about the inevitable toll, but at the time it was a staple for all teams at all levels, as much a sign that football was back as the turning of the leaves.

The rules of the Nutcracker were basic: An offensive player lined up against a defensive player. They stood between two tackling dummies set three yards apart, creating a gauntlet. A quarterback and a running back lined up behind the offensive player. At the whistle, the quarterback handed the ball to the running back, who followed the blocker and tried to get past the defender. But the quarterback and the running back were essentially props. The Nutcracker was about the collision, two opposing forces coming together, rams knocking heads. It was about setting a tone. New England Patriots coach Bill Belichick believed the Nutcracker answered some of football's most fundamental questions: "Who is a man? Who's tough? Who's going to hit somebody?"

Noll turned it into a public spectacle. The fans, watching from a hill, cheered it on like a blood sport, a modern-day gladiatorial battle. The players joined in, forming a ring around the pit and roaring their allegiances—offense or defense. The assistant coaches were ringleaders, selecting the players for combat. At one point in the 1970s, the Steelers had two coaches, Rollie Dotsch, on offense, and George Perles, on defense, who were both Michigan State grads. Perles in particular "was out of his fucking mind, and they would whip the players into a frenzy," said Stan Savran, a veteran Pittsburgh broadcaster. The two coaches, themselves in a lather, sometimes came to blows, and "even though you thought it was probably fake, you were so into the emotion of it," said Jon Kolb, the longtime Steelers tackle. "I mean, you're talking about guys with an inordinate amount of testosterone." Art Rooney Jr., the team's scouting director, said the Nutcracker was about "huffing, puffing, bleeding, farting." Once, as the team was about to run the drill, he asked a Steelers assistant, "Is this guy tough?" "Tough?" the coach replied. "He's a fighter, a fucker, a wild horseback rider."

Webster, the Steelers' fifth-round draft pick, found himself paired off against another rookie, linebacker Jack Lambert, who had been drafted in the second round. Few, if any, would have bet on Webster. Lambert was tall and lean, 215 pounds, fairly light for a linebacker. He had played at a midlevel school, Kent State, arriving one year after the protest shootings, when there was some doubt whether football, President Nixon's sport, would even survive on campus. But he was quick, tough, and smart—an intimidator and a trash-talker. "You think I'm mean, you should see Lambert," Joe Greene would later say. "He's so mean he doesn't even like himself." Lambert literally had fangs: He had lost four upper teeth playing high school basketball and would remove his bridge for football, enhancing his image of menace. Lambert's legend at Kent State included a story in which the star quarterback broke a team rule and would have to miss a game unless he accepted his punishment: running, rolling, and then crawling 100 times across the length of the field. The quarterback initially balked.

"Look, asshole," Lambert told him. "Do the drill. I'll do it with you. It may be tough, but not as tough as it's going to be if you don't do it or don't finish it. Because I'll kill you."

Upon being drafted by the Steelers, Lambert informed reporters, "I get satisfaction out of hitting a guy and seeing him lay there for a while." He confidently predicted that he would find a regular spot on a team that already had two All-Pro linebackers: Andy Russell and Jack Ham. Phil Musick, then the beat writer for the *Pittsburgh Press,* was already referring to Lambert as the Nureyev of linebackers.

Webster, in contrast, was small and slow, an obscure farm kid from the northernmost edge of the country. Rooney, the scouting director, had fallen in love with Webster's game films from Wisconsin, but even he had to admit that Webster was a reach—even as a fifth-rounder. The sense was that he might hook on as a special-teams player. The Steelers had begun to experiment with a computer for scouting, and the message the computer spit out was clear: You can't win a championship with a center as small and as slow as Mike Webster. Musick was less effusive about the Steelers' fifth-round pick than he'd been about Lambert: "In the fifth round they got a center—Wisconsin's Mike Webster—which they need primarily to snap the ball in training camp." Webster himself knew the odds. He had told his new wife to stay behind in Madison in case he didn't make the team.

It was a clear day, the temperature climbing toward the mid-eighties; back then, the punishing camp began in the middle of the sweltering summer and lasted all the way till fall. Webster squatted low. Lambert, a few feet away, bent down in a three-point stance. There was the whistle and then the explosion: Webster blasting his helmet into Lambert's chest and head, his stumpy legs churning and churning, driving Lambert first up and then back—all the way into the ground, some recalled. The crowd roared and the offense roared, and the running back easily slid past. Lambert was beaten, "tattooed," as Musick put it. They ran the play back with the same outcome: Jack Lambert destroyed. The whole thing had taken a few seconds, but it was a brief glimpse into the Steelers' future. The Nutcracker was a drill that rewarded leverage and technique and relentlessness. It was *mano a mano,* a test of brute strength and sheer will, the same battle that takes place at the line of scrimmage on every down. Lambert, of course, was a future Hall of Famer, one of the best linebackers the game would produce, but his speed and agility were of little use to him here. He was in Webster's territory.

For years to come, it was always the same matchup when the Steelers opened camp: Lambert versus Webster. "I don't remember Lambert ever making a tackle, not in the seven years I was there," said Robin Cole, a linebacker who joined the team a few years later. "He was at a disadvantage. It really wasn't fair."

Jack Lambert didn't know—would never really know—the true nature of the force that had hit him.

The story of escape—from poverty, from persecution, from violence—is timeless in American sports. But rarely has the urge to escape—and the fear of being sent back—so completely shaped an athlete as it did Mike Webster. Few Steelers would know the full extent of it, but Jon Kolb, one of Webster's best friends, got a glimpse one morning while they were driving to practice at Three Rivers Stadium. Webster and Kolb were part of the Steelers' Bible study group, and as they drove, Webster began to reflect on the "depravity" of his childhood, his shattered family, his relationship with God. Kolb would spend years with Webster on and off the field, but he never forgot the emotion of the moment, during which Webster quoted 1 Timothy 1:15: "The saying is trustworthy and deserving of full acceptance, that Christ Jesus came into the world to save sinners, of whom I am the foremost."

"We were coming down Interstate 79 and heading north toward the stadium and just coming down that hill before you get to the exit; I remember exactly where we were because it was so impactful," Kolb recalled. "There were two things that he was talking about. One, how grateful he was for God's love. But the other thing is how he really saw himself."

Years later, after examining Webster, a West Virginia clinical psychologist would write: "He indicated that he essentially had no childhood." That wasn't completely true. Later, Webster would recount many fond memories of sports, of hunting and fishing with his siblings and his friends, of working on his family's potato farm, but it was a reflection of how Webster saw himself and the long road he had traveled. Asked what drove his son so maniacally to succeed, Bill Webster said, "I don't know; maybe he just wanted to get away from it all."

Webster was born in 1952 in Tomahawk, Wisconsin, in the heart of the Northwoods, a tourist destination on the Wisconsin River where people hunt quail and deer and fish for musky, walleye, and largemouth bass. He was the second of five children: three boys and two girls. His parents met at a local bar called Tower Hill and soon afterward eloped to Michigan. "We had five kids before we even knew what was causing them," said Bill.

For a child, it could have been idyllic. Webster was raised on a farm situated in an enchanted forest of sweet-smelling timber and folklore. The name of his high school football team was the Hodags, a mythical horned creature said to roam the Northwoods. But the reality of Webster's early life was chaos, poverty, and shame. Bill Webster was a potato farmer and a local hell-raiser, a harsh disciplinarian who was quick to anger, quick to grab a belt to punish his kids. Mike Webster later told his son Colin that his father had beaten him "with sticks, switches, belts until he was black and blue." Bill Webster's own family history was riddled with turmoil and mental illness, including a brother who committed suicide. Webster's mother had mental illness on her side of the family and eventually would have a nervous breakdown. A doctor later reported that among Webster's four siblings, "all have had manic depressive illnesses, one requiring shock therapy and one who has had several suicide attempts." His youngest brother, Joey, would spend much of his life in prison for a variety of crimes; in 1978, Webster's fourth year in the NFL, Joey was convicted in Michigan on charges of bank robbery and illegal possession of firearms and sent to federal prison for 15 years.

Webster later told doctors that both of his parents were alcoholics. "My mom used to get scared and take off running with us five kids," said Reid Webster, Mike's older brother by a year, who also battled depression.

When she and her husband fought, Betty Webster would take her five kids to a motel or to her mother's house or the neighbors' houses until the storm had passed. Betty and Bill divorced in 1962, when Mike was 10. Both of his parents would remarry twice.

When Mike and Reid were old enough for high school, the two boys returned to their dad's potato farm to live with him, his new wife, and her two children. The farm, about four miles square, was in Harshaw, an unincorporated hamlet of scattered farms and dilapidated houses. On weekends and in the summers, Mike and Reid worked with their dad. They drove the tractor, sprayed the potatoes with pesticides, irrigated the soil, and harvested the potato crop in the fall. Mike and Reid would each grab one end of the 100-pound potato sacks and heave them onto trucks. By the time he reached high school, Mike could easily lift the bags by himself.

The Websters had a small black-and-white television, and when Mike was little, he announced to his father that he intended to play for the Green Bay Packers; he only needed to get big and strong. From that moment, sports became Mike's main outlet. When he and his brother finished their chores, they often played one-on-one tackle football in a hay field. As the boys grew older, the games got rougher. One afternoon before Mike's freshman year at Rhinelander High School, Reid chopped his younger brother at the knees. Mike flipped over backward and broke his wrist in two places. He had intended to play football that year, but his season was over before it started.

A few weeks later, Mike was standing on the grass in his cast, staring out at the football field. One of the players, Billy Makris, was running late for practice when he noticed Webster, stocky and blond, about 5-feet-10, big for a freshman.

"You playing football?" Makris asked.

"I can't. I broke my arm," Webster said.

It was just a fleeting image: a teenager staring longingly at an empty football field. But Makris never forgot it: "The sadness in his eyes, that's the best way to explain it, sadness in his eyes that he wasn't playing." Makris and Webster became best friends. Football, Makris believed, was Webster's refuge from his gothic childhood, almost a matter of survival.

Once Webster healed, he poured all his energy into training. To his coaches and teammates, it became clear that he was different. More than dedication, there was a kind of desperation in the way he prepared, as if he feared that the slightest letdown would lead to failure. By then, Bill Webster, already living on the margins, had moved from potato farming into a business digging for water wells. That meant more back-breaking labor for his sons, who at times were required to lift a 200-pound steel casing, slide it over the drill bar, lock it in place, and drive the casing into the earth.

Webster's only consolation was that he was able to salvage parts from the well business and use them for his training. An old piece of pipe became a weight bar. Water buckets were filled up and used as weights. Webster's weight bench was a piece of plywood resting atop two cinder blocks. By his senior year, he was lifting twice a day and wearing out the dirt roads around Bill's property.

Mike was turning himself into a small truck. It wasn't that he was so tall or imposing—6 feet, just over 200 pounds at the time of his graduation. But he was chiseled, fairly bulging out of his skin. He had large hands, "like a St. Bernard pup," said Makris. He wasn't yet an elite athlete, but what stood out was his intensity—his refusal to quit. Another injury like the one that had put him out his freshman year became unthinkable. When Webster broke his arm again, he had it fitted with an inflatable cast. Makris watched in awe as Webster blew up the cast on the sideline like a pool toy, then took his broken arm back out onto the field.

Webster was recruited to play at the University of Wisconsin. It was there that he began his transformation into "Iron Mike," the force so familiar to a generation of football fans. He anchored the Badgers' offensive line and became even more obsessive about his training. On the field, Webster adopted the habit of sprinting out of the huddle. At first, his teammates thought he was showboating, but they soon realized it was part of the same relentless package.

By his senior year, Webster was team captain and the best center in the Big Ten. He also got married. His new wife, Pam, worked in the Badgers' ticket office. Her upbringing was everything Webster's was not. She had grown up in Lodi, a small town 25 miles north of Madison, in a stable family of seven brothers and sisters. Her father drove the school bus that shuttled local sports teams to their games and worked in the heating and sheet-metal business. Her mother was a nurse. Her family led a typical Wisconsin life: "hunting, brats, and the Packers."

Pam found Mike strangely endearing. He was socially awkward and could barely dress himself, his shirts mismatched and ill fitting. Even his sense of humor seemed slightly off; he meant well but was prone to saying and doing the wrong thing. But unlike other athletes she had been around, he was a gentle soul, polite and soft-spoken, and seemed entirely unimpressed with himself. "Mike had just a really kind heart," she said. He didn't tell her much about his family, but she sensed he was the caretaker for not only his brothers and his sisters but also his mother.

"I think there was a part of him that seemed wounded to me—like his soul—that just reached out to me," she said.

Webster was part of perhaps the greatest single draft by a team in NFL history. In 1974, the Steelers took USC wide receiver Lynn Swann in the first round, Lambert in the second, Alabama A&M receiver John Stallworth in the fourth, and Webster in the fifth. All four were future Hall of Famers. Between 1969, Noll's first season as head coach, and 1974, the Steelers drafted 11 Hall of Famers, the foundation of one of the NFL's great dynasties.

Webster was the biggest long shot of them all. There were those like Rooney Jr., the scouting director and son of the Steelers' patriarch, who admired Webster. At the Senior Bowl that year, Webster had manhandled a big Tennessee State middle linebacker named Waymond Bryant, whom the Bears took with the fourth overall pick. The more film the Steelers watched, the more they were intrigued. "You gotta see this Webster," Dick Haley, the team's director of player personnel, told Rooney. "He hits like Rocky Marciano." Webster's technique seemed flawless:

He had a knack for smashing his head like a sledgehammer underneath an opposing lineman's chin, then controlling the bigger man by using his leverage. He had surprisingly quick feet, stuffing one oncoming pass rusher and then gliding over to pick up another.

But there was the lingering issue of his size. He was listed at 6 feet, 2½ inches, 225 pounds, but no one believed that. He was—maybe—6-feet-1, 215. Some people had thought Webster wouldn't be drafted at all and the Steelers could pick him up as a free agent.

Webster did make the team, benefiting from a players strike that allowed him to get a long look from the Steelers coaches. He played mostly as a backup to Ray Mansfield, a beloved veteran center known as "the Old Ranger." Webster's rookie year culminated with the Steelers winning the first Super Bowl in the team's history.

As they packed up for the year, Ralph Berlin, the team's longtime trainer, ran into Webster and asked him what he had planned for the off-season.

"I'm gonna go home and get bigger," Webster told him. "You can't play in this league where I am."

When Webster returned the next season, Berlin was stunned. Webster now weighed between 250 and 260 pounds, he recalled.

By then, Webster's dedication to his training had become so maniacal that in hindsight, his closest friends wondered if it wasn't a sign of insecurity so profound that it was almost a sickness. On most days, Webster could be found in the basement of a Pittsburgh steak house, the Red Bull Inn in McMurray, a suburb south of the city. Jon Kolb had gotten to know the manager, a power-lifting fanatic named Lou Curinga, who had turned the restaurant's boiler room into a gym. It was a lifter's dungeon, windowless and stifling, the air thick with the smell of sweat and athletic tape. Kolb recruited Webster and several other Steelers into what he called the 500 Club—players who could bench-press 500 pounds. The Red Bull Inn became Webster's second home, so central to his life that he and Pam moved closer to McMurray to cut down on his "commute."

Webster often brought his training home with him. In the winter, he would head out into the knee-deep snow with a barbell behind his head and do lunges. When the snow thawed, he put on shoulder pads and a helmet and hammered against a blocking sled he kept in his yard. Craig Wolfley, a Steelers offensive lineman, pulled up at Webster's house early one morning to find Webster "in a helmet, shoulder pads, and spikes, pushing a sled across the front yard. *Six-thirty in the morning! I said, 'Webby, do you know how crazy this looks?'"* Wolfley joked that Webster should hook up the blocking sled to a lawn mower to kill two birds with one stone. Webster pounded his blocking sled so often, it carved a trench in the yard. Sometimes his youngest son, Garrett, hopped on for the ride.

Webster's training regimen included anabolic steroids. Decades later, this would still be a matter of debate in some circles, but the evidence was conclusive. Most notable was Webster's own admission: At least two reports in his lengthy medical file contain references to steroids. In 1993, less than three years after Webster retired, a Pittsburgh doctor reported: "He took anabolic steroids for a very short time when he was in his twenties." Another report in 1993, based on a doctor's conversation with Webster, asserted that he "only rarely experimented with steroid use" during his playing career. Those reports contradicted Webster's repeated public denials and almost certainly understated the extent of steroid use.

Webster's involvement with performance-enhancing drugs coincided with their emergence in the NFL, which didn't officially ban steroids until 1983. At least two of Webster's teammates, running back Rocky Bleier and guard Steve Courson, later admitted using steroids while they were legal. Courson, who was killed in 2005 when a tree fell on him while he was cutting it down, asserted "unequivocally" in his 1991 autobiography, *False Glory: Steelers and Steroids,* that 75 percent of his teammates on the offensive line used steroids. Bleier, in an interview, said he also saw Webster take amphetamines before and during games and wondered if his drug use later affected him. "I mean, the question with Mike has always been, the effect of steroidal use on his body—did this have an effect or not—and then taking amphetamines during the game," Bleier said. "It was all legal stuff at the time, but there was still a stigma."

In truth, Webster stopped at nothing to transform himself from a high school lineman playing in the obscurity of the Wisconsin Northwoods into perhaps the finest center in history. He ingested something called spirulina—a blue-green algae taken by humans but also used as a feed supplement in the fish and poultry industries. He took desiccated liver tablets, brewer's yeast, royal honey. Colin said his father toted around a bag containing some 20 different pills. One of the side effects of this amalgam of pills and potions was flatulence, which was known to firebomb the Steelers' huddle. "Webby, was that you?" Terry Bradshaw would shout at his center.

By 1976, Webster was nearly 270 pounds. He had increased his body weight by roughly 25 percent, almost all of it muscle.

By 1980, he was literally the strongest man in the game. That year, CBS staged a made-for-TV event called "The Strongest Man in Football." Eight of the game's giants met for a weight-lifting showdown inside Auburn's Memorial Coliseum. The Red Bull Inn tandem dominated the event. Webster, listed at 267 pounds, edged out Kolb for the $10,000 first prize. Webster opened the competition by lifting 275 pounds over his head 12 times, struggling only at the finish. He clinched his victory in the bench press, pumping 350 pounds 15 times—over 2½ tons in one set. Kolb could muster only 11.

Webster "had arms like legs," Steve Courson would say, "and legs like people."

Between 1974 and 1980, the period in which the Steelers won four Super Bowls, Webster appeared in every game. To his teammates and his close friends, he was always "Webby," a nickname that seemed to fit his good-natured personality. Webster was slightly goofy, a bit of an odd duck, a locker room prankster. He left mousetraps in his teammates' lockers and rigged weights so that they stuck to the floor. During one Steelers blowout, Bradshaw walked up to the line, reached under the center, and then jumped back in horror. Webby had slit open his pants, and when Bradshaw reached down, he found himself holding his center's balls.

Webster was a conspiracy theorist who liked to regale teammates with a weekly news summary they called "Webby's Gloom and Doom Report." "Anything that was crazy, like the guy that got killed at the Indianapolis 500 when the tire went flying up 43 rows, that would freak him out," said his close friend the tackle Tunch Ilkin. A John Wayne fanatic, Webster wore cowboy boots and jeans to formal dinners and recited dialogue from *McLintock!* ("I've got a touch of hangover, bureaucrat. Don't push me.") on the field while the Steelers stretched.

To fans, Webster was simply Iron Mike. As much as superstars like Bradshaw, Lambert, Lynn Swann, Franco Harris, and Mean Joe Greene would come to define the Steelers of the 1970s, no player better represented the synergy between the city and the team.

Part of it was the times. As the steel industry collapsed, Pittsburgh was being depopulated, going from the twelfth largest city in the country to the thirtieth. An estimated 30,000 steelworkers were laid off. But Webster was indestructible. "If you wanted to see a guy who represented the city of Pittsburgh, with no fancy frills, where people just go to work and do your job, that was Mike," said Bob Stage, who for years piloted the Steelers' plane and became close with Webster. Fans hung a sign over the mezzanine at Three Rivers; it depicted a bulging biceps with Webster's number, 52.

In fact, Webster was as terrified of losing his job as everyone else in the city. "Obviously he was tough, but as I got to know Mike more and more, I realized how scared he was," said Stage. "It didn't matter if he was All-Pro every year. That was never a comfort to Mike. He was such a gentleman, such a nice person, but at the height of his career, I felt that he never really enjoyed his success." In Pittsburgh, Webster built the stable family life he had never had as a child. He and Pam had four children: two boys and two girls. They lived in a gray-and-white two-story colonial outside the city. In the morning, the kids clambered out of bed to the smell of their father's freshly baked bread. "He was like a big superhero," said his daughter Brooke, the oldest of his children, "and I was a daddy's girl." One winter, Daddy came back from the Pro Bowl bearing pineapples and grass skirts and held a luau for her second-grade class. Yet Pam agreed that her husband was never totally happy. "That was so sad for me," she said. "You know, he just never felt like happy down to your toes."

Asked what motivated Webster, one of his former teammates replied: "Total fear."

By 1978, Webster was the best center in the NFL. From that year forward, he would make the Pro Bowl eight straight seasons. If off the field he was a bit awkward, on the field Webster was totally in his element. Before the snap, the center is responsible for making the line calls, adjusting blocking assignments in response to the configuration of the defense. Webster was a master, barking out audibles, some of them decoys, assuming the role of the Steelers' field general. He studied game films endlessly—he often took them home—and came to know the Steelers' offense so well that he sometimes overruled Bradshaw in the huddle. "Ultimately he became the leader to the extent that he would call the plays," said Bleier. "Bradshaw would just say, 'Okay.'"

Webster was low to the ground, and he used that to his advantage. As the center, he often drew the gnarliest blocking assignments, the biggest and baddest linemen and linebackers. In the 3–4 defense (three down linemen) he was head up on nose tackles sometimes 50 pounds heavier. In the 4–3, he was responsible for taking on the middle linebacker. Gerry Sullivan, a former Cleveland center, recalled watching film of Webster taking on Oilers nose tackle Curley Culp, a former college wrestling champion and future Hall of Famer. Sullivan was astounded: Webster wasn't just blocking Curley Culp. He was *uprooting* him. "To me, the physics of it weren't even possible, you know?" Sullivan said. The Browns ran the film over and over, mesmerized. "You could hear a pin drop as we watched him do it like four times in a row. I don't know how he did what he did. He was just a force of nature."

One of Webster's greatest assets was his head. He used it as a battering ram, smashing it into his opponent as he exploded off the line. To stop Webster, nose tackles and linebackers tried to neutralize his head. Harry Carson, the great New York Giants linebacker, came into the NFL when Webster was in his prime. He found that his best strategy often was to bludgeon Webster as he fired off the line. "When I would explode into Mike, it was power against power," Carson said. "I would hit him in the face. That's what we were taught: to hit a guy right in the face so hard that they're dazed and stunned." Sullivan, who stayed friends with Webster for years, began to notice that a thick layer of scar tissue had formed on his forehead at the exact spot where he thrust his helmet into opposing linemen. Sullivan was jealous. It was a sign Webster was executing his block—play after play. "I was kind of disappointed that my forehead wasn't, um, disfigured," Sullivan said.

It wasn't just the games that had hardened Webster's head. Many

Steelers considered the games a break from their normal reality. "We were a collision football team," said Kolb. Years later, through collective bargaining, NFL players were able to cut down on contact during practice significantly, but not then. During training camp, the Steelers pounded one another for six weeks, often twice a day. During the season, Wednesdays and Thursdays were full-on contact. Friday brought goal-line drills—the teamwide equivalent of the Nutcracker. With the ball on the 2-yard line, the first-team offense cracked heads with the first-team defense over and over. It was one of Noll's favorite drills.

Gerry "Moon" Mullins, who played alongside Webster for six years, thought that the players had been programmed to ignore the pain caused by the continuous violence. "They'd drag you back to the huddle: 'Shake it off, man. We need your ass out here,'" he said. "Nobody knew any different. That's just sort of the way you were, sort of like the GIs when they bring in young kids and they program them: 'Rush that pillbox, that machine gun that's blazing out there!' Nobody in their right mind would do that."

Pam Webster said her husband often came home with searing headaches that he attributed to his job. When the headaches occurred, Webster would retreat to the bedroom and lie alone in the dark for hours.

If the Steelers' medical staff was aware of this condition, it was not recorded: Hundreds of pages of medical files accumulated over Webster's 15 years with the Steelers contain exactly two references to head injuries. One, dated December 19, 1982, Webster's eighth year in the NFL, indicated that he passed out after a game in Cleveland after experiencing weakness and dizziness. "He gives no history of head trauma," says the report, which attributes the blackout to low blood sugar. Webster, after his career ended, would tell one of his doctors that he absorbed several hard hits to the head in that game.

The only other reference to a head injury was on November 3, 1988: "Hit in the head during practice—complains of intermittent dizziness. No other symptoms or complaints. No nausea or headache."

The nearly blank record is not surprising. Webster rarely acknowledged his injuries, much less reported them.

There was a certain perverseness about it: The inner strength and mortal fear that drove Webster, lifting him to success beyond his wildest dreams, was pushing him to play even in the most extreme circumstances. The more he achieved, the more he pushed. Stage, the Steelers' pilot, dropped by practice one Saturday to see Webster and was told he had been admitted to the hospital. The week before, Webster had lowered his head to make a block on a screen pass and had injured his neck badly. After the game, he took an injection for the pain and had an allergic reaction, according to Stage. Webster was admitted to Pittsburgh's Passavant Hospital and told he would be unable to play that Sunday.

When Stage went to visit him, he found Webster in traction with a high fever and a lump the size of a baseball on his neck. Webster confirmed that he would not be playing the next day and asked if Stage would mind swinging by with a couple of cans of snuff.

Stage showed up as promised, but Webster was gone. He had checked himself out and taken a cab to Three Rivers, where he played the entire game. No one attempted to dissuade him. On the contrary, when Webster walked through the door, Ron Blackledge, the offensive line coach, "about started crying," Ilkin recalled.

During one six-year stretch, Webster never missed a snap—a streak of 5,871 consecutive offensive plays. That did not include long snaps on punts, field goals, and extra points or the snaps he made in preseason and postseason games. When the streak finally ended in 1986 because of a "very badly dislocated elbow," Webster estimated that dating back to his sophomore year of high school, he had played in 300 out of 300 of his teams' games. He figured he had participated in 890 out of some 900 practices in the NFL.

A s Webster was reaching the end of his career, the Steelers drafted a young running back. His name was Merril Hoge, and he had grown up in Pocatello, Idaho. Hoge was drafted in the tenth round, the 261st overall pick. His exposure to the Steelers and the NFL had come almost entirely through television. To Hoge, like most fans, the Pittsburgh Steelers were giants who roamed the earth. When he walked into the huddle for the first time, it was like walking onto a movie set.

And then, suddenly, Hoge found himself face-to-face with Mike Webster.

Hoge loved to hunt, and he thought that seeing Webster·in his natural habitat was like being startled by some fantastic animal out in the wild. He was majestic. He had an aura. *That guy's been around,* Hoge thought. *That guy knows.* He looked at Webster's helmet. The rubber was partially scraped off the face mask, exposing the metal underneath. There were cracks and deep divots in the plastic shell, "like a bear had attacked it." Webster certainly could have obtained a new helmet. He didn't want one.

Hoge was Webster's roommate that season. It was like "rooming with your dad," he said, only more intimidating: "I mean, I was scared to death." He came to understand the many ways Iron Mike was driven to succeed and survive, his toughness and the underlying vulnerability. Webster lived by one central tenet: Never come off the field. During one game, the Steelers were getting blown out in Phoenix, 31–7 in the fourth quarter. Noll pulled all his starters, but Webster refused to leave.

As the offense huddled up, Webster turned to Hoge and said, "We're gonna take the ball and we're gonna shove it down their throats. You got me?"

"You talk about inspired, I mean, I had a rocket in my ass," Hoge said.

The drive ended with Hoge catching a 12-yard pass in the end zone.

In Webster, Hoge came to see the totality of a football life.

He's the epitome of the NFL, Hoge thought. *Nobody was as tough as that dude. Nobody.*

The Steelers effectively cut Webster after the 1988 season, allowing him to become a free agent. He was devastated, having believed the team would keep him on as a player-coach. He announced his retirement and then took a job in Kansas City as a coach, but soon he was playing for the Chiefs. He lasted another two seasons. The end finally came in 1990. The Chiefs had a center of the future, Tim Grunhard, but he was struggling that year. Grunhard's father had died of cancer, and Tim was playing with a cast on his hand because of a dislocated thumb. One Sunday against the Broncos, head coach Marty Schottenheimer replaced him with Webster.

Grunhard was humiliated; he feared his career was over before it started. Then he felt a tap on his shoulder. He looked up to see Webster stripping off his gear.

"What are you doing?" Schottenheimer said.

"You gotta put this guy in," Webster told him. "I'm not playing anymore."

Grunhard never forgot the gesture. He played 11 years in the NFL.

"It was the turning point of my career," he said.

As for Webster, he was done. He was 38 years old. That year, he had played with three broken ribs, a fractured right heel that never properly mended, and bulging discs in his back that his kids could see when they splashed around in the pool.

On a medical form that Webster filled out during his last season, he was asked whether he had neck pain, such as frequent stiffness, motion limitation, and so on.

"No," he replied.

Then, in the comments section, he added, "JUST ON MONDAYS."

Some years later, Noll would mention to one of Webster's doctors that there were times in the locker room when he would look over and see his powerful center, his offensive captain, the epitome of the NFL, with his head buried in his hands, seemingly in a daze.

Webster had built a 3,000-square-foot home in Kansas City for his retirement, a monument to everything he had achieved: a successful career, a stable family life, escape from the turmoil of the Northwoods. The house had its own phone booth so Brooke could carry on her teenage conversations in private. There was a pool down the street. "It was like he wanted to make our dreams come true," said Pam.

At first, that was exactly what it looked like: a beautiful dream. Pam loved Kansas City. So did the kids. But they began to notice changes in Mike, almost imperceptible at first but growing more noticeable during his final years in Pittsburgh and Kansas City and now impossible to ignore. Before, Mike rarely raised his voice; now his temper was short. He became easily distracted and forgetful. He was often lethargic and indecisive. Where Webster once had approached his work with unrelenting focus, now "he couldn't decide what to have for breakfast," Pam said.

Webster soon became obsessed with the failings of the monument he had created. "He was *angry* at that house," said Pam. "It got built, and then he found fault with everything." Minor leaks or a problem with the tile sent him into a rage. He thought the contractor was out to screw him. Without warning, seemingly, the Websters had financial problems. Mike had led Pam to believe they were set for life, but now they were having trouble making the house payments. She couldn't understand why.

Pam was at a loss for why it was happening or what to do. She worried it might have something to do with her or the kids. As Mike's behavior grew more erratic, Pam began to think that her husband was rapidly being replaced with another person who occupied the same body.

2

PSYCH 101

Chuck Noll had a question for the Pittsburgh Steelers' brain specialist. His name was Joe Maroon, and at the time he was the only one of his kind in the NFL. Maroon had been a pint-sized running back at Indiana University back in the late 1950s. Now, in 1991, he was one of the top neurosurgeons in the country, the chairman of the Department of Neurological Surgery at Allegheny General Hospital in Pittsburgh. To reach that position, Maroon had survived nearly two decades of rigorous medical study, including residencies at Georgetown, Oxford, and Indiana. He had edited or contributed to hundreds of books and papers on everything from orbital tumors to the management of cervical spine injuries. He had served as general program chairman of the Congress of Neurological Surgeons, an international education society with thousands of members.

And now a football coach wanted to know: On what basis are you telling me that my quarterback can't play?

Steelers quarterback Bubby Brister had sustained a concussion the previous Sunday. Maroon, who moonlighted, unpaid, as the team's neurological consultant, had examined Brister and determined that he should sit out the next week against the Buffalo Bills.

Noll had gotten the Steelers job in 1969 after Joe Paterno turned it down. He was known around Pittsburgh as a Renaissance man who played guitar and dabbled in subjects as varied as photography, oceanography, and haute cuisine.

Brister looked fine, Noll told Maroon. He was throwing well. He knew the plays. Maroon, though, insisted that Brister had to rest for a week.

"Those are the recommended guidelines for this type of concussion," Maroon explained.

"Well, who wrote the guidelines?" Noll said.

Maroon informed the coach that, in fact, *he* had, along with other top neurosurgeons experienced in sports medicine. The guidelines were based on previous experiments that had examined the effects of mild traumatic brain injury, the medical term for a concussion. In one series of early experiments, professors at Wayne State University dropped dogs, pigs, pregnant baboons, and human cadavers down an elevator shaft to study the effects of concussions. In another experiment, a researcher put metal helmets on monkeys and applied pneumatic arms, which were propelled back and forth rapidly, violently shaking the monkeys' heads. The monkeys were then euthanized and their brains cut out to examine the effect.

"Were the studies double-blinded?" Noll asked. "What are the metrics? I need more information."

Maroon fumed. Noll was undeniably sharp, but who was the doctor here? But the more Maroon thought about it, the more he had to admit that Noll was right. As common as concussions were, there was not a lot of useful information about the injury he could cite to justify his opinion that Bubby Brister shouldn't play.

In the long history of brain research, the concussion was still regarded as the neurological equivalent of a stubbed toe. The injury was as underrated by the medical profession as it was by the NFL. There was little research money devoted to it and it had no glamour, particularly for an area of study whose mystery and vastness are often compared to the study of the universe. There was widespread confusion about what a concussion was, not only in the general population but also among doctors and researchers; dozens of definitions had been floated and discarded.

The fact that concussions were practically an afterthought was perplexing when one considered what actually occurred. The brain is essentially an oddly shaped sphere of Jell-O, crammed inside a box, covered in a shallow layer of cerebrospinal fluid. This gelatinous material contains a kind of electrical grid—hooked up to an EEG, the brain can power a toy train—that transmits information through the body via microscopic fibers called axons. When someone is hit in the head or stops suddenly, the brain is jolted against the skull's jagged interior, distorting or even severing the axons and interrupting the function of the synapses, the connections between the fibers of the brain. The immediate effect depends on where the connections are and the extent of the damage. Some people go temporarily blind. Others lose their memory or balance or become irritable. When the blow is particularly violent, the entire system short-circuits, like a neighborhood blackout, and the person loses consciousness.

In that context, you wondered why people hadn't taken concussions more seriously. But the focus had always been on catastrophic head injuries such as skull fractures or hemorrhages. In sports, what little research there was occurred almost by accident. One pioneer in the field was a genial, wisecracking neuropsychologist at the University of Virginia named Jeff Barth. "In the late seventies and early eighties, nobody thought mild head injury was a problem," said Barth, who resembled Hulk Hogan and liked to splice the wrestler's picture into his scientific presentations. "When you'd go to the doctor or the ER with a mild head injury, they'd say, 'Just take a couple days off, take some aspirin, and you'll be okay by Monday.'" As part of his work at Virginia, Barth saw emergency room patients from the Charlottesville area and other parts of Virginia. He and his colleagues began to notice that out of the hundreds of head injuries they treated each year, the majority were the so-called minor variety that involved either no loss of consciousness or blackouts lasting only a few minutes.

Because there were so many—Barth counted more than 1,200 concussions over a two-year period, often from traffic accidents—he decided to study them to see if he could improve treatment. He and his colleagues soon discovered that these mild head injuries often weren't so minor. "We did a three-month follow-up, and lo and behold, we found that about one-third of mild head injury patients hadn't returned to work," said Barth. "I thought, 'Wow, that's amazing! Why *is* that?'"

His findings struck a chord. The *Wall Street Journal* ran a front-page article in 1982 that described concussions as "a silent epidemic." Barth was riding high until he went to a conference and presented the study to some of his colleagues.

"It was one of the worst days of my life," he said.

As he stood at the podium, the audience bombarded him with questions and doubts. Maybe Barth was testing only people who weren't very smart. Maybe they didn't return to work because they had an excuse from the doctor. What was his control group? "I thought to myself: 'How can I get out of this?'" said Barth. "'Maybe I can fake a seizure.'"

Barth decided he needed a more rigorous study. The important thing was to find patients who were likely to have concussions and were available for follow-up. "My initial idea was we could test all of the Psychology 101 students at the University of Virginia, follow them around campus and hit them with a two-by-four, and then test them again," he joked. Other groups were considered, including race car drivers and boxers. Finally one of his colleagues, Bruno Giordani, said: "What about football players? They run and hit things."

Thus was born an entirely new field: sports neuropsychology, the study of the brain under the influence of sports. "Unfortunately, some of my colleagues who like to get at me, they don't call me the Father of Sports Neuropsychology, they call me the *Grandfather* of Sports Neuropsychology," Barth said.

Barth started to perform tests on Virginia football players to measure their baseline performance—before they got conked on the head—on tasks such as word recognition and number sequencing. He and his colleagues positioned spotters at practices and games to be on the lookout for head injuries, then tested the players immediately after an injury occurred to measure differences in brain function.

The first experiments, in 1984, were a disaster. Out of the 100 or so players who participated, there were only a few documented concussions. Virginia was terrible that year, and before he was fired, the beleaguered coach shut down Barth's experiment in midseason. But Barth persisted. The next year, he expanded his study to include the Ivy League schools and what he referred to as "a real football team," the University of Pittsburgh. This time, the results were startling: Out of 2,350 players who participated, 195, or more than 8 percent, sustained verifiable concussions. More than half still had headaches at least five days after the injury occurred. About a quarter still had signs of memory loss, nausea, and dizziness. Most of the symptoms cleared within 10 days.

What had started as an attempt to measure the effects of minor head injuries after traffic accidents had become a harbinger of football's soon to be tumultuous future. Barth's major discovery was that concussions might be regarded as "minor" injuries by coaches, trainers, and even doctors, but they weren't minor to the people who incurred them. He published his results in 1989. "Through further data review and analysis, it is our hope that we can provide the football community, and sports medicine psychologists in particular, with a brief and easily administered set of neuropsychological assessment tools that will aid team physicians," Barth wrote.

Now, two years later, Joe Maroon was faced with exactly that scenario. Chuck Noll wanted his quarterback, Bubby Brister, back on the field. Maroon, the Steelers' doctor, didn't agree. But he had no real tools to justify his assessment. As it turned out, Maroon had participated indirectly in Barth's study. In addition to his work with the Steelers, he was the neurological consultant for the Pitt Panthers—the "real football team" from Barth's experiment. Maroon didn't have enough concrete data to prevent Brister from playing, but perhaps here was a way to get at it.

Maroon went to the chief neuropsychologist at Allegheny General, Mark Lovell, and explained the situation.

"You know what, Mark?" Maroon said of Noll. "He's right."

Brister ended up playing, but that was the beginning of the story for Maroon, not the end.

To that point, the sports medical community had viewed a concussion as an invisible injury. You couldn't x-ray it or scope it or put a cast on it, so how serious could it be? Barth had shown that a player might appear normal, but if his brain wasn't functioning properly—as measured by changes in short-term memory, executive function, ability to reason, and so on—that was an indication the injury hadn't healed. As simple as it now seems, that discovery was groundbreaking.

Maroon says he didn't see a financial opportunity in the diagnosis of concussions until years later, when a colleague pointed it out to him.

This was still in the sleepy early days of the NFL's concussion crisis, and Maroon was merely looking for answers. He approached Lovell to try to figure out a way to better justify his on-field decisions to Noll and the players. But it was exactly the type of out-of-the-box idea that got Maroon's wheels spinning.

Joe Maroon was a neurosurgeon with a flair for business. He had picked it up from his father, a Lebanese immigrant who had hustled out a living in the Ohio River Valley by catering to the needs of the miners and rivermen. Charles Maroon operated Bridgeport's only bowling alley, serviced vending machines throughout the region, and built a truck stop in the northern tip of West Virginia. He owned a building that housed a strip joint called the Lucky Lady Lounge. Maroon worshiped his dad and decided to go into medicine only after thinking long and hard about whether he wanted to defy his father's wishes that he become a lawyer. Despite his size—about 5-feet-5, 160 pounds—Maroon attended Indiana on a football scholarship, started at halfback for two seasons, and was a scholastic All-American. When he was in his early forties, his wife left him and his father died in the same week. He briefly left medicine and went back to Bridgeport to run his father's truck stop, a midlife crisis that left him suicidal. Exercise helped save him. He became a health enthusiast and ran triathlons all over the world. Still competing in his sixties and seventies, Maroon wrote a book called *The Longevity Factor* in which he recommended a number of novel "secrets" to a long and healthy life.

As admired as Maroon was, there was a whiff of opportunism about him that some of his colleagues found distasteful. He seemed to combine his neurosurgery practice and his entrepreneurship in ways that pushed the envelope. Maroon touted the wonders of red wine and fish oil as the keys to staving off everything from depression to Alzheimer's disease to death itself. No one doubted that he believed what he was promoting—Maroon looked great, a trim man with a full head of graying hair—but he often seemed to have an angle. When Maroon sold his neurosurgery practice to the University of Pittsburgh Medical Center, some of his colleagues were surprised to learn in the *Post-Gazette* that UPMC had agreed to purchase real estate owned by Maroon for $6.22 million. "Joe has a lot of great qualities, he has legions of patients that legitimately adore him," said one doctor who worked with him for years. "He's done well at the professional level in all respects, including with the Steelers. But everything has to have an immediate entrepreneurial angle. You can't just appreciate it for whatever its value is, you know? There has to be: 'How can we take advantage of that?' And that's the thing that to me is a little off-putting."

Shortly after the Bubby Brister affair, Maroon sat down in the cafeteria at Allegheny General with Mark Lovell and laid out what he was thinking.

Lovell (pronounced LOVE-uhl) didn't have much experience in sports, but he had personal experience with concussions. During his junior year of high school in Grand Rapids, Michigan, he was picked up hitchhiking by a drunk driver and was thrown through the windshield when the car crashed into a parked car. "My head went through and then recoiled back," he said. "If you look at my nose, you can see that they kind of sewed it back on."

Lovell needed 120 stitches. But what he noticed over time was that the more serious problem was his head. For the next several years he had migraine headaches. "I had a concussion, but nobody called it a concussion," Lovell said.

Lovell was reserved and soft-spoken, with straight brown hair, a goatee, and an earnest manner that later made his role as one of the most controversial figures in the NFL's concussion saga seem incongruous. His specialty was neuropsychology—Jeff Barth's world—a relatively modern discipline that seemed to baffle everyone around him. Lovell's father, a Grand Rapids auto mechanic, proudly introduced his son as a "psycho neurologist." Lovell's fundamental job was to assess brain function, and Maroon had come to him with an intriguing proposition.

Maroon wanted to see if Barth's experiment could be adapted to the NFL. He wanted to know specifically if Lovell could design a neuropsychological test that could be used to establish baseline data for the Steelers and then use that test to assess changes in brain function after a concussion. If there were major changes, Maroon would have quantifiable data to present to Noll and help guide his decisions about whether a player should return. Lovell quickly agreed. The test itself wouldn't be hard. Barth already had administered it to college players, and so it was really a matter of updating the test—actually a series of tests to measure memory, executive function, and so on. The tests already existed; they were used to assess stroke patients, people with dyslexia, accident victims—any number of neurological disorders. The hardest part was devising an exam that could be administered in the heat of a game. "The thing I learned very, very quickly is that you didn't have an abundance of time to do this," Lovell said. "Neuropsychologists at that point would spend four or five or six hours with a patient. That doesn't work in sports." At most Lovell would have 15 or 20 minutes, maybe half an hour. He borrowed liberally from Barth's study and other neuropsych tests that were floating around and tried to keep it all to one sheet of paper.

Maroon went to Noll and Steelers owner Dan Rooney for approval. The test wasn't expensive—it was all done with paper and pencil—but the team needed to make the research subjects—the players—available. Noll and Rooney agreed under the condition that the testing would be voluntary. Anything more would have to be cleared through the NFL Players Association, and that wasn't likely.

The players greeted the idea with suspicion. Many thought the team was literally trying to get into their heads by assembling psychological profiles that could be used in contract negotiations. Or secretly administering IQ tests. Or looking for potential deviants. The NFL already put rookies through the controversial Wonderlic test, which Lovell described as "a test to see if you're too stupid to play in the NFL." He didn't want his test to be confused with that. "I didn't blame the players," he said. "I said, 'This has to be seen as something that's only for injury management.'"

The players were slow to come around. "Their agents called, their mothers called, everyone called until we convinced them that it was to their benefit," said Maroon. "If they had a concussion and we went by the previous guidelines, they might be out for three weeks. But if neurocognitively they returned to normal, we might be able to let them go back on the field sooner."

Twenty-seven Steeler guinea pigs ultimately volunteered after Maroon and Lovell guaranteed that the results would remain private. It was now 1993, and Maroon and Lovell were trying not to offend anyone.

"To be honest with you, I thought it was pretty cool to be nerds and get to do this stuff, to work with athletes," said Lovell. "We didn't want to get ourselves thrown out by becoming a pain in the neck." He tried to be as inconspicuous as possible. A speech pathologist administered the baseline tests during training camp. Lovell kept the data locked in a filing cabinet in his office.

The immediate hope was that the data would be used to help decide when a player was ready to return after sustaining a concussion. But almost from the beginning it went well beyond that.

One of the first guinea pigs was Webster's former roommate Merril Hoge. He wasn't totally sure why he signed up. "You couldn't be forced to do it, and I actually didn't want to do it," Hoge said. Like everyone else, he thought that on the spectrum of potential career-ending injuries, a concussion wouldn't even register. "I mean, I got a helmet on," he reasoned. But he shrugged and took the test.

In his six years since being drafted, Hoge had learned a lot about the speed and brutality of the NFL. What he hadn't learned from Webster, he had experienced himself. He found that there was a primitive quality to the pro game: Those who survived ate, paid their mortgages, and supported their kids on football. "No wonder it's so intense," he thought to himself. "This is people's livelihoods." He was astonished at how nakedly cutthroat it all was. One day at practice, an injured player violated Noll's edict to keep away from drills. The rule was a not-so-subtle message: If you're injured, not only are you of no use to us but we don't want you tainting the rest of the team. The player had wandered too close to the drill, apparently trying to impress the coaches, when Noll spotted him and said: "Go on. Get out of here."

The player moved closer, not totally comprehending. "No, get your stuff," said Noll. "You're done."

"He cut him right there on the field," Hoge said.

Hoge made his mind up that he would compensate for whatever physical limitations he had by following the rules and making himself indispensable. He made the Steelers in 1987 as a third-string fullback. His second year he started eight games but led the team in rushing. By his third year, Hoge owned the job. He was the quintessential Steelers running back—tough, a grinder. He reminded some people of Rocky Bleier, another rugged back who blocked well, caught passes, churned out yards, and, above all, never gave an inch.

At some point in his career, Hoge decided he understood why the rule makers of professional football created the huddle: "It's a chance for everybody to pause and go, 'Okay, does anybody want to quit?' It's so physically challenging that you need that 35 seconds to revisit" your decision.

One afternoon against the Philadelphia Eagles, Hoge caught a pass and turned upfield when he ran into the linebacker Seth Joyner. The two men had collided on a similar play the previous year, with Hoge getting the better of Joyner. This time the collision triggered a melee. After the two men were separated, Hoge screamed: "I'll whip your ass, Seth, you punk!" The two players returned to their respective huddles but continued to jaw across the line. Finally, the Steelers were backed up near their own goal line when Brister called for a draw play. He handed off to Hoge, who found himself staring into a human wall. It consisted not only of Seth Joyner but also of Jerome Brown, a defensive tackle, and Reggie White, one of the most feared defensive ends in the history of the NFL.

Hoge thought: I'm gonna fuck them up. I'm gonna hit them as hard as they've ever been hit in their life.

He plunged headfirst into the wall. "When I hit, I felt like my internal organs just went out my ass," he said. "It was like *poof!*"

He struggled to the sideline and sidled up to his friend Tunch Ilkin, the Steelers offensive tackle.

"Hey, Tunch, look around at the back of my pants," Hoge said. "I think I shit my pants."

Ilkin at first couldn't detect anything. Hoge lifted up his jersey.

"You shit your pants," said Ilkin.

"I played a whole quarter like that," Hoge said. "We're in the huddle, and everyone's like, 'Gawd, does it stink!'"

Hoge thought concussions were the least of his concerns. But he did notice that the effects were varied and sometimes bizarre. One Sunday at Denver's Mile High Stadium, he ran into Steve Atwater, the Broncos free safety, and found that he couldn't remember the plays or the snap count. He went to the sideline to sort it out and suddenly, without warning, burst into tears. He felt humiliated. Only later did Hoge learn that this was another symptom of a concussion: If the area of the brain that controls emotions becomes damaged, people sometimes cry unexpectedly.

Often, the most devastating hits occurred in practice. One day, the Steelers' first-team offense was playing against the first-team defense, when a play was called that required Hoge to block the strong safety Donnie Shell. Shell weighed just 185 pounds, but his technique was so refined that it was like he turned himself into a tactical missile. When Hoge heard the call in the huddle, he began to pump himself up. He weighed 225 pounds and figured that his greater mass would win the day. "I'm gonna bust that little punk in half," he thought. Hoge wheeled around end and headed straight for Shell. The two men collided in the open field at full speed.

"When I hit him, it was like a lightning bolt ran right through my body, like I'd been paralyzed and electrocuted at the same time," Hoge said. "My helmet got knocked off, and literally on the left side I was numb. I couldn't move."

Hoge was still lying there when he heard Noll's voice ring out: "*That's* it! Now *that's* how you got to hit him!"

Through his haze Hoge heard: "Run it again!"

In 1994, one year after he participated in Maroon and Lovell's experiment (and promptly forgot about it), Hoge signed as a free agent with the Chicago Bears. It would not be a long and fruitful relationship.

During an exhibition Monday-night game at Kansas City, Hoge caught a pass out of the backfield and headed toward the goal line. Several defenders closed in, including nine-time Pro Bowl linebacker Derrick Thomas. As Hoge braced himself for the collision, Thomas plowed his helmet into Hoge's ear hole.

Hoge lay on the turf, motionless. "I've never been in an earthquake, but the first thing I thought was, 'Holy cow, man, the earth is shaking,'" he said. "It was shaking so bad I couldn't get up. I had no equilibrium. I was like, 'This damn earth won't quit shaking.'" Tim Worley, a former Steelers running back who had come over with Hoge, was one of the first people to arrive on the scene. "Aw, damn," Worley said, looking down at his obliterated friend.

Worley was about to motion for the trainers, but then, amazingly, Hoge got up. His brain was on autopilot. It was as if Webster were inside his head screaming: "Get up!" Hoge made it through one more play and then stumbled to the sideline.

"Where are you?" a trainer asked.

"Tampa Bay," he replied.

Asked why he thought that, since he was standing on the field at Arrowhead Stadium, Hoge said: "Because I can hear the ocean."

The Bears sent him to the hospital for a computed tomography (CT) scan. At one point, Hoge wandered off and was found in a waiting room three floors up. He had no idea how he had gotten there.

As he prepared to board the team plane that night back to Chicago, Hoge already was thinking about the next game.

"Do you think I'll be able to play?" he asked Bears physician John Munsell.

"We'll let you know tomorrow," Munsell said.

When Hoge arrived at the Bears' training facility the next day, he looked in the mirror and was shocked. His face was white. His head was pounding "like I had been hit with a bat." But still he wanted to play even though the next game was also an exhibition. When the head trainer, Fred Caito, informed him he'd have to sit out on Munsell's orders, Hoge asked if he could call the doctor and try to talk him out of it. The trainer said no.

Hoge came back the next day.

"Did you guys change your mind?" he asked Caito.

The answer was still no. Hoge now set his sights on the season opener, two weeks away. He desperately wanted to play. The Bears, who had just signed him to a three-year, $2.4 million contract, wanted that too, of course. Unlike Pittsburgh, the Bears had neither a neurological specialist like Joe Maroon nor a diagnostic test to measure how Hoge's brain was functioning. It was all an educated guess as to whether Hoge, chomping at the bit, was fit to play again.

And so one week after Hoge thought he heard the ocean in Kansas City, he rejoined the Bears in preparation for the regular-season opener against Tampa Bay. Hoge knew he wasn't right. He still had blinding headaches and sometimes forgot the snap count. "I mean, most people now when I tell them, it's like, 'How stupid are you?' " Hoge said. "Listen, I didn't go to school to be a neurological doctor."

Hoge played in the season opener and three more games after that. Then, on October 2, the Bears took on the Buffalo Bills at Soldier Field. Early in the game, Hoge bent low to make a block. What happened next is a blur. When Hoge reached the sideline, his chin was sliced open and his face mask caved in. A Bears assistant had to pry it off to treat him. Hoge was unresponsive, staring into space, and so the Bears sent him to the locker room.

He was sitting on the training table when he heard someone say, "Man, are you all right?"

His eyelids fluttered, and he fell to the floor. Hoge had stopped breathing; doctors later told him that 20 seconds passed before he was revived.

He was taken to Northwestern Memorial Hospital in an ambulance. The Bears initially didn't disclose the extent of his injury, announcing only that he had sustained his second concussion in six weeks and a lacerated chin that required stitches. Hoge held out hope for another quick return. He was released from the hospital the next day and went straight to Halas Hall, the Bears' practice facility, wearing the same clothes he'd worn to Sunday's game. He told a reporter for the *Chicago Tribune* that he hoped to play the next week.

In reality, Hoge was in a fog. There were many things he could no longer remember, including his two-year-old daughter's name. A few days later, he went for a doctor's appointment and was found wandering aimlessly in a hospital corridor. The doctor, sensing his confusion, asked him: "Who's the President of the United States?" Hoge didn't know that, either. By the end of the first week, the Bears were saying that Hoge was out indefinitely. The team sent him to specialists and put him through a battery of tests and scans.

When Hoge realized he wasn't getting any better, he decided to return to Pittsburgh to see Joe Maroon and Mark Lovell.

- - -

The concussion test that Lovell and Maroon had created was designed to assess exactly this type of injury: How badly hurt was Merril Hoge's brain? Lovell pulled out Hoge's baseline scores from the original Group of 27 and administered the exam to Hoge again.

When he saw the results, Lovell did a double take; he had never seen a football player so impaired. It had been almost two weeks since Hoge had sustained his second concussion, but his scores were half of what they'd been a year earlier.

One of the tests, the Wechsler Memory Scale, measured short-term memory in a variety of ways. One involved repeating a random sequence of numbers forward and backward. A year earlier, Hoge had tested in the sixty-first percentile on the backward test and the twentieth percentile on the forward test. This time, he tested in the eleventh percentile backward and the second percentile forward.

Lovell then administered the Controlled Oral Word Association Test, in which the subject is asked to list as many words as possible from a specific category—words starting with the letter B, for example. Profanity was allowed. Some players called it the "Fuck Ass Shit Test."

Before his concussion, Hoge listed 43 words in 60 seconds. After: 21.

Hoge then took the Trail Making Test, a measure of mental flexibility in which he was asked to connect a set of 25 dots as quickly as possible. He couldn't complete it.

Lovell showed the results to Maroon. The neurosurgeon was shaken. It was as if Hoge had run his car into a wall at high speed. Maroon's first thought was: "I don't want anybody to die following a football game on my watch."

He summoned Hoge to Allegheny General. Maroon's office was packed with Steelers memorabilia, plastic brains, neurological textbooks, and dozens of papers Maroon had written on brain science.

He laid it out bluntly: "You do this to your brain again, I can't help you. Whatever happens, it's done, it's final, it's finished. If you drool or you can't speak or you can't function, I can't do anything about that. I wouldn't be able to sleep at night if I allowed you to play again."

"Do you understand what I'm saying?" Maroon asked.

Hoge did. More than anyone, he was painfully aware of how hurt he was. The inside of his head was broken. He was incapable of living his life, much less playing professional football. For nearly a decade, Hoge had ignored pain and injury to keep himself on the field. It was part of what had made him so successful. Even in that final game, Hoge had been playing with a broken hand. After the concussion, doctors had fitted him with a cast, reasoning that he wouldn't be playing again for a while. But there was no cast for what he was dealing with now.

"You're just gonna take this?" Hoge thought to himself. "You're not gonna put up a fight or question him? You're just gonna go: 'Okay'?"

But that was exactly what he did. Hoge flew back to Chicago, notified his teammates, and officially announced his retirement from the NFL. He was 29.

O ver the next several months, as Hoge's memory slowly returned, Maroon would get phone calls in the middle of the night. He knew who it was before he answered. "Hey, you know, Doc, I feel great!" Hoge would say. "There's nothing wrong with me!"

Maroon would patiently walk Hoge through it all over again. There was no telling what might happen if he got hit again. He could lose his memory permanently, even his life. And there was always the chance that he would accelerate the process that led to a series of devastating diseases: Parkinson's, Alzheimer's, dementia.

Hoge would let it pass until the next time he ached to get back on the field. Then he'd call Maroon again.

One night, Hoge went to make a personal appearance in Pittsburgh. It was a wine tasting, of all things. Hoge didn't drink wine, but he had committed to going, and so he showed up and pretended he cared or knew anything about wine. He commented on how one wine was bold and one was dry and one was wet.

"Here, try this one," someone said.

"So I did the little swirling thing; I was gonna be a smart-ass and take a little sip," Hoge said. He pressed it to his lips. And then the world went black.

"Everything shut off," he said. "I mean, there was nothing. I scratched my eyes. I blinked my eyes, and I couldn't see a thing."

For ten seconds Hoge couldn't see. When his sight came back, he called Maroon in a panic. The Steelers were in New York playing the Jets, and Hoge reached Maroon at the team hotel. Maroon told him it was an indication that part of his brain was still traumatized.

"This is what I'm trying to tell you, Merril," Maroon said. "You're not healed. Are you willing to risk your vision to play?"

Hoge understood.

"I won't be calling you anymore," he said.

3

"DAD IS IN OHIO"

The dream house had turned into a nightmare. Besides the leaks and the minor flaws, real and imagined, that Mike Webster constantly complained about, the reality was that he couldn't afford it. Pam didn't know where the money had gone. Mike had earned more than $1 million over the last three years of his career. The Websters needed to move on, but Mike was paralyzed—*mentally* paralyzed. For two decades he had been the forceful leader of his household, his every decision creating comfort and stability for his wife and his children, but now he changed plans every hour. Pam woke up wondering: Am I staying in Kansas City? Am I going back to Pittsburgh? Am I going home to Wisconsin?

For most professional athletes, retirement is like falling off a cliff. Webster was 40. He had played 17 years in the NFL, 245 regular-season games. It had provided him with a militaristic structure for his life: train, practice, play; his work schedule was so rigid that it was printed up in the newspaper every fall. Now all of that had been ripped away. It was a struggle all professional football players went through: After so much violence, the transition was a form of post-traumatic stress. Most had trouble coping on some level, but this was different. People who came in contact with Webster found him delusional about both his career prospects and how and where he and his family would survive.

Bob Stage, the Steelers' pilot and his close friend, flew out to Kansas City to spend a weekend with Webster. In some ways, he was the same old Webby; Mike still called him Robert, using the faux French pronunciation, and was generous to a fault. Stage knew that some of the financial problems could be traced to people who had treated Mike like an ATM: "They took his generous heart and took advantage of him."

"You're the only friend who's never asked me for money," Mike once told Stage. But in Kansas City, Stage found Webster totally unrealistic about his future. One warm evening, Webster decided he wanted to throw a baseball around. "Mike had so much nervous energy, he about wore my arm out," said Stage. "The sad part is, he wouldn't listen to anybody. That night when we were playing catch he told me: 'I'm gonna become an agent.' I said, 'Mike, you didn't even get your degree at Wisconsin. How are you going to do that?' He would come up with these ideas, but the dots didn't connect."

"I think I'm gonna sell RVs," Mike said to Pam one morning. The next day he announced: "I think I'm gonna go to chiropractor school."

Pam ended the indecision by persuading Mike to sell the dream house at a steep loss. The Websters put their belongings—furniture, sports equipment, almost everything they owned—in a storage unit and moved back to Wisconsin to start over. They eventually bought a four-bedroom house in Lodi, Pam's hometown, not far from her parents. When they were living in Pittsburgh, Mike and Pam had imagined a simple life after football, with trees and open space, maybe even a log cabin. But the new Mike spent indiscriminately. He bought a speedboat and a pair of Harley Softail Fat Boy motorcycles, toys for his retirement. Where the money came from—and where it went—remained a mystery. Pam later learned that Mike had opened some two dozen checking accounts, stopped paying taxes, and drained three annuities that had been set up for their retirement and the kids' college fund.

Instead of settling on a career, Mike became nomadic, not a traveling salesman but a man on the road in search of a deal—a dreamer and a schemer. He disappeared from the Lodi house for weeks at a time. Unpaid bills began to show up in the mail. Many seemed related to business endeavors that Pam had never known about and that had gone nowhere. Then one day the phone rang.

"Is this Pam Webster?" a woman asked. "I have some of your stuff."

"What do you mean you have some of our stuff?" said Pam.

"Well, we were at an auction, and we bought one of your buffets. It had some of your personal items in it. I'd like to send them to you."

Mike had stopped paying the rent on the storage unit in Kansas City. The company had auctioned off the contents—almost all of the Websters' possessions.

On the occasions when he returned home, Pam and the kids were never certain which Mike would show up. There was Good Mike—gentle with the kids, a loving husband, relatively normal—and Bad Mike— irrational, even destructive. Usually his anger was directed at Pam. She figured out a way to gauge his moods: If her picture was upright on Mike's desk, everything was fine. If it was turned over, she knew to stay out of his way. His eruptions were almost always followed by profuse apologies and profound sorrow over his lack of control.

Each week seemed to bring another low point in Webster's accelerating transformation. One day, Pam returned from a trip to the store to find all the photographs and portraits of Mike as a player dumped on the floor. The pictures were slashed, the frames broken to pieces. As bad as it was, Pam thought it was worse because she was unable to shield the kids from what was happening to their superhero dad, who now seemed to be lashing out at everything he had been. "It was horrible for the kids to see their dad destroying pictures of himself," she said.

One afternoon, Webster took his seven-year-old son Garrett into Madison to pick up some medication. In addition to his deteriorating mental state, Webster was in constant pain: ice pick headaches, throbbing knees, gnarled hands, an aching back. To relieve the pain, he took whatever he could get his hands on: Vicodin, Ultram, Darvocet, Lorcet. When they pulled up at the drugstore, Webster told Garrett to run in and get the medication. He told the boy that in no circumstances was he to let anyone know he was outside. But of course, when Garrett looked up from the counter and asked for his father's painkillers, the pharmacist explained that he couldn't give pills to a little boy.

"Is your dad here?" he asked.

"Yes, he's out in the car. I'll go get him," Garrett said.

When Garrett told his father what had happened, Webster frantically drove off.

"He just started yelling for probably 35 minutes straight," Garrett said. "I'm seven years old at the time, he just started yelling, hitting the dashboard of the car, stuff like that, talking about how now everybody's gonna know he was there. That's where we really noticed he was becoming paranoid. It was always, 'Somebody's following me, or somebody's going through my garbage or listening on the phone line.' " Within ten minutes of the outburst, Webster had apologized and bought Garrett a toy.

And then, like a passing storm, Webster would be gone again, his whereabouts unknown. The Websters soon developed a dark inside joke to explain his long absences: "Dad is in Ohio." It was an all-encompassing catchphrase to be used at missed family functions, school events, important meals. *Dad is in Ohio.* Sometimes the phone would break the silence, like a radar blip revealing a lost ship or plane. It would be Mike, calling from the road about some new scheme. Or it might be the police in Columbus, Wisconsin, a little town east of Lodi, calling to say that Mike had been sleeping in the train station for two days. Would someone please come get him?

Mike sent just about every dime of whatever money he earned back to Pam and the kids, but it came in a trickle. Ultimately, the Lodi house went into foreclosure, and Pam scrambled to get a job and a modest apartment.

Finally, in 1994, Webster returned to Kansas City. Carl Peterson, the team's president and general manager, had tossed him a life preserver. Webby would be the Chiefs' strength and conditioning coach. In normal circumstances, it would have been the perfect assignment. But later, few people recalled him playing much of a role. Marty Schottenheimer, the head coach, would say he didn't even remember that Webster had been around.

For much of the season, Webster lived in a storage closet above the weight room at Arrowhead Stadium. "It was pretty spartan," said Bob Moore, then the team's public relations director and now the Chiefs' historian. "It consisted of a cot and broken weight machines. It was sad, but he was never down about it. He wasn't complaining about it."

Moore had the impression that Webster was either estranged from Pam or divorced; it was obvious that Peterson was trying to help him through a tough time. Webster sometimes appeared at practices, snapping the ball during drills, and also worked with players in the weight room. But he was as much a hanger-on as he was a coach. No one was entirely sure what to make of his presence, this living legend just four years removed from playing in the NFL but seemingly dropped in from another galaxy.

Tim Grunhard was now the Chiefs' starting center. Webster had mentored him during his rookie year, and the two men were close. During his rookie season, Grunhard had noticed some fits of irrationality, but he thought Webster was just quirky. Now, four years later, he saw that Webster was a changed man. "I can't put my finger on what it was, but he wasn't the same guy," said Grunhard.

Webster spent a good chunk of that season with the Chiefs. One day, Moore noticed that he hadn't been around for a while.

"Where's Mike?" he asked.

He's got some other opportunities in some other places, came the response.

What those opportunities were, nobody seemed to know.

When Sunny Jani first heard that Mike Webster was sleeping at the Greyhound bus station in downtown Pittsburgh, he couldn't believe his good fortune. The wheels started spinning immediately. Jani wasn't really that curious about Webster's fall from grace. Rather, he was plotting how he could befriend the former Steeler and make some money off him.

Sunny Jani was his given name. Born outside Bombay, he'd moved to Pittsburgh with his family when he was 12. His parents settled in McKees Rocks, a hardscrabble former steel enclave on the other side of the Ohio River. Sunny's father opened the Blue Eagle Market on Broadway, and when Sunny wasn't at school, he could be found hanging out at the family convenience store, stealing packs of trading cards from his dad. Like most Indian boys, Sunny grew up around cricket and soccer; he found American football difficult to comprehend—Wow, they're killing each other for a little frickin' ball, he thought—though it wasn't hard to pick up on the religious fanaticism that surrounded the Steelers. Jani stole so many packs of trading cards—his father looking the other way—that he eventually accumulated enough to open his own card shop next door to the market.

Sunny knew that Webster had played "a million years" in the NFL, possessed four Super Bowl rings, and was one of the most beloved Steelers of all time. For an enterprising young memorabilia dealer, it was a rare trifecta. After hearing about Webster's plight, he drove to the Greyhound station, and sure enough, there he was, disheveled but unmistakably himself. Webster was sitting alone on a bench, his long, unkempt hair spilling out of a dirty cowboy hat. He was surrounded by a half dozen duffel bags filled with clothes and books. No one appeared to notice the legend in their midst.

Sunny introduced himself and made his pitch.

"Mr. Webster, would you like to come sign autographs? I would pay you for it."

"You're gonna pay me for my autograph?" Webster replied.

Thus was born the Mike Webster–Sunny Jani partnership. Mike followed Sunny out of the bus station—a homeless former Steeler and his spindly twentysomething Indian guide. Jani got Webster a haircut, took him to Kmart to buy new clothes, and rented him a room for a month at the Red Roof Inn—at a discounted rate, since Sunny immediately was able to trade on Webster's name to get a good deal.

Sunny was using Webster, but he seemed to drain some of the sleaziness out of the transaction by being so outrageously transparent about his motives. Every day, people try to turn a celebrity or a sports star into their meal ticket, but seldom do they announce it to the world. Sunny didn't take a percentage from the first deals he made for Webster. That was part of his strategy. "I wanted him to trust me and build up a relationship with him," Sunny said. "My hidden agenda was I wanted to get famous. I said, 'You know, this is my meal ticket, but I have to take care of him.'"

Webster, perhaps the most guileless man in the world, especially in his addled state, wouldn't hear of it. He insisted that Sunny get his fair share. Jani suggested a 10 percent cut. Webster countered with a 50–50 split, and there wouldn't be any negotiating. Sunny knew it was ridiculous, unfair even. He used much of his proceeds to buy groceries for Webster or pay off some of the bills Webster was ignoring.

Sunny secured appearance fees for Webster all over Pittsburgh: $150 to sign autographs at a bowling alley here or a flea market there,

$5,000 to give a speech at Sears. Sunny once arranged an appearance in a friend's garage, where Webster signed autographs for $10 a head. He cut deals for Webster at restaurants, persuading the managers to let the Steelers great eat for free or at a discount. He exchanged Webster's autograph for rent, for cars, for medical expenses, for whatever he could conceive.

"You know, now I feel bad, but I kind of whored him out," Jani said years later.

One client, a meter reader named Dennis, became a cash cow for Sunny and Mike. Dennis was massively overweight, and Webster was entertained by watching him inhale a meal. "He made love to food," Sunny explained. They would go to all-you-can eat buffets at Ponderosa or a Chinese restaurant, with Dennis, of course, paying the freight.

On occasion, Dennis would pay $300 to have Webster come to his apartment and watch a game. Sunny set up this unusual business transaction perhaps a half dozen times until Webster began to feel guilty. Because Dennis liked to hang around, Sunny recruited him into the motley collection of people he employed to keep Webster's life from completely falling apart. Jani dubbed it Team Webster.

Sunny had become the center of Mike Webster's universe. Their relationship, born of exploitation, had shifted until they were now more like a patient and his deeply loyal caretaker. Webster often needed help just getting through the day, his body and mind deteriorating rapidly in opposite directions: Physically, he was an old man. Mentally, he was becoming a child.

As much as Jani tried to keep Mike's life stable, Webster remained perpetually on the move, as if he couldn't sit still. He spent hours driving all over the Midwest, sometimes sleeping in the homes of old friends, or in his cluttered Suburban, or in bus or train stations. By 1996, Webster would estimate he had spent about a year and a half of the last five sleeping in his car.

Webster made the drive from Pittsburgh to Wisconsin and back dozens of times without incident. But suddenly it became an adventure. He was practically living out of his truck, hauling around all his belongings, mainly clothes and books. To the very end, Webster loved to read and write, and the truck was filled with piles of books: Louis L'Amour novels, historical tomes on JFK, Winston Churchill's works, Patton's greatest quotes, which he used to prop up his flagging moods. "He knew his story wasn't gonna end well," Webster's youngest son, Garrett, would say.

Sometimes on those drives, Webster would call Jani in the middle of the night, lost and out of gas, with no money.

The conversations all went something like this:

Sunny: Mike, what do you see around you? What's the mile marker? What highway are you on?
Webster: I see a lot of trees.

It became such a regular occurrence that Jani started hiding money—$20 here, $50 there—inside different books. He always put the money on page 52, Webster's number with the Steelers.

"Mike, I put $50 on page 52 of *Remembering JFK*," Jani would tell him.

Not long after he met Webster, Jani got married; he and his wife had a baby girl. But Webster came to consume so much of Jani's life that Jani was perpetually on call. He finally gave Webster the garage code to his home so that Webster could let himself in and sleep in the basement. Other times, Webster could be found sleeping in the back office at the Blue Eagle.

"You love Mike more than you love me," complained Jani's wife, Marsha. Whenever Mike called, Sunny jumped.

Soon Jani was divorced.

"We built up a great relationship of trust and love," Jani said.

He was talking not about his wife but about Webster.

So much of Mike's life was coming apart in 1996. In May, Pam, with little choice, filed for divorce; Webster was so out of it, he didn't realize until years later that his marriage had been dissolved. The IRS slapped him with a $250,000 tax lien. His health continued to get worse. In the six years since his retirement, Webster had experienced fainting spells. He was hospitalized with heart problems and colitis. During one inexplicable stretch, he lost 20 pounds in three days. Doctors informed him he had lymphoma—until it turned out to be an infection; no one was able to explain why it occurred or went away. Even a minor cut on his leg wasn't simple. Where a Band-Aid would suffice for anyone else, blood spurted out of Webster's leg to the point that he began applying Super Glue to stanch the bleeding.

When Webster showed up at the offices of Dr. Stanley Marks on September 5, 1996, Marks, who had treated him for years, reported that his patient's life had "really deteriorated." Marks continued: "He has had major problems with depression and obsessive compulsive behavior and is currently being treated with Ritalin and Paxil. . . . He also has frequent stress headaches."

One morning that summer, a manager at the Amtrak station in downtown Pittsburgh called the Steelers' offices: Webster had been there all night. Joe Gordon, the team's longtime public relations director, said he would be right over. The Rooneys had hired Gordon in 1969, the same year they had hired Chuck Noll, in an effort to upgrade the previously dismal franchise. Gordon was a Pittsburgh native who had played varsity baseball at Pitt and whose hard-knuckle attitude fit perfectly with the brawling team. In the days preceding the 1976 AFC Championship Game against the hated Raiders, Gordon decked an Oakland TV reporter. Asked the next day if his team was ready, Noll said, "I don't know, but Joe Gordon is."

Gordon had developed great respect for Webster during his 15 seasons with the Steelers. Like everyone, he was wowed by the center's work ethic and was well aware of the brutal childhood that drove him. As the PR director, Gordon also was impressed by Webster's generosity.

"He was always very accommodating, never ever turned down an interview request or to visit a sick kid or go to Children's Hospital," Gordon said. "Mike was always there."

When Webster earned $500 for doing a print ad that Gordon helped set up, Webster tried to give him half the money.

"If it wasn't for you, I wouldn't have had this opportunity," Webster said.

"Mike, that's part of my job," Gordon replied.

Before Gordon left for the train station, he stopped by owner Dan Rooney's office to tell his boss about Webster. Gordon said he planned to take $200 out of petty cash to help Iron Mike. Rooney agreed that was a good plan. Gordon found Webster sitting at a counter, hovering over a pile of photographs of great athletes such as Muhammad Ali and Mickey Mantle. Webster looked messy, his clothes wrinkled, but Gordon didn't think he appeared all that different from the way he often did. When Webster saw Gordon, he seemed unsurprised that the two old friends were meeting in the train station or that one of them seemed to be sleeping there.

"It was just like I'd seen him two or three days ago," Gordon said. "It was a normal meeting with him."

Webster explained that he had acquired the rights to distribute the high-quality photos of sports greats. He told Gordon he was going to make a fortune. Gordon quickly deduced that the business, or at least its prospects, was a figment of Mike's imagination.

"Well, come on, you've got to get out of here," Gordon said. "Where are you staying?"

"I've got a place to stay," Webster said, mentioning the Red Roof Inn.

Before home games, the Steelers stayed at the Hilton, and Gordon suggested that the team could put him up there for the weekend. Webster agreed. He stayed on through the weekend and well beyond that, with no one pressing him to leave. Occasionally, Gordon would stop by, and it appeared as if Webster never left the room. Clothes, towels, candy wrappers, the remains of two-day-old room service were strewn everywhere. Webster assured Gordon he would let the maids clean up. Finally, three days having turned into three months, Rooney had to put his foot down: Webster couldn't live on the Steelers' dime indefinitely. The bill had reached more than $8,000. Gordon was dispatched to tell Webster he had to move on.

Then, with Webster's condition rapidly deteriorating, it was announced he had been elected to the Pro Football Hall of Fame.

The announcement, of course, was not unexpected; Webster was one of the greatest linemen in NFL history. But it presented an uncomfortable dilemma. Webster's struggles had become an open secret in Pittsburgh and parts of Wisconsin. As preparations for the induction ceremony unfolded, those closest to Webster wondered how he would get through it.

In early July 1997, weeks before the ceremony, ESPN aired a story that laid bare Webster's postretirement life. The story noted the loss of his home, his car, and "most of his worldly possessions." Pam was quoted saying, "As good as times got, they got bad. We've gone through times when we didn't have toilet paper, where we did not have heat in the house."

Webster said doctors believed he might have Parkinson's disease or a form of post-concussion syndrome. During a subsequent interview in which he suggested that the ESPN story had overstated his problems, Webster described visiting a doctor in Philadelphia who ran tests that revealed head and chest problems.

"Have you been in a car accident?" the doctor asked Webster. "Have you been hit lately? And how often?"

"Oh, probably about 25,000 times or so," Webster responded.

By the time Team Webster arrived in Canton for the Hall of Fame induction ceremony, the tragic tale of the fallen hero had been published across the country:

Houston Chronicle:
WEBSTER'S INDUCTION COMES AMID CHAOS

Atlanta Journal-Constitution:
HUMBLED HERO; WEBSTER FIGHTS TO OVERCOME DESPAIR

Pittsburgh Post-Gazette:
A LIFE OFF-CENTER

St. Petersburg Times:
A MAN OF STEEL CRUMBLES

Still other papers picked up a story from the Associated Press titled "From Super Bowls to Sleeping in Bus Stations"—a story in which Webster insisted, "I'm not as bad off as people say."

Of course, he was worse. But as humbling as it had been to see the demise play out so publicly, Sunny and Team Webster viewed the Hall of Fame induction more than anything as a business opportunity. At signings, Sunny could now eliminate the word *Future* from *Hall of*

Famer; that had to be worth more money. Webster was in no mood to celebrate, not that he ever was. He had come to view the Hall as a sick ward inhabited by former players discarded by the league, their bodies and minds left to wither and rot, just as his were. He approached the event with two main objectives: dispel the rumors that his life was a train wreck and persuade several other Steelers Hall of Famers to join him in a new business venture. They would market themselves collectively: merchandise, signings, personal appearances.

"This was gonna be his big weekend: 'Hey, I'm not a loser. I'm not a homeless guy living under an overpass like everyone says and addicted to pain medicine,' " said his son Colin. "That and 'Here I am. Look, I made it.' It was gonna be his weekend and the start of a new era."

But none of his former teammates would sign on to his business plan. Some wanted to help, but no one was going to go into business anytime soon with Webby, not in his current state. Webster asked Bob Stage, the pilot, if he would introduce him before his acceptance speech. Stage was touched, but he thought the choice was a reflection on how sick Webster was. "Mike, I'm honored, but you need somebody who had an impact in your career, not Joe Blow," he said. Webster asked Stage if he thought Bradshaw would do it. Of course he would, said Stage.

In fact, Bradshaw did more than that. During the weekend, the retired Steelers quarterback pulled Webster aside and handed him a check for $175,000. Webster tore it up. "Nooooo!" Sunny cried. "Mike, we need it!" Webster's pride in such matters was as erratic and malleable as his mental state. One minute he was living in the Pittsburgh Hilton on the Rooneys' dime, and the next he was ripping up a $175,000 check from his quarterback of over a decade. As the years went on, Webster repeatedly rebuffed offers from his friends and former teammates, eventually alienating many of them. He developed an irrational loathing of the Steelers, blaming the team for a variety of his ills.

The ceremony on July 26, 1997, was delayed by rain; it was sticky and humid, with temperatures reaching the eighties. Webster was the last to be inducted into a class that included Raiders defensive back Mike Haynes, New York Giants owner Wellington Mara, and Dolphins coach Don Shula, who, tanned and youthful, looked like he had just arrived from the Bahamas, especially compared with Webster, sitting next to him, who was pale and disheveled.

Webster fidgeted through the ceremony, adjusting his gold Hall of Fame blazer and tie, which he wore over a dark blue golf shirt, its collar half up and half down. The inductees sat in a row behind the podium. At one point, in the middle of Mara's speech, Webster got up and left, returning after a few minutes. When Bradshaw finally took the podium to a loud ovation, his introduction was more of a sermon than a speech. Bradshaw rarely had set foot in Pittsburgh after his career ended, apparently because of his resentment over the abuse he endured early in his career. But for 10 minutes—longer than even the inductees were supposed to speak—Bradshaw talked largely about himself, a homespun tale of his dream to play football and how God had not only granted him that dream but allowed him to share it with some of the greatest players ever—Swann, Stallworth, Harris, Bleier, Greene, Lambert, Ham, Kolb, Holmes.

Finally, Bradshaw reached the powerful climax:

"But what good is a machine if you ain't got a center? And oh, did I get a center! I didn't just get any ol' center, no sirree. I got the best that's ever played the game, the best that ever put his hand down on a football. I loved him from the first time I ever put my hands under his butt."

As Bradshaw continued, Webster, aware that he was about to speak, removed his tie.

"There has never been or there never will be another man as committed, totally dedicated to making him the very best that he could possibly be," Bradshaw continued. "There's never been a man who was so loved. He was the background on which we were built around. He was our spine. There never has been, never will be, another Mike Webster!"

At Bradshaw's own induction in 1989, he had yelled, "What I wouldn't give right now to put my hands under Mike Webster's butt just one more time!" And so as he completed his introduction, Bradshaw reached into a paper bag, pulled out a football, and shouted, "One more time!" Webster rose, with the Steeler faithful delirious, took off his blazer, and limped over to Bradshaw. He grabbed the ball, somehow managed to hunch down as low as he ever did when he was playing, and snapped a bullet to Bradshaw.

The two men hugged, Webster approached the podium—and Team Webster held its breath.

By this point in Webster's life, Ritalin was one of his best friends, a drug he came to depend on to get him through the day. He used it to focus and take the edge off his spiraling depression. A psychostimulant, Ritalin had grown popular for treating children with attention deficit disorder. Though it sparked the release of dopamine in the brain—the chemical most associated with pleasure and reward—the drug had the effect of honing an ADD patient's concentration. Some doctors saw its potential with Parkinson's patients and with adults who had experienced brain trauma. It was clear to Webster that Ritalin worked for him. Before taking the podium in Canton he gulped down 80 mg.

Even then, his rambling speech lasted 21 minutes—13 more than his allotted time. Speaking without notes, Webster was conversational, occasionally inspiring, and funny. But he was also all over the place. He opened with a slightly awkward joke: "Giving Bradshaw a forum and a microphone is like giving Visine to a Peeping Tom." He added another later: "His dad says he was so ugly, his mom carried him around for two weeks upside down, thought he only had one eye." Webster left the stage briefly to hug Pam, the kids, and other family members. He bounced in and out of messages about failure and success, briefly quoted Longfellow, and lost his train of thought several times.

Sometimes it appeared as if he were giving a talk to a group of middle-school students:

"Don't give up, don't be afraid to fail. No one is keeping score. All we have to do is finish the game, and we'll all be winners."

Other times he sounded like a man trying to save his country, though it was unclear what he was trying to save it from:

"I'm talking about things that are going on today that have been ignored for a long period of time. And yeah, we're addressing them now because we have a history of only addressing them only when they jump up and bite us in the ass. And not until we do that. But we can change that. We can change, but we're in this, we gotta care about one another, we gotta care about our kids, we gotta care about a lot of things. And we do care about a lot of things, but we gotta have enough people caring and working together. And we can get that done, it's not impossible. Hell, nothing else is working. You know, maybe it's idealistic, but nothing else is working, folks. And I'm just appreciative that I had the opportunity to play with these men both in Pittsburgh and Kansas City, and against the jerks on the other teams."

As he watched Webster struggle, Bob Stage cringed. The Steelers' pilot had enjoyed Webster's company for years and considered him one of the most decent men he had ever known. The man he was now watching was being honored for his greatness on the football field, which was fitting, but it was no longer Mike Webster.

"It made no sense," Stage said. "It broke my heart."

Perhaps most notable in Webster's speech was who he didn't thank—and who didn't attend. There was no mention of Steelers owner Dan Rooney or Joe Gordon or anyone else from the team's front office except for the beloved and deceased Steelers patriarch, Art Rooney Sr. No one from the organization attended. Dan Rooney said he was in Dublin preparing for the team's American Bowl preseason game the next day against the Bears. "I expected more," Pam told the *Post-Gazette*. "It's a shame. They could have sent someone or sent a telegram. It would have been the classy thing to do."

By this time, Webster's festering enmity toward his former team was obvious to those closest to him, though its origins were never clear. Part of it was Webster's belief that the Steelers had never offered him a coaching job at the end of his career, although Dan Rooney later said they had. Part of it certainly was his growing paranoia and, with that, his lasting belief that Rooney had somehow betrayed him. Why he came to hate Joe Gordon, no one really could say. Just a year earlier, Gordon and Rooney had rescued Webster from the Pittsburgh Greyhound station. But hate was what it was, and as Webster got sicker, that hate consumed him.

There was, however, one moment of astonishing lucidity in Mike Webster's Hall of Fame speech, a moment that seemed to capture the essence of the sport that had broken him. "You know, it's painful to play football, obviously," he told the crowd. "It's not fun out there being in two-a-day drills in the heat of the summer and banging heads. It's not a natural thing."

Seated behind Webster was the NFL commissioner, Paul Tagliabue. This remark, as truthful as any that Webster would utter that day, seemed to provoke in Tagliabue neither awareness nor reflection as he sat next to Bradshaw watching an NFL legend unravel. Instead, the commissioner and Bradshaw seemed to be laughing at something.

4

FUCK YOU, JERRY MAGUIRE

In March 1996, about a year and a half after Merril Hoge announced his retirement, some of the nation's leading experts in sports medicine gathered during a spring snowstorm at Allegheny General Hospital in Pittsburgh. By the standards of some medical conferences, it wasn't a huge gathering: about 200 brain specialists, team doctors, and trainers, mostly from across the Northeast. The conference was billed as "the first cross-disciplinary attempt to confront the many difficult issues regarding evaluation and treatment of sports-related concussion." Maroon, who cohosted, used his Steelers connections to put together an "experts roundtable" of doctors and retired players, including Hoge, New York Giants linebacker Harry Carson, Steelers quarterback Mike Tomczak, and Buffalo Bills safety Mark Kelso. The moderator was former Steelers great Lynn Swann, whom Maroon introduced as "a master chef, poet, and good friend."

What followed was an eye-opening dialogue about the realities facing the NFL when it came to brain injuries. The players told the audience of doctors that they had spent their entire careers essentially ignoring them, playing through pain and injury out of fear of letting down their teammates and losing their jobs. During one exchange, Swann asked Carson, a future Hall of Famer and one of the best linebackers of his generation, a leading question: Do players feel their "livelihood" is threatened when they come off the field?

"Very much so," said Carson. "Football players are very insecure people. Players are interchangeable parts. Someone played your position before you, and when you leave, someone else is going to be in your place. You are only there for a short time, so you want to make as much as you can in the time given you. You do not want to give anyone else a shot at your job. Football players understand that if they give someone the opportunity to do the job better, their days are numbered."

Perhaps the most startling admission came from Tony Yates, the Steelers' team doctor, who said he was essentially powerless to bench a highly motivated player. He cited as an example Greg Lloyd, a Steelers linebacker who once said, "I know I haven't played a good game unless my hand has been stepped on or if somebody somewhere isn't bleeding." Yates told his fellow doctors, each of whom had taken the Hippocratic oath ("Do no harm"), that the ultimate authority for getting Greg Lloyd off the field was not him, the doctor, but the head coach. "Many times it is just physically impossible," Yates said. "Only a head coach can pull a player off. When we finally reach the head coach and impress upon him the seriousness of an injury, the players come off."

Sitting in the audience, mesmerized, was a Michigan State graduate student named Michael (Micky) Collins. He had made the five-hour drive down from East Lansing with his faculty adviser, mostly out of curiosity. Collins felt like he was at a personal crossroads. A former pitcher and outfielder at the University of Southern Maine, he was in his second year studying for a master's degree in clinical psychology. But Collins had no idea what he wanted to do with his life. He missed sports and had thought about coaching or perhaps a career as an athletic trainer. He had traveled to Pittsburgh at the suggestion of his adviser, who thought the combination of sports and brain research might stir Collins's interest.

Collins was attentive to what the players had to say, but for him the real stars were the doctors and the scientists. He watched as Joe Maroon and Mark Lovell presented their latest findings on concussions. "These are the coolest guys in the world," Collins thought. During the drive back to East Lansing, he told his adviser: "This is what I want to do with my life."

At this point in the looming concussion crisis, Merril Hoge was no

longer a professional football player; he was a case study and a caution-
ary tale. During the conference, Lovell had presented slides showing
how Hoge's brain function had fallen off a cliff after the hit in Chicago.
Lovell's concussion test already was becoming known in neuropsych circles as the Pittsburgh Steelers Test Battery, although the Steelers didn't
own it and the test was not yet the marketing juggernaut it would come
to be. Collins was fascinated. After watching Lovell's presentation, he
approached him and asked if he could use the Steelers Battery as the
basis for his own research into football-related concussions. Lovell readily agreed. Thus began the steep upward trajectory that within five years
would turn Collins into one of the leading concussion experts in the
country and a member of a partnership with Maroon and Lovell that
would shape the NFL concussion saga in huge and controversial ways.

Collins was nothing if not enterprising. He first used the Steelers Battery on the Michigan State football team, having secured permission through a trainer. Collins baselined a Spartan a day for months,
all the while thinking to himself, No way this is gonna work. Then one
day a lineman named Chris Smith came off the field with a concussion.
Collins tested him the next day. "He looked normal, he talked normal,
he acted normal, and he went right back to play," said Collins. There
was one problem: The test indicated that Smith was a walking zombie;
he shouldn't have been playing at all. "I was thinking to myself, 'Wow.
This really works,'" said Collins. At that point, he was in no position
to influence whether Chris Smith played or sat out, but he was emboldened. He secured a small grant to study other colleges. He traveled to
the universities of Utah and Pitt and then got an internship to study the
University of Florida football team.

When he was done, Collins wrote up his findings. He submitted the
paper not to some minor publication for young researchers but to the
Journal of the American Medical Association, or *JAMA,* the most widely
circulated medical journal in the world. "'What the hell, it's a sexy
topic, isn't it?'" he thought. Collins titled his sexy paper "Relationship
between Concussion and Neuropsychological Performance in College
Football Players." He cold-called a *JAMA* editor, who agreed to take
a look. The fact that the paper was accepted, he later acknowledged,

was a tribute less to its quality ("It's probably the worst paper I've ever published") than to the sudden appetite for a subject that researchers had ignored for years but that now seemed critically important, an issue whose time had come, like the dangers of nicotine or cholesterol. The paper's major findings, published in 1999, were that neuropsychological testing was an effective tool to assess concussions in athletes and that those with a history of multiple concussions or learning disabilities were far more likely to fail those tests.

"Quite honestly, and not to sit here and blow, but this paper was seminal," said Collins. He seemed dismissive of the earlier work of researchers such as Jeff Barth, who had reached similar conclusions but had published his research as a chapter in a book called *Mild Head Injury*. Years later, that book was still available on Amazon, delivered to your doorstep within days, but Collins would say: "The other article published on this stuff was published in some obscure journal, and there was very little. You had to dig deep to find it." Collins's own article, in contrast, was big-time: "This was *JAMA*!"

Collins had short blond hair, an angular head that squared off at its crown, and the wiry physique of a distance runner. He was tightly wound and argumentative and sometimes came off as being about as charitable with his peers as he was with Barth. Collins had particular contempt for neurologists, for example, believing that most of them failed to grasp the intricacies of his particular specialty: "There are some incredible neurologists, but ninety percent of them have no clue how to manage a concussion, ninety-five percent of them," he said. When explaining his work and the science of concussions, he had a habit of punctuating his sentences with a quick check to make sure his listeners were able to keep up: "You following me? Does that make sense?" He was the opposite of his mentor, Lovell, who projected a kind of sleepy calm. But when Lovell went to work at the new sports medicine center that had been established at the University of Pittsburgh Medical Center, joining Maroon at UPMC, he brought Collins with him.

Collins worshiped Lovell. "Mark Lovell is probably the smartest human being I've ever met in my life," he said. "He has vision. He's a tinkerer. He's the mad scientist in the room. Smoke comes out from under the door. I'm the guy that sees all the patients and runs around."

After decades of neglect, concussions were taking off as a research subject that merited serious attention. As Collins had correctly pointed out, examining the brains encased in football helmets adorned with the team logos to which millions of Americans had sworn allegiance was suddenly a sexy topic. There was money to be had and, equally important, prestige. There were headlines and careers to be made. The researchers who got in early—Jeff Barth, Joe Maroon, Mark Lovell, and a few others—soon begat other researchers, and they too began to make discoveries, many of which would prove highly problematic for one of the nation's leading concussion factories: the National Football League.

Julian Bailes was a rising star when Maroon recruited him out of Northwestern University in Chicago to join him on the neurosurgical staff at Allegheny General Hospital in 1988. The two men could hardly have been more different in background and temperament. Maroon had grown up in Bridgeport, Ohio, a striver in the blue-collar image of his hustling father. Bailes was the son of a Louisiana Supreme Court justice. He had spent much of his early life in New Orleans and other parts of Louisiana and exuded the easy charm of a southern patrician, a stout handsome man with a slight drawl and thick dark hair that he swept back from his forehead.

Bailes had been ambivalent about beginning his career in sleepy Pittsburgh. But Maroon possessed one particularly attractive chit: In addition to performing brain surgery, Bailes could join him working the sidelines with the Pittsburgh Steelers, learning from the man who had watched over the brains of Terry Bradshaw and Jack Lambert. Bailes had been an all-state linebacker in high school and had gone on to play at Northwestern State University, a small Division I school in Natchitoches, Louisiana. He still lived and died for football. "I said, 'Shit, that sounds like as good a reason as any to move to Pittsburgh,'" Bailes recalled. "I'm in." He quickly adapted to his surroundings. "You know, there was no greater feeling than being a single neurosurgeon in Pittsburgh and going to the Porsche dealership and writing a check for $120,000 and driving this Porsche out and not even caring," he said. "I went through about five of them."

In the mid-1990s, around the same time Maroon and Lovell were developing the Steelers Battery, Bailes was introduced to Frank Woschitz, a longtime official with the NFL Players Association. Woschitz had just conducted a health survey on retired players that he hoped would persuade the union and the league to give the players lifetime health insurance. It was a huge problem: Players often left the game so battered that they were unable to qualify for health insurance. But the league refused to provide it.

Bailes had agreed to look at the data for Woschitz—hundreds of questionnaires stacked in cardboard boxes—expecting that it would focus on mundane issues such as arthritis, back injuries, and heart disease. But when Bailes took a closer look, he was stunned. "Yes, they had hyperlipidemia [high cholesterol] and joint pain and cardiac disease, as expected," he said. "But they were also having all kinds of cognitive problems. It was way out of line for what you would expect."

Bailes shared this curious piece of information with a New York neurologist named Barry Jordan. In neuroscience circles, Jordan was already something of a legend. While attending Harvard Medical School in the late 1960s, Jordan, one of the few African Americans in his class, had decided to make up his own concentration: sports neurology. "All my classmates laughed at me," he said. By the time he connected with Bailes, Jordan was one of the preeminent experts in sports medicine in the country and the chief medical officer of the New York State Athletic Commission.

Jordan agreed that the survey findings were off the charts. He wasn't entirely surprised. Jordan had done a lot of research into boxing, in which the issue of chronic brain damage had been known since the 1920s, and had been expecting to see it show up in other contact sports. As early as 1999, he wrote that chronic brain damage "has been described primarily in boxers, but it may be anticipated in other sports such as American football, ice hockey and perhaps soccer."

Now, if Frank Woschitz's survey was correct, retired football players were showing dramatically elevated signs of incipient dementia in huge numbers. Bailes and Jordan followed up with a survey of their own. To avoid tipping off the players that they were specifically looking at brain damage, Bailes and Jordan asked questions about a broad spectrum of injuries. Again, the numbers were dramatic.

In May 2000, Bailes and Jordan presented their findings at the

American Academy of Neurology's annual meeting in San Diego. Out of 1,090 former players, 60 percent reported that they had sustained at least one concussion during their careers; more than a quarter reported more than three. The players with concussions, most in their fifties and sixties at that point, were reporting significant neurological problems: memory loss, confusion, speech or hearing problems, and headaches.

The news, preliminary as it was, was in many ways worse than what researchers such as Barth, Lovell, and Collins were uncovering. Those studies had shown that concussions had to be taken seriously, with symptoms that often lingered for days or weeks or even longer. But it was assumed that with time those symptoms eventually went away. After the release of his first paper in *JAMA*, Collins told the *Detroit News*: "If you give the brain time to heal, there's no reason to see long-term deficits."

But Bailes and Jordan were suggesting that that wasn't necessarily the case. They were saying something quite ominous: that the head-banging endemic to the NFL might have far-reaching—even permanent—consequences.

Bailes vowed to study the issue further. He believed "a trove of information" was contained in Frank Woschitz's cardboard boxes, a researcher's gold mine. Later, those early results would remind Bailes of another health crisis he had witnessed. "It's like when HIV started coming out; I was here in Chicago, and we didn't know what it was," he said. "There were these young men, 22, 23 years old, showing up with Kaposi's sarcoma and other weird things that you shouldn't get when you're 23. It was the HIV suppressing their immune system."

Looking back, Bailes believed that he and Barry Jordan had stumbled onto "the first whiff" of another new disease.

The early scientific breakthroughs of the 1990s involved almost exclusively men who toiled in white lab coats beneath the fluorescent lighting of hospitals and universities. But there was a connection between the growing interest in concussion research and the carnage unfolding in stadiums across the country. In many ways, the research was being fueled by the dawning awareness of football fans, who began to notice that the big hits they so relished seemed to produce a sobering by-product: the vacant stares of their heroes lying motionless on the field.

In the tenth week of the 1992 season, the New York Jets traveled to Denver to play the Broncos. The Jets' premier receiver at the time was Al Toon, an elegant contortionist whose jazzy surname perfectly fit his improvisational style. Toon stood 6-4 and once made the Olympic trials in the triple jump. He frequently hurled himself into space to make impossible catches, climbing above defenders who lacked his speed and balletic grace. Toon often paid for it: The Steelers' Lloyd once knocked him out cold, then slapped the turf with his palm next to Toon's splayed body as if he were counting him out.

In Denver, Toon caught a pass and was falling near the sideline, his head about a foot off the ground, when linebacker Michael Brooks flew over him, catching the back of his head with his elbow. It was not a particularly dramatic hit—Toon would later say that Brooks "grazed" him—but the effect was like "a cannonball hitting me on the back of the head," he said. From that point forward, what Toon recalled about the play was gleaned largely from film and information he picked up from the Jets' trainers.

As he lay on a training table in the dank basement of Mile High Stadium, Toon found that there were many gaps in his memory. They included: How old am I? Do I have kids? What am I doing here? What year is it?

"I had to go through a process of remembering who I was," he told ESPN's Greg Garber.

Toon's symptoms—the headaches and disorientation, the projectile vomiting—had always dissipated, but this time they didn't: They grew worse. The concussion stayed with Toon like a "lingering flu." Loud noises, bright lights, the motion of a passing car, all made him swoon. He spent the next two weeks "in bed, in a dark room, curtains drawn, no noise, no kids, no conversation." As he lingered in his cognitive netherworld, the Jets put out an estimate that the concussion was the fifth of his eight-year career. Toon believed it was more like 10. He confided to Garber that he had contemplated suicide.

The team sent him to multiple neurologists. The one who led the case, Ira Casson, like Barry Jordan, had studied boxers and chronic brain disease and had even examined Muhammad Ali's CT scans, determining that Ali had had brain damage even before the end of his career. Casson knew as well as anyone the ravages of the injury, what someone with an overpounded brain looked like. A decade earlier, Casson had led a landmark study that examined 10 boxers who had been knocked out. He discovered "cerebral atrophy" in half of them, an indication of chronic brain damage. Toon already had decided to put his fate in the hands of his doctors, and Casson, for one, had grave doubts: "I'm not sure that you should do this anymore," the neurologist told Toon. "I don't know what the next concussion is going to do to you." Toon interpreted this to mean that he might never wake up.

Toon had an economics degree from Wisconsin, making the dean's list his last two years, and was known as one of the smartest players in the league. He had recently signed a three-year, $4.1 million contract but was already financially secure, having acquired his real estate license and used it to expand his own business. He and his family lived on a horse farm outside Madison. That made the decision easier. Weeping softly, Toon, still five months shy of his thirtieth birthday, announced his retirement on November 27, 1992, three weeks after his injury.

By the time Hoge went down two years later, writers were proclaiming 1994 the "Season of the Concussion." One bloody Sunday in October, three quarterbacks were knocked out: Troy Aikman, Chris Miller, and Vinny Testaverde. That season, an idea was floated to send defensive players to an NHL-like penalty box for flagrant hits on quarterbacks. Aikman's concussion had been caused by Wilber Marshall, a 240-pound linebacker. Marshall, then playing for Arizona, plowed the crown of his helmet into Aikman's chin, splitting it open and lacerating his tongue. Aikman, a bloody mess, made it to the sideline, where he was asked three questions by the Dallas doctor: What day is it? What month is it? What year is it?

"I think he scored 33 percent," said the doctor, J. R. Zamorano. Aikman was aware only that it was Sunday.

As the grisly episodes were recounted, one phenomenon was not lost on the fans and the media: The current generation of players was noticeably bigger, stronger, and faster than the one that preceded it. The prototypical new player was Giants linebacker Lawrence Taylor, a tornado of violence who single-handedly launched a nationwide search for unique specimens who embodied the same combination of size, speed, strength, and, more inexact, ruthlessness. Wilber Marshall, in fact, was one of those people.

The physical consequences of this new phenomenon were obvious: As the game got bigger and faster, the destructive force behind the hits grew. Any fan could see this, but one of them happened to be an atomic physicist. Tim Gay liked to boast that he had played football at Cal Tech ("La Verne College used to kick our ass on a routine basis"). At the University of Nebraska, where he worked, his primary focus was polarized electron physics. Gay's works included *Use of Partial-Wave Decomposition to Identify Resonant Interference Effects in the Photoionization-Excitation of Argon,* but Gay also had carved out a niche as the resident expert on the physics of football. On Saturday afternoons, with a voice like a carnival barker, the bow-tied, bespectacled professor delivered one-minute lectures on the science of the spiral to 75,000 Cornhuskers fans who watched him on HuskerVision.

Gay eventually turned his side project into a book, *Football Physics,* in which he explored, among other things, changes in kinetic energy as football players got bigger and faster. He focused on the line of scrimmage, the Pit, where the battle for territory is most pronounced and the biggest players smash into one another on every down, creating huge amounts of destructive force. Hoge called it "the Box," a qualitatively different world from the perimeter, the place where "the big boys play." Drawing on figures from the NFL Hall of Fame and other sources, Gay calculated that the average mass of a lineman had increased by 60 percent between 1920 and 2000, reaching almost 300 pounds (that figure would climb to 310 by 2011). The average speed had increased by about 12 percent. Gay didn't want to limit himself to the static force elaborated by Newton's second law of motion (force = mass × acceleration). He wanted to measure the potential for destruction inside the Pit; hence his focus on energy. "Energy is actually what goes into breaking bones and causing concussions," he said. "It's how much I crush him."

By Gay's calculation, the amount of kinetic energy unleashed in the Pit had effectively doubled as modern players evolved. Kinetic energy is a measure of combined mass (in pounds) and speed (in feet per second).

The figure Gay arrived at was 1,875 units of kinetic energy. "To put all of this in perspective," he wrote, "a bullet fired from a .357 Magnum handgun has about 300 [units] of kinetic energy, so we would need to unload a full revolver chamber into the defense in order to expend the same amount of energy on them. We might even suggest that the result would be no more deadly than getting hit by some of the offensive lines that Dallas put on the field in the mid-1990s."

For its part, the media seemed not entirely certain how to respond to this new old injury and whether to take it any more seriously than a strained hamstring or a groin pull. Greg Garber's piece for ESPN had been groundbreaking. The frank admissions by players like Toon, Hoge, and Harry Carson about their post-career suffering were poignant and, in many ways, harrowing. Yet when it came time to edit the piece, Garber, a decorated reporter who had written the script along with his producer, Christine Caddick, found that ESPN was reluctant to use the term *brain damage*. That's exactly what had occurred, of course: The players' brains had been damaged for weeks, months, and even years. Garber and Caddick met with the network's highest-ranking executives, who told them they couldn't use the phrase. Only at the last minute did it make it in the feature. In the back of his mind, Garber wondered how much of the debate had to do with ESPN's contract with the NFL, which at that point was worth not $15.2 billion but a little over $500 million.

Sportswriters described concussions with a mix of the old jocularity and newfound seriousness. There were scattered calls for reform. After watching Testaverde, then the Browns' starting quarterback, lose consciousness and, for a time, his senses, Cleveland columnist Bill Livingston pronounced the NFL's concussion problem "a disgrace." He decried the league's lighthearted treatment of the injury, its business strategy of "making money on pain." "Pro football doesn't just lovingly detail mayhem, it has helped create a mass culture that thrives on it," he wrote. Dave Anderson, the *New York Times'* Pulitzer Prize–winning sports columnist, warned that the NFL was courting "a tragedy" reminiscent of the hit that had left Darryl Stingley paralyzed in 1978.

- - -

The NFL, in a refrain that would seem eerily familiar years later, downplayed the crisis. Greg Aiello, the league's director of communication, repeatedly told reporters that the rate of concussions since 1989, when the NFL began to keep track, was unchanged: one concussion every three or four games. The data, Aiello said, had been collected by the teams and passed on to an epidemiologist who had crunched the numbers for the NFL's competition committee. "In the big picture, when you consider the number of times the head is impacted [in pro football], the number of concussions is relatively small," said Aiello. "But hey, they do occur. And maybe there's more we can do."

But of course it depended on how you counted concussions. The league, Aiello acknowledged, was counting head injuries as concussions only when a player lost consciousness or was seriously dazed. Garden-variety concussions were not part of the program. Joe Maroon did his own calculations and estimated that two to four concussions occurred in *every* NFL game.

That discrepancy perhaps should have raised red flags. At minimum, there was a 156 percent difference between the rate of concussions reported by the NFL and the rate reported by the senior neurological expert in the league. Maroon said that he, for one, was quite concerned. But few people seemed to notice.

Late in the Season of the Concussion, Tagliabue appeared with two other commissioners, the NBA's David Stern and the NHL's Gary Bettman, in the auditorium at Manhattan's 92nd Street Y to discuss the state of their respective leagues. The panel's moderator was the journalist David Halberstam, who had gone on to a career of writing books, including several about sports, after winning the Pulitzer Prize for his coverage of the Vietnam War for the *New York Times*.

After dispensing with questions about labor relations and league finances, Halberstam turned to the NFL's growing concussion problem. Tagliabue quickly dismissed the matter as a "pack journalism issue" and then used the league's dubious statistics to try to deflect concern. Tagliabue repeated the claim that the NFL experienced "one concussion every three or four games," which he said came out to 2.5 concussions for every "22,000 players engaged."

For Halberstam, it was a moment of déjà vu. He seemed to be taken back to the days of the Five O'Clock Follies, the name the Saigon press corps bestowed upon the surreal, statistics-crammed U.S. government press briefings. Halbertstam compared the NFL commissioner to the former U.S. defense secretary: "I feel I'm back in Vietnam hearing McNamara give statistics," he told the audience, which howled.

Sports Illustrated, covering the exchange, lit into the commissioner: "Tagliabue's head has been spared this season's spate of bruising hits; on this issue he ought to be making better use of it."

Not long afterward, the NFL announced its own scientific initiative. At Tagliabue's behest, the league said it was assembling a subcommittee of experts to study concussions. Tagliabue's initiative would be called the Mild Traumatic Brain Injury Committee.

The NFL's most influential voice on concussions belonged not to the news media or a player or perhaps even the commissioner. It belonged to an agent.

Leigh Steinberg represented almost every major quarterback in the NFL. At a time when free agency was finally coming to football in a significant way and TV money was helping the NFL realize its full financial potential, Steinberg had emerged as one of the league's most powerful men. His reach extended into the commissioner's office, the networks, the front offices, and beyond. In December 1993, the seven-year-old Fox Network had paid $1.58 billion to broadcast the NFC, a staggering bet that had knocked out CBS, the league's network and partner for the previous four decades. The transaction underscored how television was shaping the modern NFL. Steinberg derived his outsized power from his near monopoly of the stars of the show.

Steinberg had come out of Boalt Hall, UC Berkeley's prestigious law school. He had fallen into "sports agentry," as the nascent profession came to be known, after a friend, Cal quarterback Steve Bartkowski, asked him to represent him in his contract negotiations with the Falcons. Bartkowski was the number one pick in the 1975 draft, and Steinberg landed him a deal for $650,000 over four years, at the time the richest contract given to a draft pick in the history of the league. Steinberg was 26, not much older than his client. When he and Bartkowski touched down at Atlanta's Hartsfield Airport, Steinberg was astonished to find the tarmac lit up like a movie set, a crowd pushing against a police barricade. "I looked at Steve like Dorothy looked at Toto when they got to Munchkin Land and said, 'I guess we're not in Berkeley anymore.'" For Steinberg, who was still trying to chart his own career path, it was a moment of epiphany: "I saw the tremendous idol worship and veneration that athletes were held in, how they were the movie stars, they were the celebrities. I saw the power that athletes had to potentially be cultural symbols, and I could see that football—although baseball at that time was still the most popular sport—was going to fit the new media, was gonna fit television and grow up together in a unique way."

By the mid-1990s Steinberg was at the height of his power. He brought a mixture of naked ambition, self-promotion, and Berkeley-style activism to the job. He insisted that his athletes take seriously their power as role models. He and his clients donated tens of millions of dollars to charity, setting up personal foundations and volunteering in their communities. Steinberg titled his best-selling autobiography *Winning with Integrity: Getting What You're Worth without Selling Your Soul*. He became sports' first true superagent. The writer-director Cameron Crowe trailed him for two years and then hired him as a consultant on *Jerry Maguire,* the 1996 movie about a brash sports agent who grows a conscience overnight.

The movie's plot turns on a scene in which an athlete who suffered a concussion wakes up to see his wife, his son (who appears to be about 12), his doctor, and his agent at his bedside. After the player, with his wife's assistance, remembers his name ("Wait, it's coming . . . my name is Steve Remo") and identifies his family, his freckle-faced son confronts Jerry Maguire, played by Tom Cruise, in the hallway.

"This is his fourth concussion," the boy says. "Shouldn't somebody get him to stop?"

"Hey, hey, hey," says the agent, checking his cell phone. "It would take a *tank* to stop your dad. It would take all five Super Trooper VR Warriors to stop your dad. Right? Right?"

"Fuck you," says the boy, flipping off the agent as he walks away.

The scene resembled a real one that had taken place three years earlier. Steinberg had Dallas quarterback Troy Aikman among his clients. When the Cowboys beat the 49ers in the 1993 NFC Championship (played January 23, 1994), a defensive lineman accidentally kneed Aikman in the head during the third quarter. Afterward, the Cowboys said Aikman had a "mild" concussion. J. R. Zamorano, the team doctor, predicted: "He'll be ready for the Super Bowl. There's no contact in practices this week, so I don't foresee a problem." But it was enough of a problem for the Cowboys to put Aikman in the hospital for evaluation.

That night, Steinberg stood by Aikman's bed at Baylor University Medical Center. The city was still celebrating the Cowboys' second straight trip to the Super Bowl. As Steinberg describes the scene, Aikman is "in a darkened hospital room, alone, no doctor and this incredible celebration is going on which you can hear in the background—horns honking, people screaming. He looked up at me with a puzzled look on his face and said, 'Leigh, why am I here?' "

"Well, you suffered a concussion," Steinberg replied.

"Did I play?" Aikman asked.

"Yes, you played."

"Did I play well?"

"Yes, you threw some touchdown passes."

"What's that mean?"

"Well, it means you're going to the Super Bowl."

"He was happy, his face brightened," Steinberg said. "I sat there, and about five minutes later he turned to me with a confused look on his face and said, 'Leigh, why am I here? Did I play today? Did I play well?' The same exact questions. So I answered him, and about 10 minutes passed, and he looked back with the same puzzled expression and said, 'Why am I here?' It terrified me. I saw how tenuous the bond was between consciousness and dementia and realized that this young man who I cared for and loved was sitting alone as a result of a concussion and we had no idea what the consequences were."

The immediate consequences were that Aikman walked out of the hospital the next morning, not having slept, and got on the team plane for Atlanta, where Super Bowl XXVIII would be held. By Wednesday, he was practicing, and although his teammates said he was sluggish, he laughed it off and proclaimed himself fit to play. Steinberg knew better. Throughout the week, Aikman was dizzy, sometimes vomiting, and at one point led Steinberg to believe he thought he was still playing for his Oklahoma high school team, the Henryetta Mud Hens. By Sunday, Aikman was coasting through the Cowboys' 30–13 blowout of the Buffalo Bills. A year later, he remembered almost none of it.

For Steinberg it wasn't much of a victory. He had become convinced that he was guiding his clients to ruination. He had reached his own turning point.

"I'm an enabler," he thought to himself. "That's all I'm doing."

Steinberg thought most agents were so beholden to their clients that they would indulge any fantasy, no matter how outrageous, to avoid endangering their fat commissions. "I used to say that if a player was on the ledge of a 90-story building about to jump, he would have a whole coterie of fans and his agent saying, 'The law of gravity, it doesn't apply to you! Go ahead, you can fly!'"

Steinberg, at least at the time, did not have that problem. He controlled 21 quarterbacks in the NFL and had written hundreds of millions of dollars in contracts. On the one hand, taking on the concussion issue was self-evidently bad for business. Neither the owners nor the players wanted to hear it; one client, Warren Moon, said to him: "You're probably right, but I wish you'd shut up." On the other hand, his activism could prolong careers, generate more contracts, and, at the very least, soothe his conscience.

He knew the first order of business was to gather more information. Steinberg had been setting up more and more of his players with neurologists, and he asked the doctors pointed questions to try to get to the heart of the matter: How many concussions are too many? What is the point at which an athlete risks long-term brain damage? Are there any methods to prevent those problems and, once they've occurred, treat them? "There were no answers," Steinberg said. Steinberg, whose battle with alcoholism later derailed his career, thought the whole era reminded him of how people once viewed public drunkenness as slapstick comedy and "there were people like Red Skelton and Foster Brooks and Dean Martin, a whole series of people who laughed and laughed about drunk driving. No one talked about the fatalities or the effects of alcoholism."

His solution was to set up informational seminars on the effects of concussions. He would bring in his high-profile clients and a panel of concussion experts to educate the players and the public and put pressure on the league to address the issue. Steinberg invited Tagliabue, or at least a representative of his new Mild Traumatic Brain Injury Committee, to attend the first meeting in 1995. The response from the NFL was silence. Steinberg spoke privately to league owners and appealed to their pocketbooks, if not their humanity: If a brain-damaged player of Aikman's caliber could no longer take the field, he reasoned, not only would the team lose the player, but his salary would be counted against the newly instituted salary cap. But there wasn't much interest. Steinberg felt that the culture of denial was so embedded in the NFL that it was as if he had "asserted that the world was round instead of flat" and he was "one of the heretics."

Of course it wasn't just the league: Many of his own players refused to take the issue seriously. Steinberg held the first seminar at the Newport Beach Marriott, not far from his famous office, a memorabilia-stuffed museum to pro football that made a cameo appearance, along with Steinberg and Aikman, in *Jerry Maguire*. In addition to his superstar quarterbacks—Aikman, Warren Moon, Steve Young—he invited some of the less heralded athletes in his stable. One was a 49ers linebacker, Gary Plummer, who like Steinberg had gone to Cal, the main reason the superagent agreed to represent him.

Plummer's view of the seriousness of the concussion issue was best expressed by his response when a trainer once asked him how many fingers he was holding up. "*One,*" replied Plummer, extending his middle finger.

To Plummer, just raising the issue contradicted pretty much everything he had been taught and believed about pro football. It was not that he wasn't aware of concussions; he had both experienced and inflicted them. But he viewed them as minor nuisances. When Toon and Hoge retired, his reaction was neither concern nor pity. Plummer thought simply: "They're pussies."

"I had been playing football since I was eight years old, and there is nothing more revered in football than being a tough guy," he said. "I prided myself on being a tough guy. I encouraged others to be tough guys. I did some horrendously stupid things in my career—like having surgery on Tuesday and playing on Sunday twice. I would never give you specific names, but there are hundreds of guys who had more talent in one hand than I had in my entire body, but because they weren't tough, they couldn't play in the NFL. The coaches have euphemisms. They'll say: 'You know, that guy has to learn the difference between pain and injury.' Or: 'He has to learn the difference between college and professional football.' What he's saying is the guy's a pussy and he needs to get tough or he's not going to be on the team. It's a very, very clear message and literally hundreds of guys that I played with were just pussies."

Plummer's solution to pain was not rest or retirement but Toradol, a painkiller that had come on the market in 1989 and soon swept through the NFL like a miracle drug. In a 2002 academic paper first mentioned in the *Washington Post,* 28 team doctors reported injecting Toradol every Sunday, some to as many as 35 players. Plummer, like many, injected the drug preemptively, "literally right before the game," to mask his injuries. "It's like an overall body analgesic, and it dulls the pain," he said. Plummer and another ex-49er, the center Ben Lynch, said that as the season wore on, players lined up 10 or 20 deep before games to get their injections. "I mean, it really was like a production line," said Lynch, "a line of guys that would just pull their pants down, show their butt cheek, and the doctor would give them a shot of Toradol. It wasn't, 'Come in and shut the door. Hey, how ya doin?' It was just *boop, boop, boop, boop.*"

The drug lasted "almost exactly four hours," Plummer said, after which "it feels like literally a gang of thugs had just taken a baseball bat to your body." That included his head: "When the Toradol wore off, I'd just get this unbelievable headache for somewhere around six hours. It felt like somebody had hit you in the back of the head with a two-by-four." The pain revealed one of the more insidious aspects of Toradol: The drug masked the actual injury to allow players to play, increasing the likelihood of making the injury worse.

Plummer resisted attending the seminars but was finally "convinced" after two of Steinberg's assistants enticed him with "a car service to pick me up, a hotel room, and ordering $2,000 worth of stuff out of a Nike catalogue."

Now, in a conference room at the Newport Beach Marriott, Plummer listened to the medical experts Steinberg had assembled describe the dangers of concussions. Mark Lovell was there from Pittsburgh, explaining his new concussion test. So was Julian Bailes, talking about the potential risks of long-term brain damage. Plummer sat in the back of the room next to Steve Wallace, a 49ers tackle who had sustained so many concussions that he had taken to wearing a kind of helmet for his helmet: a half-inch-thick Styrofoam "ProCap" that made him look so much like an alien that his teammates called him Gazoo after the big-headed character on *The Flintstones*.

"They're up there giving their spiel, and I wasn't even paying attention because I'm like, 'You know, this is my *job*: to freaking smash people. I really don't care that these quarterbacks get hurt,'" Plummer said. "So all of a sudden this guy—I don't know who he was, some doctor—he says: 'Many of you don't understand that there are three grades of concussions. A Grade I concussion is seeing stars, being slightly disoriented. If you had one of those, you need to get evaluated on the sideline. And if you've had them back-to-back, you probably need to sit out for a week or two.'

"I had been bored stiff, but now I literally jump up out of my chair and I say: 'I don't know where you're getting your data from, but you've obviously never played in the NFL.' The guy's kind of startled, and he says: 'Excuse me? What do you mean?' I said: 'If I didn't have five of your so-called Grade I concussions a game, that meant I was basically inactive. And by the way, there are some plays when you get *two* of those on the same play.'"

Plummer was on a roll: "You try putting your forehead underneath a 330-pound offensive guard and then get off of him to take on a 220-pound running back," he told the doctor. "Trust me, you're going to see stars just like the cartoons with the little birdie flying around your head. I'm in my thirteenth year of professional football, and I have five of these a *game*. So according to your theory I've had over 750 concussions, and you know what? I'm pretty lucid.'

"The guy started to get argumentative, and I told him to take his clinical studies and put them where the sun don't shine because he's full of crap."

That, of course, was not the public message that came out of Steinberg's seminar. The agent announced that he intended to produce a white paper on concussion assessment and treatment and present it to the NFL. It would call for the elimination of AstroTurf fields, a study of helmets, and the creation of an independent "medical referee," preferably a neurologist whose sole job would be to determine whether a player should return to play. Some of the players in attendance, mainly the quarterbacks, seemed to take the discussion seriously. Aikman admitted that he barely remembered the details of the previous year's Super Bowl. He noted that the NFL benefited from videos that showed particularly vicious hits and that the revenue "goes right into NFL Properties' pockets. They're kind of straddling a line there."

"I've had concussions, and I've come back too soon," Aikman said. "People this year were asking me, 'When is enough enough?' The next one could maybe be my last one. I've said before if it comes to the point that I'm worrying about concussions, I will get out."

Aikman would play five more years.

Steinberg believed he was "dancing on the edge of the apocalypse to raise these issues. No one wanted it to be true. No one wanted concussions to pose a threat to the NFL. No one wanted there to be long-term ramifications." When word from the league eventually got back to Steinberg through a team official or someone else connected to the commissioner, the response was always the same: "Show us the studies. There are no studies." But Steinberg felt he was making progress. He had aligned himself with the people who believed the world was round, people such as Lovell and Bailes and Barry Jordan. Those men had produced studies, and soon there would be more. Steinberg thought the force of his argument eventually would win the day, and the NFL—the commissioner, the players, everyone—would wake up to the reality that the sport needed to change drastically. At least that was what he thought.

5

THE MIKE WEBSTER
HEALTH CARE SYSTEM

Team Webster's two-pronged strategy for the Hall of Fame had failed miserably. Webster's rambling acceptance speech, even delivered on 80 mg of Ritalin, only reinforced the perception that he was to a large degree unhinged. His latest moneymaking scheme, the Steelers Hall of Famer collective, also went nowhere. Having ripped up Bradshaw's $175,000 check in a grand gesture of pride and pique, he returned to Pittsburgh, where he was now living with his oldest son, Colin, in a two-bedroom apartment furnished with camping utensils and furniture culled from yard sales and the Dollar Store. Colin and Mike ate sparingly: "We'd have a little pasta or just sliced bread and toast," Colin said. "Once in a while we'd get some cheap Italian sausage or hamburger and throw them in the sauce and kind of stretch it."

Colin sarcastically referred to those lean times as "my bachelor pad years." He was 19, just out of high school, his life a 24/7 job of looking after, caring for, and chauffeuring around his famous father. But what else could he do? He had been living in Wisconsin with his mom and his siblings when they received a call one day that his dad was in trouble in Philadelphia. Colin and his sister Brooke immediately hopped on a train. When they arrived in Philly, they found Webster nearly catatonic and living in a suite at the historic Warwick Hotel.

"He looked like death," Colin said. "He was just very addled." Webster was holding a bottle of large oval-shaped pills, which Colin understood to be muscle relaxers. "He would take some of these horse pills and lay down. Then he'd take some more 15 minutes later. I'd be like, 'Dad, no!' " Colin and Brooke somehow got their 250-pound father into the shower. A moment later, they heard a crash. "I thought he was going to be dead when I went in there because the smack was so loud; he tripped over the tub line and it was just *boom!*" said Colin. "It was a marble floor, and the sound was just sickening. I can hear it to this day." He found his father sprawled on the floor but otherwise okay. A couple of days later, Colin took Mike back to Pittsburgh and moved in with him.

At that point, it was hard to say which was more alarming: Webster's mental or physical deterioration. He was 45. His hands and feet were swollen and disfigured; his perpetually aching right heel tormented him. Webster seemed susceptible to grotesque and inexplicable afflictions; one day, without warning, dozens of red, open sores erupted across his arms and his back. As often as not, Webster would ignore those myriad ailments or treat them himself with a variety of medieval coping mechanisms that combined the creativity of alternative medicine with Ace Hardware.

Between his sparse meals, Webster subsisted on junk food—Coke, Dots, Little Debbie Cakes, pecan swirls—and ever-present tins of snuff. Soon his teeth began to fall out. He couldn't afford a dentist, and so "he'd Super Glue his teeth back into his head," said Colin. Webster lost—and reset—about 10 teeth this way, according to Colin. "It was kind of awesome in a not necessarily so awesome way." The bottoms of Webster's feet were cracked—long fissures that made it painful to walk. This he solved by wrapping them in duct tape. Webster slept erratically; because of his constant back pain, he shunned beds and often nodded off in a chair. When that didn't work, he walked outside and tried sleeping behind the wheel of his truck.

When that didn't work, Webster took more drastic measures. He had acquired a number of mail-order stun guns. "One was real long, like a police baton," Colin said. "It had the two prongs, and you could see a clear blue spark; it'd make that *crack, crack, crack* sound. And then he had one that was called the Myotron, which he was really excited about because it was guaranteed to put somebody out for thirty minutes." Sometimes, Webster put himself to sleep with the Myotron, calling it soothing. Colin, who inherited his father's love of reading and penned science fiction novels, joked that his dad had "a primordial nervous system that allowed him to absorb energy" like a superhero.

One day, Mike asked Sunny Jani, his booker and caretaker, to put him out. "He had really bad pain, and he just wanted to go to sleep, you know?" said Sunny. "I did it only once. I didn't know if he wouldn't wake up and I'd have to go to jail." Sunny winced as he gingerly applied the Myotron to Webster's thigh. Mike was jolted unconscious. "I'm like, 'Oh, fuck, what the hell just happened here?'" Sunny said. "I'm like, 'Holy heck, wake up, man! Wake up!'"

Mike came to about a half hour later. Sunny, standing over him with a glass of water, felt his heart pounding.

"Man, that was the greatest nap I've ever had," said Webster.

"Please, Mike, don't ever ask me to do that again," Sunny told him.

Sunny came to refer to Webster's various methods of self-treatment as the Mike Webster Health Care System.

Team Webster clearly needed a doctor. Shortly after the Hall of Fame induction and Webster's scattered acceptance speech, James Vodvarka, an internist in Wintersville, Ohio, was talking with one of his hunting buddies, former Steelers lineman Steve Courson.

Courson was concerned about Webster. "You know, there's something wrong with him," he told Vodvarka.

"What do you mean?"

"Well, he's living out of his truck, and he's not able to function. He can't hold a job. He's just not able to function in society."

Like Sunny, Vodvarka had grown up in McKees Rocks. He was a die-hard Steelers fan who worshiped Iron Mike as a leader on those fabled teams. He could still see him sprinting out of the huddle, his bulging biceps exposed in the subfreezing weather, or delivering measured, articulate analysis after the game. When Courson asked if he'd be willing to examine his friend, Vodvarka said he would be delighted.

Almost from the moment Webster came through the door, Vodvarka could tell something wasn't right. Although he was an internist,

Vodvarka knew a lot about brain dysfunction. His father had had a stroke years earlier, and more recently his son had been born with a slightly deformed skull and a brain bleed.

Vodvarka noticed that Webster had a "Parkinsonian stare." "You know, when you watch somebody, it's like at times there's no expression?" he said. "There's no emotion, and it's like somebody's looking right through you when they talk to you." Tracing his hands over Webster's skull, Vodvarka discovered a cluster of knots on his forehead: scar tissue that he thought was indicative of trauma. Vodvarka had seen this in car-crash victims, but typically there was one lump where the head had hit the steering wheel or the dashboard. In Webster's case, there were lumps everywhere.

Vodvarka thought immediately there could be only one source of Webster's problems. "Here's a guy that's pretty discombobulated, beat up physically, and played the position of center in football," he said. "I mean, it didn't take much thinking to think that football was the main cause."

Vodvarka told Webster he wanted him to return for regular follow-up appointments. Webster did, although it was never clear if he would show up on the right day, much less the right time. In many ways it was an ideal arrangement: Webster had neither money nor health insurance (besides the Mike Webster Plan); Vodvarka was only too happy to treat him for free. In that regard, Vodvarka was like many people hanging around Webster, basking in his former greatness. When they went out to eat, Vodvarka invariably picked up the tab. "He'd be stopping people on the way out of the restaurant going, 'Hey, do you know who this is? This is Mike Webster,'" said Colin. "It was just really awkward."

But Vodvarka also was indispensable, the perfect doctor for Team Webster—on call at all times and a trusted and reliable source when Mike ran out of his meds. Webster called him Jimbo and soon was making regular one-hour drives between Pittsburgh and Wintersville, often to pick up prescriptions for Ritalin or Ultran, a pain pill.

It was clear to Vodvarka that Mike was disabled; no way could he hold down a job. But Webster had never filed for disability benefits with the NFL. The league had a program, the Bert Bell/Pete Rozelle NFL Player Retirement Plan, that granted benefits to retired players and their families. The plan was administered jointly by the players and the owners; three reps from each side ruled on disability claims. But many former players viewed the plan with contempt. It was the place where their pleas for help went to die or at least remain in perpetual limbo. They complained of a byzantine application process, of being sent to doctor after doctor, of their claims being stretched out interminably. A decade later, when the NFL and the players union were called before Congress to answer questions about the league's commitment to retired players, officials would acknowledge that only 317 out of more than 10,000 eligible players were receiving benefits.

Brain injuries were viewed as the hardest sell. It was as if the NFL's disability board was channeling the views that Tagliabue had articulated to Halberstam at the 92nd Street Y. Some players and lawyers came to believe that the board simply did not award benefits for any neurocognitive impairment—*ever*. Brent Boyd, a Minnesota Vikings offensive lineman who had been diagnosed by several doctors with football-related brain damage that prevented him from working, told Congress that the board was using "tactics of delay [and] deny" in the "hope that I put a bullet through my head to end their problem."

But Vodvarka believed that if anyone deserved disability benefits—to help him solve at least a few of his myriad problems—it was Webster. Vodvarka knew it would be an immense challenge. Webster certainly couldn't handle it himself. He decided Webster needed a lawyer who was smart and tough enough to stand up to the NFL. Vodvarka called a judge he knew in West Virginia.

"What if you had an NFL player that's hit rock bottom, but there's a reason for it and nobody will listen?" Vodvarka asked the judge without naming Webster. "Who would be an attorney that I could get that would be able to go against one of the biggest entities in our country and not be intimidated?"

The judge replied without hesitation: "Bob Fitzsimmons—he's the best."

Mike Webster and Bob Fitzsimmons had one major thing in common: Neither of them slept. On most nights, up until midnight and often beyond, Fitzsimmons could be found in his office, a

converted firehouse on Warwood Avenue, one of the main thorough-
fares in Wheeling, West Virginia. As a grace note, Fitzsimmons had
kept the fireman's pole, which ran between the first and second floors
next to a mahogany staircase. When Mike and Sunny first went to meet
him, Fitzsimmons penciled them in for 10. "Mike, what kind of lawyer
works at 10 at night?" Jani asked.

In fact, Fitzsimmons was the kind of lawyer who with a single
glance conveyed the impression, "You do not want to fuck with me."
That happened to be an accurate impression, because Fitzsimmons had
carved out a considerable reputation in the Ohio River Valley as the
man to turn to on the biggest cases involving medical malpractice, coal-
mining accidents, toxic exposure, and so on. The region, the heart of
the nation's rust belt, produced enough litigative fodder for generations
of personal injury attorneys, and Fitzsimmons was now bringing his
sons into the business. Fitzsimmons's father had been a plumber, and
Fitzsimmons had worked his way through high school, college, and law
school as a member of Local 83 of the United Association of Plumbers
and Pipefitters. He was neither tall nor particularly imposing, but he
projected a coiled intensity that seemed to lie just below the surface.
One thing was crystal clear: If Bob Fitzsimmons joined Team Webster,
he would be nobody's sycophant.

Fitzsimmons didn't normally take disability cases, and so he wasn't
initially certain how he could help. But as Webster began to talk,
Fitzsimmons realized that (1) something was very wrong with the legendary player and (2) Webster's case was not totally dissimilar to other
personal injury cases he had handled. Fitzsimmons had already read and
heard some of the stories about Webster, that he was "some nut case
running around out there." Instead, he found him intelligent and well
read, instantly likable, but with no apparent ability to focus. Every two
or three minutes, Webster would change the subject. Fitzsimmons tried
to obtain his medical history—Have you seen a doctor? What have you
been treated for? Who did you see?—but Webster was no help there.
There were long pauses as Mike hunted for words. "He was a total
blank," said Fitzsimmons. "It was like he had amnesia."

Fitzsimmons thought it was obvious: Webster had some sort of
closed-head injury. This was Personal Injury Law 101: Client gets in car

crash, lawyer brings in psychologist to do workup, damages are awarded. "It's been a common thing," Fitzsimmons said. "It's been common now for years and years and years."

This case would prove slightly more complicated than that. If Fitzsimmons didn't fully grasp the complexity of the journey he was about to embark on, he soon would. It would involve not only the all-consuming and unpredictable care and feeding of Mike Webster, a client who would end up all but living with Fitzsimmons, but the most powerful entity the lawyer had ever confronted: the National Football League.

But that was later. For now, Fitzsimmons spent much of 1998 setting up a series of psychological exams for Webster. He sent him first to see Fred Krieg, a Wheeling psychologist and professor at nearby Marshall University. Just getting Mike to the doctor could be a slapstick adventure. He canceled several appointments, and then, on the day he did show up, he was two and a half hours late because he got lost getting to an office that was less than three miles from Fitzsimmons's office. Webster was off his Ritalin when he saw Krieg, and so an evaluation that should have taken only a few hours ended up lasting two days. Without Ritalin, Webster admitted to the doctor, "I can't think straight."

Krieg took Webster's personal history and performed a battery of tests. He was moved that even though it was to Webster's advantage to do poorly—the better to make his case to the NFL—he tried hard to impress the doctor. He sugarcoated his problems and focused on his physical ailments rather than his mental and emotional ones. "He is obviously a very proud man who is somewhat embarrassed by his present situation," Krieg observed.

Krieg concurred with Vodvarka: Football had given Webster irreparable brain damage. He wrote: "I believe that Mr. Webster's condition is caused by many years in the NFL and the repeated blows to the head he received as a center." Krieg compared Webster's condition to that of a punch-drunk boxer. "It takes very little time to realize that he has fallen from the position of hero to one of pity," he wrote.

Fitzsimmons also sent Webster to see Charles Kelly, a local family practitioner and social worker who also dealt with mental health cases. Among other things, Kelly worked as a ringside physician at West

Virginia boxing matches. To Kelly, like Vodvarka and Krieg before him, the situation was obvious: Football had given Webster chronic brain disease. "It is my opinion that Mr. Webster suffers from encephalopathy caused by head trauma," he wrote.

Fitzsimmons turned finally to a forensic psychiatrist at the University of Pittsburgh Medical Center named Jonathan Himmelhoch. Himmelhoch would examine Webster six times over three months, more extensively than any other doctor except perhaps Vodvarka. He then wrote a devastating six-page summation of how football had destroyed Webster mentally and physically.

Himmelhoch described Webster as a confirmed "encephalopath"—a person with chronic brain injury—whose "totally disabling" condition was the primary reason he was now living like a "vagabond, often using his old pickup truck as a home." In Himmelhoch's opinion, part of Webster's desperate condition derived from the fact that his medical treatment had been compromised from the start of his career. His care, he wrote, "has been delivered by doctors working for two masters—1st the Pittsburgh Steelers and second, Michael L. Webster." Those doctors repeatedly allowed or encouraged Webster to play hurt, essentially refusing to save him from himself to advance the interests of the team. "Full recovery of subtle head injury is a necessity before resuming any job," Himmelhoch wrote. "If there is no recovery period, subtle, then manifest cortical injury is insured. One can conclude, therefore, to reasonable medical certainty that Mr. Webster's progressive deteriorating encephalopathy began while he was still playing NFL football."

Webster, Himmelhoch concluded, "suffers from a traumatic or punch-drunk encephalopathy, caused by multiple blows while playing center in the NFL."

The disability case became Webster's obsession. It was a forum to show the world how football could destroy a man's mind. At the same time, the case fed Webster's growing hatred of the Steelers' brass and the NFL.

Webster came to believe it was his destiny to restore the dignity of thousands of battered players and avenge the league's sins of abusing and discarding them. As Fitzsimmons gathered evidence, Webster raged against those he perceived as trying to stop him, including Steelers owner Dan Rooney, PR man Joe Gordon, the Steelers' organization, and the retirement committee itself. He became convinced that the Steelers had burned his medical records and paid off doctors to torpedo his case. In fact, the opposite was true. Fitzsimmons would later say that Rooney called him personally to ask how he could help and notify him that he had lobbied the league on Webster's behalf. Even in the worst of times—and they would soon get very bad—Fitzsimmons had nothing but good things to say about Dan Rooney and the Pittsburgh Steelers.

Here was the essential, sad truth about Mike Webster. His cause was just. He was leading a fight that eventually would lift the secrecy and shame that shrouded an untold number of former players sustaining the devastating effects of head trauma and other football-related injuries. His struggle would significantly advance the science of concussion and the search for the truth about the connection between football and neurodegenerative disease (Fitzsimmons called him the "father of the whole thing"). Yet the disease now ravaging Webster's brain was plunging him into a world of delusion, incoherence, self-loathing, and rage. It was an increasingly dark world.

Webster through the years had collected an array of firearms: a .357 Magnum revolver, a Sig Sauer P226 semiautomatic pistol, an M1911 semiautomatic pistol, riot shotguns, stump shotguns, hunting rifles. He kept them under his bed and in his truck. Now, when he launched into a particularly intense rant, he told his son Colin that what he would really like to do was kill Dan Rooney or Joe Gordon or the many people connected to the Bert Bell retirement plan.

"He wanted to go shoot these guys in the head," said Colin. "They don't know how close I guarantee you it came to happening on many occasions. Dad literally wanted to go and shoot these guys, some of them that were messing with him."

Colin, while living with Webster, had absorbed his father's rage and in many ways came to share it. He said he understood the desire for revenge. The only thing that held his father back, Colin believed, was his fear that such an act of violence would reflect badly on his family.

Webster thus poured his emotions into legal pads and notebooks, which he toted everywhere in a heavy satchel. Webster's fingers were so mangled, his knuckles so swollen, that he couldn't hold a pen for very long. To write, he used the same duct tape that held his feet together and wrapped it around his fingers. He holed up for hours at Kinko's or Barnes & Noble, at rest stops during his wanderings along the highway. He sent the letters to almost everyone he came in contact with: his doctors, his friends, his children. Fitzsimmons received letters almost daily, some hand delivered, some faxed from wherever Webster happened to be writing. Fitzsimmons cleared out a storage room in the basement and let Mike use it as an office where he wrote and sometimes slept. Webster bathed himself with paper towels, leaving water all over the floor of the basement's tiny bathroom. Fitzsimmons would leave late at night, only to find yet another letter stuck to the windshield of his car. Some were 20 or 30 pages long. By the end, the lawyer had collected hundreds. Some went unread; there were simply too many to keep up. Others were incomprehensible, depending on Webster's mental state.

Almost always, the letters revolved around the disability case. His bitterness was palpable:

> *Dear Bob,*
> *Thank you for Taking the time to See me Today. I know you are Busy and I Expected that the Burt [sic] Bell People under the Direction of Dan Rooney and His Associates will Drag this out and Deny me a Thing so that I Never make it out of my own Personal Hell!*

Often they were jumbled and despairing:

> *No Money Poverty Worse Every day. No money many weekends almost everyone sit can not do anything or Go anywhere. No source of Help and Where to Turn So I do not know when last time any Fun & Enjoyment and Cost of Medical and other Costs has been staggering.*
> *My goddamn writing and mind are going to shit. Wow.*

Occasionally they were hopeful:

> *Restoration of my Past my name and the lives and future*
> *of my kids, my mind, body, honor and to have a chance to*
> *live out my life in a little peace and harmony, then I can go*
> *to work for you, Robert, investigating and cracking the case,*
> *underground secret investigation and super snooper, sergeant*
> *Columbo. That's me!*

Often they were delusional, starting with precise lettering and dissolving into a looping, incomprehensible scrawl. In one, Webster even attacked Carl Peterson, the Chiefs' general manager, who had given him a job a few years earlier when his life was falling apart. Webster had once considered having Peterson introduce him at the Hall of Fame induction. Now he referred to him as "another S.O.B Brownnose FemeNazi" and railed against the system that he believed had used him up:

> *It would Be the same as Having you come in my House*
> *Bend my wife over the Couch Fuck Her in The Butt and,*
> *Beat up abuse my Kids etc while I tell them It's O.K. Family*
> *These Guys Gave Me The privilege of working For Them and*
> *Getting the shit Beat out of myself and Despite Helping Them*
> *and The Coaches have High Percentage of winning Records*
> *and multiple championship that sell out every Game excess*
> *profits etc and can always get Jobs, They Want Just a Little*
> *Free Liability To Keep Taking from Us!*

Webster, ominously, often quoted from Revelation 6:8:

> *Then Behold a Pale Horse*
> *The Man Who Rode Him Was Death*
> *And Hell Followed With Him*

"No Revenge, No Sir," Webster scrawled on a scrap of paper ripped from a small daily planner. "Not Revenge, But <u>Reckoning</u>!"

Webster regularly threatened to become the first player to quit the Hall of Fame to protest the plight of the retired players, many of whom he believed also had brain damage. He thought the Hall had come to represent the exploitation of the men who had built the league, including and especially him. Webster swore many times that he intended to sell his Hall of Fame ring and his four Super Bowl rings to raise cash and get rid of the valuable keepsakes he claimed he no longer cared about.

Sunny had turned the Super Bowl rings into yet another money-raising scheme—not by selling them but by *renting* them to collectors; at one point he used the rings to obtain a $90,000 line of credit from an Altoona lawyer. But Webster still insisted he wanted to sell them. Once he claimed to have lined up a deal for $100,000—$25,000 for each ring. Sunny called Fitzsimmons in a panic. By now, Fitzsimmons was Team Webster's head coach, the one man who could tell Mike what to do. Sunny thought Mike held Fitzsimmons in the same regard in which he once held Chuck Noll. Fitzsimmons called a meeting for 11 P.M. at his office. Sunny managed to get Webster there early.

Webster was agitated, pacing around the conference room.

"I don't need these fucking things!" he screamed. "They aren't any good to me, okay?"

Webster said he needed the money to send to Pam and the kids. Sunny implored him: "Mike, your legacy is more important than $100,000."

Three men in black trench coats ("Straight out of central casting," said Fitzsimmons) showed up to consummate the deal for the Super Bowl rings. It seemed that there was no stopping it. Then Fitzsimmons tossed a Hail Mary: "Mike, I can get you $200,000!" he said. "I know people who will buy these." The trench coats left. Webster kept his rings for another day.

Despite all the insanity that his condition engendered, Webster was acutely aware of what was happening to him. In addition to the mainstays on Team Webster, Mike had become good friends with Charles Kelly, one of the doctors who had evaluated him for his disability case. Kelly was kind and soft-spoken, with the same small-town upbringing as Webster. When Mike was on Ritalin, in the quiet of Kelly's home outside Wheeling, it could be hard to tell that he was even sick. He would bring over Kentucky Fried Chicken and a collection of tomahawks he had acquired and show Kelly's son how to fling them against a tree. Webster and Kelly would sit around the table for hours and talk politics and history and life.

Often the conversation turned to brain trauma. Webster saw himself as an advocate for the issue, particularly as it related to football. He brought Kelly textbooks on brain damage, marking them up as if he were a medical student. One was titled *Traumatic Brain Injury: Associated Speech, Language, and Swallowing Disorders*. On page 235, Webster underlined several sentences, including: "Difficulty in establishing psychosocial well-being following [traumatic brain injury] represents a pervasive impediment to the social reintegration of individuals with TBI and affects their quality of life."

Mike told Kelly that once he won his disability case, he wanted to use the money to start a foundation to offer legal and medical support to players with cognitive issues.

"He talked to me about that a lot," said Kelly. He would come to see that as Webster's legacy.

On Saturday, February 20, 1999, a few days after dropping off a Ritalin prescription to be filled at an Eckerd Pharmacy in Rochester, Pennsylvania, about 25 miles north of Pittsburgh, Webster returned to pick up the drugs. Federal agents walked up to him and said: "Mr. Webster, you're under arrest."

The pharmacist had called the authorities after learning that the doctor listed on the prescription no longer practiced in Pennsylvania. The Drug Enforcement Administration alleged that Webster had forged Ritalin prescriptions on dozens of occasions all over the Pittsburgh area: Rochester, Center Township, Kennedy Township, McKees Rocks.

Exactly how Webster committed his crimes was not totally clear. The fact that he had been writing his own prescriptions was not in dispute. Sunny said a sympathetic doctor/Steelers fan had issued Webster a blank pad, but that was never pursued. Sometimes Webster apparently changed the numbers on valid prescriptions so that 90 magically became 190.

Regardless, the arrest was a PR disaster and a sign that his drug use was out of control. "If you'd let Mike pop Ritalin all day, he probably would have done it," said Vodvarka. "If he'd had an unending supply, he'd have taken one every hour." In fact, Vodvarka's files bulged with hundreds of prescriptions he himself wrote for his friend. Webster couldn't function without Ritalin. Himmelhoch, the University of Pittsburgh psychiatrist who evaluated Webster for his disability claim, helped get him out of the charges with only probation by persuading the judge that Webster had forged prescriptions "for a drug that was and is appropriate treatment" for his brain damage. Ritalin "lifts the scales of [his] confusion," Himmelhoch wrote. But it was an exceedingly sharp double-edged sword. Ritalin is a stimulant, like cocaine; among other things, it clearly was fueling Webster's manic literary life. "He'd stay up several days and take it round the clock and write you these notes," said Vodvarka, who received numerous letters. After the arrest, Vodvarka decided to cut Webster off. By enabling his addiction, he worried, he could jeopardize his medical license or, worse, Mike might overdose.

Fitzsimmons scrambled together a press conference at a Holiday Inn outside Pittsburgh to make the case that Webster wasn't responsible for his actions, that football had altered his brain. He brought in the doctors: Vodvarka, Kelly, and Krieg. Some of Webster's former teammates, including Rocky Bleier, Mel Blount, and Randy Grossman, were recruited to show support. But behind the scenes, some players argued that jail might be the best option for Webster, if only to get him off the streets and free him from his addiction.

Team Webster gathered in a room to prepare. Fitzsimmons had written a statement for Webster, but Vodvarka and others worried that he couldn't deliver it in his condition. Webster sat in the middle of it all in disgrace. "Everyone's gonna think I'm a criminal," he told Colin. It was the lowest point of his entire soul-shattering post-career ordeal. "You could see it just clobbered him," said Colin. Now, between Webster's obvious depression and his erratically functioning brain, Vodvarka, Fitzsimmons, and others tried to figure out how to get him through the humiliating press conference.

Vodvarka and Fitzsimmons pulled Webster aside 30 minutes before it started.

"Listen, take your Ritalin now so it kicks in and you can organize your thoughts," Fitzsimmons told him.

Thus it came to pass that shortly before offering a contrite apology to the city of Pittsburgh for forging Ritalin prescriptions, Webster gulped downed 80 mg of Ritalin with a cup of water.

"I want to apologize very specifically for any embarrassment and sadness these allegations have brought," Webster said. He choked up twice while reading the statement. "I am not seeking your pity or sympathy. I'm not seeking a pardon for my actions, and I'm not really asking for your understanding—even though grown men need understanding."

The press conference was largely successful. Webster came off as sympathetic, a hero brought low by his overreliance on an obscure drug he needed for injuries related to the years of profound joy he had given to Pittsburgh. The focus quickly shifted from his crimes to his head. But this had an unanticipated effect: The discussion of Webster's brain touched off a mini-debate over whether football had actually caused his problems.

On one side were doctors such as Vodvarka, Kelly, Krieg, and Himmelhoch, who made their views known that the repeated blows Webster sustained during his illustrious Steelers career had turned him into the damaged man he was today.

"Mike has the football version of punch-drunk," Krieg said.

But there was another side. Curiously, it was led by Joe Maroon, the Steelers' longtime neurological consultant. Five years earlier Maroon had advised Merril Hoge to retire because of the fear that repeated concussions would leave him permanently impaired. Now Maroon told the *Post-Gazette* that such long-term injuries were rare. Of the claim that football gave Mike Webster brain damage, Maroon said: "That's not confirmed." Maroon, of course, was one of the doctors Himmelhoch had accused of working for two masters: first the Steelers and then Webster. He was at least indirectly responsible for the player's medical file, which showed hardly any signs of brain injury during his 15 years in Pittsburgh.

The *Post-Gazette* story went on to tout what it called the "Pittsburgh Steelers Test Battery," a neuropsychological exam developed by Maroon and his University of Pittsburgh colleague, Mark Lovell, as an indication of the team's commitment to treating concussions. Maroon explained that the test was now used by every team in the National Hockey League and a dozen teams in the NFL. An affordable software version soon would be available for high school trainers, the story said.

Maroon wasn't the only doubter. The Bert Bell/Pete Rozelle NFL Player Retirement Plan had gotten back to Fitzsimmons with a response to Webster's disability claim. Four doctors weren't enough, the NFL told Webster. The board wanted a fifth doctor: an independent neurologist who would examine Webster on the league's behalf. This tactic was familiar to many retired players, who regarded it as a sham, part of the league's callously indifferent bureaucracy, which they believed was designed to keep them from getting what they deserved. The "independent" doctor invariably came from a list of physicians compiled by the NFL. The doctors on that list, it was thought, frequently sided with the league.

Coming on top of the Ritalin arrest, this news was greeted by Team Webster with overwhelming despair. As addled as Webster was, there was a growing feeling among Fitzsimmons, Sunny, Vodvarka, Colin, and the others that Webster was right: The NFL intended to let him rot. Their paranoia was such that even the location of the independent doctor the NFL had recommended—Cleveland, the home of the Steelers' archrival—was viewed as part of a magnificent setup.

Nevertheless, on June 21, 1999—four months after his arrest—Webster traveled to the offices of Edward Westbrook, the NFL's handpicked neurologist. Westbrook, a distinguished-looking man with silver hair and wire-rimmed glasses, had an Ivy League education and worked at University Hospitals Case Medical Center in Cleveland. He had played football in high school until he broke his collarbone, after which his coach advised: "Don't play college football. They'll kill you." Westbrook then had rowed at Harvard.

By the time Webster came to see him, Westbrook had examined perhaps a half dozen former NFL players on behalf of the league. Whatever was going on inside the Bert Bell/Pete Rozelle NFL Player Retirement Plan, Edward Westbrook was not in denial. He had found himself "impressed and maybe horrified" by the degree of brain damage he encountered in the players he examined. One young former player had Parkinson's disease, which Westbrook thought was probably connected to repeated hits on the field. The rest of the players had varying degrees of severe cognitive dysfunction.

Westbrook didn't look at the reports from Fitzsimmons's doctors before he examined Webster. He did go through the medical reports from the Steelers and Chiefs and was surprised to find almost no mention of head injuries. Webster complained about headaches, some of which, he said, felt like the top of his head would blow off, and also memory loss. But what really struck Westbrook was Webster's demeanor. He was "like a five-year-old child who was amazed by the whole situation," Westbrook said. Webster tried to be helpful, but Westbrook struggled unsuccessfully to obtain even the most cursory medical history.

"I mean, he was very pleasant, very charming, but didn't have the drive and direction and decision-making ability," Westbrook said later. "And this is what gets destroyed in this process of repetitive brain injury. He was pretty much at sea in an open boat unless somebody directed him."

Westbrook thought it was an "easy case to decide." He wrote to the disability board: "With the history of multiple head injuries that all football players have and the history that the patient has predominately problems with what appears to be frontal lobe function, I think we can be pretty comfortable that this is related to injury."

"I don't think it's rocket science to say that there's chronic injury from head injury in football," Westbrook said. "I mean, we've all talked about it."

It would be years before it was known publicly what Edward Westbrook had concluded about Mike Webster, a period in which the concussion issue would sweep over the NFL like a giant wave and the question of what the league knew about the connection between football and brain damage—and when it knew it—would potentially be worth millions, if not billions, of dollars.

On October 28, 1999, on Westbrook's recommendation, the retirement board granted Webster "Total and Permanent" disability benefits on the basis of his injuries. A few months later, Fitzsimmons received a letter from Sarah E. Gaunt, the plan's director, explaining the decision: "The Retirement Board determined that Mr. Webster's disability arose while he was an Active Player." The medical reports, including one from the NFL's handpicked neurologist, "indicate that his disability is the result of head injuries suffered as a football player with the Pittsburgh Steelers and Kansas City Chiefs." The league's own disability committee—chaired by a representative of the NFL commissioner and managed in part by the NFL owners, who elected that commissioner— had determined that professional football had caused Mike Webster's brain damage.

A decade later, as thousands of former players were suing the NFL for fraud, Fitzsimmons, who by then had nothing to do with the lawsuit, would describe that 1999 letter as "the proverbial smoking gun."

The decision was a hollow victory for Webster. The league didn't dispute that pro football had caused his brain damage, but the retirement board disagreed on when he became so disabled that he couldn't hold a job. All five doctors—Westbrook included—concluded that that happened immediately after Webster's career ended. The board determined that it was several years later, even though Webster's only full-time employment was his truncated season with the Chiefs in which he lived in a storage closet. Financially, the retirement board had made a hairsplitting—but life-changing—distinction. It was the difference between $42,000 a year and hundreds of thousands.

Webster, of course, was apoplectic, and so was Fitzsimmons. The attorney whipped off letter after letter to the board in "an attempt to correct an obvious mistake." He recruited more doctors. He filed more forms. But no change was forthcoming. "Needless to say, I am disappointed and also frustrated," Fitzsimmons wrote. "I have now written to you . . . on 38 separate occasions. I have submitted the reports of at least ten independent doctors. Mike has filed three affidavits and we have obtained all of the available records you have requested."

Vodvarka, who continued to bear witness to Webster's decline as his personal physician, sat down and wrote Fitzsimmons a letter to try to make sense of it all. For much of his life, Vodvarka had worshiped Mike Webster, the Pittsburgh Steelers, and the National Football League. He couldn't get over the injustice, how the NFL had honored Webster by putting him in the Hall of Fame, how Webster was frequently named to the all-time teams that experts put together. Yet the league had abandoned him. "I am and could only be appalled," Vodvarka wrote Fitzsimmons. "We are dealing with a unique situation where a human being has lost his well-deserved dignity, respected reputation and most importantly his family. The Pittsburgh Steelers and the National Football League have turned their backs, and have done nothing but try to destroy one of their most prolific players. I can only imagine what misery some of the National Football League's lesser players must suffer. Are they [the NFL] afraid to set a precedent? Do they expect the common people/taxpayers to fund their casualties while paying to watch them occur?"

Fitzsimmons concluded he had no alternative except to sue the Bert Bell/Pete Rozelle NFL Player Retirement Plan. Thus began an entirely new battle, one that Webster would not live to see concluded.

His life was now in free fall. As soon as the disability checks started rolling in, the IRS garnished most of the payments; after taxes and the levy, he was getting $641.67 a month. His ability to remember people and places was fading rapidly.

One night he and Colin took a drive to the local convenience store, just down the block from their apartment. They had made the trip dozens of times. Suddenly Webster made a wrong turn.

"What are you doing, Dad?" Colin asked. "The convenience store is that way."

"What are you talking about?" said Webster.

Colin tried again, but Webster started arguing. For 10 minutes they went back and forth, with Colin trying to convince his father that he was mistaken.

"I think you're crazy; I don't know what you're telling me, but all right, let's look," Webster said.

When Webster came upon the store, he was shaken.

"That was the scariest look I've ever seen on his face," Colin said. "It was like, 'Oh, my God, I just lost how to brush my teeth or tie my shoes.' The confusion and horror that was in his eyes, it was like, 'Oh, man!' I think that was really the worst for him, that he knew he was losing it."

One night Colin went to get a snack in the kitchen only to discover his father standing in front of the oven, the door open, his pants down, pissing into it.

"What are you doing, Dad?" Colin asked.

"Oh, Jesus, I thought I was going in a urinal," Webster said.

Eventually, two years out of high school, with no money and no career prospects, Colin decided to join the Marines. When he left, his younger brother, Garrett, not yet 16, came down from Wisconsin to assume the role of son/caretaker/roommate. In Garrett's case, it was more roommate and caretaker than son. If Colin and his father had been like bachelor pals, Garrett and Webster were more like high school buddies. Garrett was huge, nearly 6-8, bigger than his dad. He played football even though his heart wasn't in it, saddled by the burden of being the son of a Hall of Fame center.

But Garrett, like Colin, loved hanging out with his dad. They browsed around Kmart at two in the morning, went to WWE wrestling matches, watched many of the same movies over and over: *The Princess Bride, Tombstone, Goodfellas, Happy Gilmore,* and, of course, any John Wayne flick. He and Garrett were *Star Wars* nerds, so they made sure they were there when *Episode II—Attack of the Clones* opened in spring 2002. Near the end of the movie, when Yoda strikes a pose with his light saber, ready to fight for the first time, Webster leaped out of his seat, screaming, "Yeah, yeah!"

But where once Team Webster could expect maybe 15 or 20 good days every month, he was down to perhaps 3 to 5. Sunny said Mike often sniffed ammonia late at night to stave off sleep, fearing he wouldn't wake up. "I don't want to fall asleep, little buddy," Webster would say.

Webster's demise was reflected in his incoherent letters.

One read:

What is NOW what every one Family Kids Poor mother wives all more trouble Terrible situation Every one poverty worse & worse use more more our own Property Saving Every Penny still not enough

From a Kinko's in Madison on March 15, 2002, Webster faxed a nine-page letter to the Brain Injury Association of America. It was written in the third person in Webster's hand. One passage read:

To Levery all but a pathetic $800 from all Mike's monthly assets He has Levied Then about $14,000 per month and hHas Virthually Causes The Collapse of all the Good and Beneficial Polciies That had Mike making His own Way, meeting the oblgations and

Honroing the Dependents Needs and also Paying out on Thos obli-gations Which he has been Determoin and resolute to Fullfill.

One night, Bob Stage, the former Steelers pilot, ran into Webster at a convenience store in Moon Township. The two men had once been close. Stage had attended Pro Bowls in Honolulu with Webster. The two men had gotten their families together, had prayed together and shared their faith. But now Webster had cut himself off—from old teammates, old friends, nearly everyone.

Stage walked up to say hello. Webster was gaunt and frail; he looked like he was 70.

"Mike, it's *Robert!*" said Stage, using the faux French pronunciation the way Webster used to.

"You could see a little flicker of recognition," said Stage, "and then it was like a light going out in his eyes."

Stage was destroyed. He went home and wept.

Three months later, around 11:30 P.M., Garrett called Sunny from the Walmart parking lot at Robinson Township. He said his father was having chest pains and trouble breathing. Sunny joined them and called Charles Kelly, the Wheeling doctor who had become Mike's good friend. By then, Webster's lips were turning blue. Kelly told Sunny to give Mike aspirin "in case he's having a heart attack" and drive him to the emergency room. Garrett went into the store and came back with Tylenol. His dad cussed him out. "Are you trying to kill me?" Webster said. "That's not the right stuff."

Garrett went back to the store and fetched some aspirin, which Mike gulped down. His condition wasn't improving. Sunny drove him to the emergency room at Heritage Valley Sewickley Hospital.

"I got Hall of Famer Mike Webster in my car; he's not feeling well," Sunny told the nurse. "Can you please help him?"

Webster was talkative and upbeat. He asked Sunny to take Garrett to school in the morning. As a nurse went to insert a catheter, he joked: "This is the first time a woman has touched me like that in ten years." The nurse injected him with morphine, and Sunny and Garrett could hear him saying behind the curtain: "Oh, yeah, baby, that's the good stuff."

They thought everything would be fine. And then suddenly it wasn't.

Tests revealed two fully blocked arteries and two that were partially blocked. Webster's heart was failing. He was transferred to Allegheny General in an ambulance. Webster was still optimistic and reassuring. When he saw Sunny, he reminded him of their plan to buy a pair of motorcycles someday.

"Don't worry," Webster told him. "When I get better, we're going to get those Harleys. We'll go out and make some money on some signings and do some different things."

But not long after the surgery, Garrett and Sunny were told they should call the rest of the family. There was too much blockage. Webster's body was shutting down.

Garrett and Sunny were stunned. Like everyone who had known him or watched him, they believed to the end that Iron Mike was indestructible. But he wasn't. In the early morning hours of September 24, 2002, Mike Webster was pronounced dead. He was 50. Sunny, the memorabilia collector, recalled being struck by the time of death: 12:52 A.M.

Bradshaw wore 12, Webster 52.

The Steelers paid for the funeral: $5,000. Two hundred people attended, including a Who's Who of Steelers greats: Bradshaw, Swann, Harris, Blount, Noll. And the owner, Dan Rooney. Sunny had called Joe Gordon to ask the team for help; he had never really understood Webster's hatred of the Steelers. Colin was at Camp Lejeune, about to be deployed to Iraq, when he got the terrible news that his father was dying. At the funeral, he watched with disgust as Garrett greeted Rooney and the other Steelers. At one point, two of Rooney's assistants approached Colin to ask if he would come over to see the owner and receive his condolences. "Fuck you!" Colin shouted at Rooney. "My dad loathed you till the day he died. You have no business here."

Pam found herself looking around at all of Webster's ex-teammates and their wives. She wondered: Why aren't you all having to deal with this? Why just Mike? What did we all do to deserve this? Why are your husbands all fine?

Noll's wife, Marianne, came up to offer her sympathies.

"I didn't know Mike was sick; he didn't appear sick," she told Pam.

"Mike didn't appear sick because his injuries were inside his helmet," Pam said.

A few days later, the phone rang at Bob Fitzsimmons's office. The caller introduced himself as a pathologist with the Allegheny County coroner. Fitzsimmons could hardly understand him. The caller had a thick accent, and Fitzsimmons was tired and grief-stricken. He had lost a client who had become his friend. Fitzsimmons had grown to love Webster, and Mike's death had only made him more committed to confronting the NFL, to trying to recover what Mike was owed on behalf of his family.

Fitzsimmons wasn't totally sure he understood what the doctor wanted. He asked him to repeat himself, and the pathologist explained that he had read about Webster's problems before his death.

Then he repeated his odd request: Could he please study Mike Webster's brain?

6

THE VANILLA GUY

Leigh Steinberg's Marriott brain seminars were causing a cultural shift in the NFL. Steinberg knew that the tradition of players laughing about their head injuries or hiding them from trainers and doctors would never be fully eradicated; expecting otherwise was "somewhat akin to asking a drunk driver whether they're drunk," he thought. But the culture was definitely changing. Exhibit A was Steinberg's biggest client.

"The flippancy went away in that time period," said Steve Young.

Steve Young was not like most football players, and it went well beyond his use of words like *flippancy*. He was the great-great-great-grandson of Brigham Young, patriarch of the Mormon Church and founder of the university where Young played college football. Young was born in Salt Lake City but raised in Greenwich, Connecticut, after his father, a corporate lawyer and former BYU fullback, got a job in New York City. He was a National Merit Scholar and a great high school quarterback with a suspect throwing arm. Young decided to attend BYU, at the time a quarterback factory, even though he had no guarantee he'd get to play quarterback there.

Young took a long and circuitous path to NFL immortality. He started out eighth on the depth chart at BYU and spent much of his time there in the shadow of Jim McMahon before emerging as a star his senior season. Instead of going to the NFL, he signed a $40 million contract with the Los Angeles Express of the short-lived United States Football League, a decision he immediately regretted. Within a year, Steinberg had wrangled Young out of his contract. Young landed in 1985 with the lowly Tampa Bay Buccaneers, where his record as a starter was 3–19. Tampa Bay then traded him to the 49ers to make room for Vinny Testaverde. In San Francisco, Young became embroiled in the mother of all quarterback controversies, a rivalry with Joe Montana that lasted six years.

Young was almost 32 when the Niners finally traded Montana to Kansas City. Still, he remained in the legend's shadow, respected by his teammates but viewed as a curious case: cerebral, proper (the Brett Favre part in *There's Something About Mary* was originally written for Young, but he turned it down because he felt the humor was inappropriate), the kind of quarterback who picked up his law degree in the off-season and might someday run for president or Congress. That changed one afternoon when head coach George Seifert pulled Young in the third quarter with the Niners losing badly to the Philadelphia Eagles. Young went nuts—confronting the stoic coach on the sideline, unleashing a stream of un-Mormonlike expletives in front of his stunned teammates and a TV audience. To himself, Young was merely frustrated: He felt Seifert had unfairly singled him out. But his teammates were energized. Some believed that Young threw off the yoke of Montana's legacy that day and became the true Niners QB. "When Steve Young told Seifert to fuck off, he became a leader," said Gary Plummer, who was on the sideline that day. "It was literally at that point that guys on the team started embracing him. That tough-guy thing, that mentality that we all started learning at 8 years old, Steve really didn't see that as a beneficial character trait of a quarterback in the NFL until he was 32 years old."

By the time Young was 37, he was regarded as one of the toughest quarterbacks ever to play the game. He once scrambled nine yards after his helmet was knocked off—in a preseason game. He also was one of the league's most battered quarterbacks. As he grew older and the 49ers dynasty was fading, he was a half step slower, and defenses seemed to land shots more cleanly. Young had two concussions in 1996, then another on the fifth play of the 1997 season when Tampa Bay's Warren Sapp kicked him in the head. Young was so averse to coming out of games that he sometimes hid behind offensive linemen to avoid his coaches. When Sapp drilled him, he managed to talk coach Steve Mariucci, Seifert's successor, into putting him back in. But it had reached the point where San Franciscans worried about Young's long-term health; people openly feared that the next hit would be his last. In 1999, during a win over New Orleans, Young was hit 21 times—"his impression of a pinata," one writer called it—with the Saints swarming over him, including a helmet-to-helmet shot that briefly left him inert. His own linemen feared for his safety. "It's basically got to stop," said guard Derrick Deese. "We were way over in volume of hits that he was taking."

The next week, the Niners traveled to Arizona. Young's fiancée, a former model named Barbara Graham, had invited her family to the game. Near the end of the first half, Cardinals cornerback Aeneas Williams blitzed from the right—Young's blind side. Williams, untouched, blasted Young, who went down so fast and so hard that it was difficult to tell what had happened—even on film. In fact, Young had been turned into a human pinball: On his way down, the back of his head hit tackle Dave Fiore's knee and then the hard turf. Plummer, by now a broadcaster, watched the play from the press box. "I was easily 300 feet away, and you could hear not only the helmet-to-helmet contact, you could hear his helmet hit the back of the *ground*. It was brutal." Whether Young was unconscious would become "a personal debate between my wife and me," he said. "I honestly don't remember whether I was knocked out or whether I just laid there." In any event, he wasn't moving. After several tense moments, Young rose and made it to the sideline.

At halftime Young told Mariucci: "I know you're not going to believe me, but I feel pretty good."

In an earlier time, perhaps, Young would have gone back in. But not now. The mood of the league and his own case history were working against him. Bay Area newspapers had begun printing time lines of Young's concussions dating all the way back to college, including one at BYU in which he was assisted off the field and then returned to lead a game-winning drive against Utah State. Now he was the quarterback who cried wolf. "We went in the locker room, which is a long walk from the old Tempe stadium, and I remember being asked, 'How you feeling?'" Young said. "I felt fine. But that's the first time I'd ever felt, 'You don't believe me.' That's where the injury for me became different than other injuries. This was the first time I felt not completely trusted."

Young had been planning to stay in Arizona with his fiancée and her family. That was now out of the question. Mariucci and the medical staff ordered him back to San Francisco for tests. The 49ers first indicated that Young might miss only a week. Then a week became two. By the third week, Young's head had become part of the national sports conversation, with some commentators imploring him to retire. Greg Garber, who had done the story for ESPN after Al Toon's and Merril Hoge's premature retirements, wrote a piece for the *Hartford Courant* under the headline "Young Should Quit While He Still Can." "The emperor is wearing no clothes, but no one will tell him he is naked," Garber wrote. Mariucci didn't dispel the speculation that Young might have to retire. When the 49ers' coach spoke of his quarterback now, it was in the mournful tones reserved for someone with a terminal illness. "I keep thinking and hoping he's going to be back eventually," Mariucci said. "But we're being realistic. This is lasting longer than we all thought."

Young was seeing a Stanford neurosurgeon named Gary Steinberg (no relation to Leigh). Young liked and admired him, but he felt the doctor was in an impossible situation, an "innate conflict" in which as an independent physician he was being asked to either bench the most beloved athlete in the Bay Area or risk, what, killing him? "I was feeling a little bit trapped," said Young. "It was just a red-hot situation, a tender situation." Young couldn't go to the store without getting advice. Elderly women would clutch his face and tell him: "*Please* be careful." "I promise. I will," he'd respond. For his part, Gary Steinberg said it was still too dangerous for Young to play. "The reason he hasn't been cleared to play up until now is that it's my opinion and the opinion of the 49ers that it's in the best interest of Steve Young to allow his brain to recover," he said during the third week of the crisis.

The 49ers were also conflicted. Mariucci was just six years older than Young, and the two men were like brothers. Young was so close with 49ers doctor Jim Klint ("a dear friend"), he later spoke at Klint's funeral. The conversations between Young and Mariucci began to take on a Shakespearean character. Each day, Young would beg Mariucci to let him back on the field. Each day, Mariucci refused. The discussions took place anywhere Young could corner Mariucci: in the coach's office, on team buses, as Young stood idle on the sideline. Then, of course, there was Leigh Steinberg, who had turned concussions into a national health issue. The decision about whether Young would play had moved beyond the calculus of professional football. The main decision makers—the coach, the doctor, the agent—were like extended family members mounting an intervention to save Young from himself. "They kind of became the Italian grandmother, you know what I mean?" said Young. "The Jewish grandmother. The Mormon grandma. As I melt it down and think about it, those opinions are the ones that carried the day. Not the opinions on the street or even the intense scrutiny of concussions at the time. What held me back from getting back on the field? It was trying to convince people who truly loved me."

"Mooch, you've lost all perspective," Young told Mariucci. "You're too close to this. You've got to be practical. This can't be emotional."

"I'm not emotional," said Mariucci.

But of course he was. At times, the coach was in tears.

As the season wore on, it became clear that at least from the 49ers' perspective, Young was done. The team, with Jeff Garcia at quarterback, was on its way to a 4–12 season, including at one point eight straight losses. "I could have run sprints and recited *War and Peace* and they would have said, 'You're out,' " said Young.

That off-season, the question of Young's retirement hung over San Francisco like the summer fog. To Young, it became clear that of the many hurdles he faced, one was the most significant: No one in the Bay Area would let him go back on the field—not Steinberg (the neurosurgeon), not Mariucci, not Klint, not Bill Walsh, then the team's vice president and general manager. Walsh was a big fight fan, and he publicly expressed his fears that Young could end up punch-drunk.

Young had one prominent ally: Mike Shanahan, the head coach of the Denver Broncos. Shanahan had been Seifert's offensive coordinator during the transition from Montana to Young. His quarterback in Denver, John Elway, had just retired, and no one was more prepared to succeed a legend than Young. Young was faced with a brutal decision: play in Denver, rejecting the advice of pretty much everyone who loved him, or retire.

One of his more interesting advisers during this period was Plummer. Two years earlier, Plummer had retired and taken a job as a 49ers broadcaster. The transition was chastening. Shortly after he left, Plummer was walking the sidelines and found that he had a whole new perspective on pro football. "I remember seeing the violence and laughing to myself, saying, 'I can't flipping believe I did this.'" He was no longer the same Plummer who had stood in the back of a Marriott conference room heckling a neuroscientist. On the contrary, he was embarrassed. "It's still remarkable to think how uneducated I was," he said. "I mean, I went to Cal; I didn't go on a scholarship, I got in because of my grades. I thought I was a pretty smart guy. I mean, now I look back at what a fucking moron I was to be mocking some of the most brilliant minds in the country on their specialty. I'd love to go back and say, 'I'm sorry, I was a moron.' But that was the attitude at the time."

Plummer, like almost everyone, urged Young to get out. "This isn't about your teammates anymore, this is about your life," he implored him. "This is about having kids and being able to play with them in your backyard and not wanting you to be a mush mouth."

On June 12, 2000, Young announced his retirement at the 49ers headquarters in Santa Clara—grudgingly and defiantly. "For the record, I know I can still play," he said. That was undoubtedly true. He said he had been cleared. That was partially true. Walsh said: "The San Francisco 49ers, we considered the risk factor really to be too much for us to overcome." Young was now married, and he and Barb were expecting their first child. "The fire still burns," Young said, "but the stakes were too high."

Thirteen years later, Young sat behind a desk at a nondescript office complex in Palo Alto, where he runs his charitable foundation, Forever Young; manages a hedge fund; and juggles car pool assignments. It was the first time he had talked extensively about the issue that now tormented the league. Young was not entirely comfortable with his association with the NFL's concussion crisis. "I've danced away from concussions because I don't think it was that vital to the big picture for my career," he said. "But the truth is you're coming to me because that's a practical reality: the perception that part of my career is concussions."

Young drew a distinction between himself and some of the horror stories that had come out. He said he once took a desperate call from a "prominent player" holed up in his basement, in tears and depressed, seeking guidance and empathy. The player essentially was looking to swap stories, compare their struggles, but Young was at a loss. It was true that the issue came to dominate his last couple of years in the NFL, but he felt that others had had it much worse, that he had become more of a pawn in the politics of concussions than a true casualty.

"Concussions didn't drive me out of the game," Young insisted. It was a combination of factors, including the changing nature of the 49ers organization and, in the end, his desire to finish his career in red and gold.

"I'm not the one that's going to be a real compelling story," he said. "I'm an expert on vanilla concussions: I felt tired, I rested up, and about a week later I felt 100 percent. That's my history. I'm the vanilla guy."

In reality, though, the message couldn't have been any less vanilla to the NFL and its fans: Steve Young, a certain Hall of Famer, had been forced from the game by concussions. The league had a burgeoning crisis.

By the late 1990s, Pittsburgh had become ground zero for concussion research in the United States. Nearly all the major players were connected to the University of Pittsburgh Medical Center, where Jonas Salk developed the polio vaccine, or the Steelers. Many of the specialists were connected to both the university and the team, whose training site was next door to the UPMC sports medicine facility. Mark Lovell continued to tinker with the concussion test he had created for the Steelers, bringing in a software developer who enabled him to administer the test on the computer. To that point, each exam had to be done with pencil and paper, a laborious process that made it time-consuming to administer and thus less attractive to the volunteer research subjects—the players—critical to making it work. The migration to computers made the exam faster, more accurate, and, not insignificantly, more marketable. What previously had been known to a small circle of neuropsychologists as the Pittsburgh Steelers Test Battery was soon rechristened as ImPACT: Immediate Post-Concussion Assessment and Cognitive Testing. ImPACT later received funding from UPMC, which maintained a financial stake in the new company. Its founders were Lovell, his protégé Micky Collins, and Joe Maroon.

Julian Bailes, the smooth Louisiana neurosurgeon who had produced the ominous survey on NFL players, broke away from Maroon and moved to Orlando to run a neurosurgery ward and continue his own research. Bailes was still in possession of the raw data from the survey: the questionnaires compiled by Frank Woschitz and the union. He decided to bring in another researcher with Steelers connnections to help sort through the data and plot future research.

Kevin Guskiewicz was more steeped in Steelers lore than any of his fellow neuroscientists. He had grown up in Latrobe, Pennsylvania, a small city east of Pittsburgh that in the late 1800s fielded one of the first professional football teams. The Steelers held their training camp each fall at Latrobe's Saint Vincent College; as a kid, Guskiewicz would ride his bike to the school to watch his heroes, players such as Webster and Mean Joe Greene, from a hill overlooking the field. Guskiewicz's father designed kitchens and bathrooms and, with Guskiewicz's uncle, ran the Southside Inn, a bar that catered to steelworkers. When Guskiewicz was old enough, he worked the Saturday morning shift, pouring boilermakers at 7:30 A.M. At West Chester University near Philadelphia, Guskiewicz studied sports medicine and journalism. He wrote for the school newspaper, *The Quad,* and worked as a freelancer for the *Philadelphia Inquirer.* After he graduated, he applied to the prestigious Columbia University School of Journalism but was wait-listed. To say this minor setback was fortuitous for Guskiewicz would be the understatement of his life. At the last minute, he decided to apply to Pitt, which had a new master's program in exercise physiology and sports medicine. Within a few years, newspapers would be a dying industry. The concussion business was booming.

Guskiewicz had sandy hair, blue eyes, and an earnest, down-to-earth manner that allowed him to fit in with everyone from players to trainers to brain surgeons. People found him immediately disarming. (Later, when Guskiewicz received a $500,000 MacArthur "genius grant," he admitted he had heard of the award only because he'd seen a reference to it on an episode of *Friends.*) While studying at Pitt, Guskiewicz landed a job as an apprentice to the Steelers' longtime trainer Ralph

Berlin, aka the Plumber. As Berlin's second assistant, he learned how to treat elite athletes and served as a gofer and ankle taper. The Steelers put Guskiewicz through graduate school. He thought about continuing on as a Steelers trainer, but he was about to get married and concluded that it was a difficult life in which to raise a family. On the advice of his mentor at Pitt, he applied to get his doctorate at the University of Virginia, where Jeff Barth, the "Grandfather of Sports Neuropsychology," was waiting for him.

At Virginia, Guskiewicz worked with a local high school team and was immediately appalled by the way it treated concussions. "We were handling ankle sprains better than we were handling brain injuries," he said. "It was scary." Most of the research to that point had focused on cognition (Barth, Lovell, Collins, et al.); Guskiewicz, with the encouragement of another researcher, Dave Perrin, started to examine how concussions affected balance and motor skills. He found that the effect was often profound. He devised his own diagnostic tool to measure the connection between brain injuries and balance, and soon he too was publishing concussion research. Years earlier, when they had both been with the Steelers, Bailes and Guskiewicz used to hang out on the sideline during games—Bailes as an understudy to Maroon, Guskiewicz as an understudy to the Plumber—and now Bailes began inviting Guskiewicz to Florida to appear at concussion conferences and collaborate on research.

By then, Guskiewicz had finished his doctorate—his dissertation was titled *Effect of Mild Head Injury on Postural Stability in Athletes*—and was working as an assistant professor at the University of North Carolina in Chapel Hill. One afternoon during a conference in Florida, Bailes handed Guskiewicz a stack of papers: Woschitz's questionnaires. Bailes had something big in mind. The data had suggested to him that the plight of retired NFL players, particularly their mental health, was far more desperate than had been known previously. His idea was to set up a research institute to examine the long-term health effects of playing professional football and other sports, and he wanted Guskiewicz to run it. If the idea sounded far-fetched and perhaps overly ambitious, it's because it was—essentially an entire research institution born out of a bunch of six-year-old questionnaires stuffed into cardboard boxes. The players union agreed to provide some of the seed money, roughly $75,000, though that concerned Guskiewicz. He feared the center would be perceived as a vehicle for the union, the research it produced a tool for getting players more benefits. That was certainly one goal of the union, but not necessarily of the researchers. Guskiewicz bought some independence by persuading UNC's vice chancellor for research to kick in $200,000. The fact that the center would be at UNC and not at the union offices in New York also helped. Still, three officials from the Players Association, including Frank Woschitz, were listed in the directory for the newly born Center for the Study of Retired Athletes.

Guskiewicz's first task was to update Woschitz's survey. "It was poorly constructed. I mean, it wasn't anybody's fault; it was probably just done by some office staffer that said, 'Oh, here are the kind of questions I think we want to know about,'" Guskiewicz said. He decided to start from scratch, constructing a 10-page survey that would turn into the most comprehensive health study in the history of the NFL. The survey was divided into seven sections: Football History, Medical History, Concussions, Musculoskeletal Injuries, Health Status, Nutritional and Substance Use, and Personal Information. The hundreds of questions included:

> *How much bodily pain have you had during the past 4 weeks?*
> *Have you felt downhearted and depressed?*
> *Do you currently have a mental or physical condition that limits*
> *your ability to do the things you want to do?*

In the Concussions section, the survey first defined for the former players what a concussion actually was:

A concussion is a blow to the head followed by a variety of symptoms that may include any of the following: headache, dizziness, loss of balance, blurred vision, "seeing stars," feeling in a fog or slowed down, memory problems, poor concentration, nausea, or throwing up. Getting "knocked out" or being unconscious does NOT always occur with a concussion.

The survey went out in 2001. The response was overwhelming, an indication of how badly the players wanted to be heard. Guskiewicz sent out surveys to all 3,683 living members of the NFL Retired Players Association; 2,552—over 69 percent—sent it back. The survey highlighted more completely what the original had only hinted at: More than 60 percent of the players reported sustaining at least one concussion during their careers; nearly a quarter had had at least three. More than half said they'd lost consciousness on the field or experienced memory loss at least once. But perhaps the most disturbing finding was the apparent correlation between the number of concussions and depression. Players who reported concussions were three times as likely to report that they were depressed. Guskiewicz wasn't immediately sure why this was so, but he theorized that the concussions or the *symptoms* of the concussions—perpetual headaches, memory loss, erratic moods—were causing it.

Guskiewicz knew more than anyone the implications of where his research was headed. He was a former NFL trainer, albeit an apprentice, and a die-hard Steelers fan. Bailes, his colleague, was a former NFL doctor. "We're not here to paint an ugly picture of life in the NFL," Guskiewicz told the *Los Angeles Times*. But he added: "These injuries are a hazard of their occupations."

Guskiewicz continued to drill down. He followed up that survey with one that focused on mild cognitive impairment—the interim stage before full-blown dementia, characterized by memory loss, erratic behavior, and language difficulties. This time, 1,399 former NFL players and their close relatives participated. The results were even more ominous: Players who reported at least three concussions were *five times more likely* to be diagnosed with early signs of dementia. Part of the reason this finding was so devastating was the nature of the way concussions occurred. Guskiewicz had looked at college football players and found that those who experienced one concussion were much more likely to incur another one and then another. There was something about the initial trauma that primed the brain for further injury, especially when it had not had time to heal. The structure of Guskiewicz's NFL study— a survey conducted largely by mail—raised some questions about its accuracy. The players were self-reporting, after all, some many years after they had played. But the surveys were anonymous, and experience suggested that players *under*reported their injuries. Most were like Gary Plummer, who upon hearing the definition of a mild concussion concluded that he'd had hundreds.

The study's conclusion was blunt: "Our findings suggest that the onset of dementia-related syndromes may be initiated by repetitive cerebral concussions in professional football players."

Guskiewicz kept going. He now focused on the earlier finding suggesting that concussions triggered depression. He isolated players reporting at least three concussions and found that they were three times more likely to be diagnosed with clinical depression.

Guskiewicz observed these results with pity and sadness. What had happened on the field to players such as Al Toon, Merril Hoge, and Troy Aikman was certainly powerful. But Guskiewicz—in his lab at UNC, away from the fans and the pressures of the NFL—was discovering something even more profound: a persuasive argument that concussions were not only an inevitable part of professional football but often led to misery and torment later in life—not only for the players but for everyone around them. The results were "daunting," he wrote, "given that depression is typically characterized by sadness, loss of interest in activities, decreased energy, and loss of confidence and self-esteem. These findings call into question how effectively retired professional football players with a history of three or more concussions are able to meet the mental and physical demands of life after playing professional football."

Guskiewicz, Bailes, and their colleagues made it clear that they believed that the game itself was causing something destructive and insidious to occur deep inside the brains of huge numbers of retired players. Football-induced concussions, they wrote, "can result in diffuse lesions in the brain. . . . These lesions result in biochemical changes, including an increase in excitatory neurotransmitters, which has been implicated in neuronal loss and cell death. A potential mechanism for lifelong depression could be this initial loss of neurons, which could be compounded by additional concussions, eventually leading to the structural changes seen with major depression."

Translated, their hypothesis was this: Football causes brain damage. Guskiewicz and his colleagues were laying out a scientific explanation for all the ominous research that had preceded it: why concussions were hardly "minor" brain injuries; why they seemed to repeat themselves and come in clusters, inflicting more and more damage; why they led to devastating consequences such as depression, memory loss, and dementia, in much higher rates than in the general population; and why those symptoms sometimes never went away.

A more explosive theory was hard to imagine. But at this point it was just that—a theory. Detecting those changes in the brain of a retired professional football player would require one key missing element: The player would have to be dead.

Beyond Leigh Steinberg's awareness campaign and the disturbing science that continued to emerge, there was another—largely unspoken—reason the NFL's concussion culture was changing: In 1996, in Waukegan, Illinois, Merril Hoge was suing the Chicago Bears.

Technically, Hoge was suing only the team doctor and his primary employer, an Illinois hospital, but his complaint was an indictment of the way the Bears had handled his treatment before he was driven out of football. After his retirement, Hoge had plenty of time to ponder what had happened to him. As his brain recovered, he had taken a job as a football analyst for ESPN, a job at which he excelled. Still, he felt he wasn't the same person. At home, trivial matters set him off—his kids whining, the smallest mishap; one day his wife asked to borrow his toothbrush, and it was all he could to do keep himself from exploding. Bright lights tormented him, and so he installed dimmers in every room of his house. His ESPN colleagues knew that the film room had to be dark when he entered. "Managing my state is every day," he said.

One day, Hoge was working at a football camp when a woman walked up and berated him.

"You should be ashamed of the example that you set by going back and playing with a concussion," she said. She grabbed her son and walked away.

Hoge sat for a moment, stunned. He thought: "She's right, but she's wrong." Hoge believed that if he had been aware of the potential consequences of his injuries—brain damage, even death—he would have been wrong to go back on the field so quickly after his concussion in Kansas City, the one that had caused him to believe he could hear the ocean. But he didn't. At that point, he still thought a concussion was like an ankle sprain or a pulled hamstring; no matter how bad it was, he could play through it. Five weeks later, when he was concussed a second time, it was too late. His career was over.

Hoge desperately missed football, and he soon directed his anger at the Bears' team physician, John Munsell. Munsell worked primarily as an internist at Lake Forest Hospital. He had been the Bears' doctor since 1978, sharing the duties with another physician. Munsell conducted preseason physicals and split time on the sidelines during home and away games. For this, the Bears paid him and his colleague an undisclosed retainer. Munsell treated not only the players but also, on occasion, coaches, team officials, and their families.

What transpired in Hoge's lawsuit was a preview of the NFL's troubles in the years ahead. Hoge was accusing Munsell of malpractice, but it went deeper than that. He argued that Munsell should have been aware of the latest developments in concussion research and applied them to his care. Instead, Hoge alleged, he was kept in the dark and allowed to continue to play despite his lingering symptoms. Hoge brought in the Pittsburgh Steelers brain trust—Maroon, Lovell, and Bailes—to explain the seriousness of concussions and the recent advances in diagnostic testing. Munsell argued that his treatment was state-of-the-art and that Hoge had had an obligation to inform the Bears' medical staff of his symptoms.

"It was a difficult case; there was no real precedent," said Robert Fogel, the Chicago lawyer who represented Hoge. "It isn't like a lot of other football players were suing doctors over their mistreatment of concussions."

Munsell was not an ideal witness for the defense. He acknowledged under oath that despite his role as team doctor he had no specialized training in sports medicine, nor had he read any medical literature on concussions. Before 1994, when Hoge's injury occurred, "I don't recall when I read an article in a book about a concussion," he said. He seemed unaware of the most recent protocols for allowing concussed athletes to return to play.

Munsell did not take notes or keep records on Hoge's brain injuries. Speaking of the night of the concussion in Kansas City, he said:

"I didn't carry a notebook or notepad or paper and pencil on my person, but I certainly would have had it been available to me."

That night on the team plane, Munsell informed Hoge that he would not play the next week. After touching down in Chicago, he never examined Hoge again.

Hoge's injury had occurred on August 22, 1994. Under questioning from Fogel, Hoge described the extent to which his injury was monitored:

"Merril, were you examined by any doctors from August 23rd till you returned to play August 29th?"

"No."

"Did you have any conversations with any doctors from August 23rd to return to play on August 29th?"

"No."

"Did you ever speak, and I mean in person, or on the telephone, with Dr. Munsell between August 23rd and August 29th when you returned to play?"

"No."

"Merril, after August 22, 1994, did Dr. Munsell ever examine you before you returned to play?"

"No."

"Did any doctor examine you before your return-to-play?"

"No."

Munsell's lawyers tried to show that Hoge had hidden his injuries from the Bears' medical staff. This was the crux of Munsell's argument: How could he be held responsible for failing to treat Hoge when he was never informed that the player still had symptoms when he went back on the field? Didn't Hoge bear some of the blame? Hoge knew football was a violent sport, yet he wanted so badly to continue playing that sport, he hid his injuries from the team doctor.

"We are dealing here with an intelligent man, not a child, not a person of suboptimal intelligence, but an intelligent adult," Munsell said. "I believe there was a responsibility to be shared there."

Munsell's lawyer went through a long windup before raising this issue with Hoge on the witness stand.

Hoge seemed to be waiting for it like a power hitter sitting on a fastball.

"We could probably save a lot of time here: Nobody told me anything about my concussion," he said. "Nobody told me about the signs and symptoms and what to be aware of. Had I known those things, you're darn right: I would have told him. Would have been more than happy to tell him.

"But at that time, I knew nothing. I did not know what I was risking. We talk about fatality and brain damage; I should have known about that, you're darn right I should have known. If I feel like I can perform and I'm doing everything possible to perform, I will perform. But we're not going to compare knees and ankles here. We're talking about a brain, far more important than any other part of our body. And I did deserve that.

"Dr. Munsell took me over as his patient; that is his obligation. Not to stick me on a plane, send me home, and have nothing to do with me again."

The jury awarded Hoge $1.55 million—the last two years on his contract plus $100,000 for pain and suffering.

Not long afterward, the judge threw a wrench into Hoge's celebration. He ruled that Fogel had failed to disclose a key piece of evidence: a letter from a Chicago neurosurgeon who believed that Munsell should not be held liable. A new trial was ordered, at which point Hoge and Munsell settled out of court.

Still, it was a devastating defeat for the Bears and, by extension, the NFL. It put the teams, its doctors, and the league on notice. Fogel suddenly found himself getting calls from lawyers around the country. They represented not only football players but athletes from other sports as well. The NFL's mushrooming crisis now had legal implications.

The league, of course, was aware of the lawsuit. An indication of its concern came late in the case, when Munsell's lawyers produced a new witness. According to a letter filed with the court, this witness, in contrast to the leading concussion experts in the country, would testify that "at all times Dr. Munsell acted within the standard of care" for the National Football League. *At all times*—the letter emphasized that point repeatedly. Munsell's treatment met the standard of care for the NFL from the moment Merril Hoge heard the ocean in Kansas City. His treatment met the standard of care for the NFL when Hoge was allowed to take the field a week later without Munsell or any other doctor examining him. Munsell's treatment met the standard of care for the NFL right up to the moment five weeks later when Hoge bent down to make a block and his world went black, ending his career.

It turned out that Munsell's lawyers produced this expert witness too late, and so he was not allowed to appear in court in support of the Bears' team doctor. But Fogel always wondered how the witness suddenly materialized. "I just got the sense, you know, some of this went to another level."

The witness's name was Elliot Pellman. He was the head of the NFL's Mild Traumatic Brain Injury Committee.

PART TWO

DENIAL

7

GALEN OF PERGAMON

Even though they were on opposite sides of Merril Hoge's lawsuit, Mark Lovell and Elliot Pellman knew each other well. One day back in 1994, Pellman had called Lovell in Pittsburgh, identifying himself as the chairman of the NFL's Mild Traumatic Brain Injury Committee. Pellman explained that the new entity had been created by Commissioner Paul Tagliabue to study concussions. He told Lovell he was familiar with his new concussion test—of course he would have been, since that test had been used to end Hoge's career—and invited him to participate in the committee's first meeting in February 1995 at the NFL Combine in Indianapolis.

As skeptical as Tagliabue was about the NFL's concussion problem ("a pack journalism issue"), the MTBI committee was a logical response to a mushrooming public relations crisis. The retirements of Toon and Hoge, Troy Aikman's erased memory after the 1993 NFC Championship Game, and the spate of head injuries league-wide had left fans with a growing impression that the entire sport was concussed. The Mild Traumatic Brain Injury Committee—some researchers said the name itself suggested the NFL's benign view of the problem—promised to take a scientific approach to concussions and come up with a series of measures to make the game safer than ever.

Lovell traveled to his first meeting of the MTBI committee with the trepidation befitting a novice entering the seat of power. He had started baselining the Steelers just two years earlier and was still unfamiliar with the world of pro sports. His innate shyness didn't help. Accompanied by the Steelers' doctor, Tony Yates, Lovell put on his best suit for the occasion. "What are you trying to do, embarrass me?" said Yates. When they walked into the hotel conference room where the first meeting was held, the dozen men who greeted Lovell were a picture of casualness in both manner and dress; some wore sweat suits emblazoned with their team's logo, as if they had just come off the sidelines. "I'm the only guy wearing a suit," Lovell recalled of the moment. "I feel like a jerk." Most of the men seemed to know one another, but Lovell didn't recognize any of them, nor did they seem to have any clue who he was. He suspected that they probably had no idea what a neuropsychologist was, much less how one might treat a concussion.

Lovell, of course, was involved in some of the most cutting-edge research in the emerging science of head trauma—he was one of Steinberg's people who believed the world was round. With the NFL's power and resources, he imagined he would be joining a veritable dream team of concussion experts to attack the problem. In fact, there were very few. The contemporary researchers whose studies were reshaping the entire conception of what a concussion was—men such as Jeff Barth, Julian Bailes, Joe Maroon, and Barry Jordan—were nowhere to be found. Instead, Tagliabue's concussion committee was made up almost entirely of NFL insiders. Nearly half the members were team doctors, the same men who had been sending players back on the field for years. There were two trainers, a consulting engineer, and an equipment manager. The committee did have one neurologist, Ira Casson, who had studied boxers and had made the fateful recommendation to Al Toon that he retire, and a neurosurgeon, Hank Feuer (pronounced FOY-er), who had done an internship at Indiana Medical School at the same time Maroon was there and worked for the Colts. Reflecting years later on his status as the committee's lone neurosurgeon, Feuer, measuring his words, said: "That was always, to me, ah, I just thought it's an *interesting* committee. The best way I could put it." The MTBI committee's epidemiologist—the man charged with analyzing much of the committee's research—was John Powell, the number cruncher behind the NFL's claim that concussions had held steady at one every three or four games.

The most perplexing choice was Tagliabue's handpicked chairman: Pellman. With the endorsement of the powerful commissioner, Pellman had instantly become one of the most influential concussion researchers in the country, yet he had not produced a single piece of scientific literature on the subject. This almost certainly was due in part to his medical specialty, rheumatology, which deals primarily with bone and joint disorders such as arthritis. Pellman was genial and stout, a balding man, then 41, routinely described by colleagues as "a good administrator." Through his contacts with the NFL, Pellman came to work as a top medical adviser with other leagues, including the NHL and Major League Baseball. One executive who worked closely with Pellman described him as a kind of medical "concierge" whose primary responsibilities were to administer flu shots and recommend specialists. "If an individual employee has a bad back, Elliot is great in New York about getting you in to see the best back guy," the executive said. He described Pellman as "honestly, a nice man" and suggested he was kept around because of his pleasantness.

The most complete professional biography of Pellman would be assembled years later by the *New York Times* after the newspaper discovered in 2005 that he had exaggerated his credentials in a biography he sent to the House Committee on Government Reform. This came as Pellman testified before the committee, offering effusive praise of baseball's steroids policy, the same policy that had done nothing to prevent Barry Bonds from shattering the career home run record. Pellman had claimed in his biography, which he circulated widely, that he obtained his medical degree from the State University of New York at Stony Brook. In reality, Pellman had attended medical school in Guadalajara, Mexico, and received his medical degree from the New York State Department of Education. Pellman also reported that he was an associate clinical professor at the Albert Einstein College of Medicine, when, in fact, he was an assistant clinical professor, an honorary position held by thousands of doctors, and didn't teach at the school. He told the *Times* the errors were minor. "In a way, I thank you," he said, "because those discrepancies are not important enough to be there, and they have all been fixed." Pellman explained he had enrolled at the Universidad Autónoma de Guadalajara, which had lower admissions standards, because he received poor grades as an undergraduate biology major at NYU. He attributed his poor academic record to his complicated life at the time, including his father's death and a busy schedule working in his family's flower shop in the Bronx and as a cab driver. Pellman blamed the errors on his secretary and the New York Jets, where he had worked as team doctor since 1988. "So SUNY said he didn't get an MD from there?" Jets vice president Ron Colangelo told the *Times*. "Oh my goodness, oh my goodness gracious."

When Pellman first came to the NFL, he was practicing rheumatology at Long Island Jewish Medical Center. As the Jets' doctor, he had treated Al Toon after the concussion that ended Toon's career. When Pellman went to look for a neuropsychologist to test Toon's brain function, he approached a colleague, Bill Barr. "I don't know who any neuropsychologists are; I've never worked with one," Pellman said, according to Barr, who recounted the conversation to ESPN's Peter Keating. "But somebody said Al Toon should see a neuropsychologist, so I asked around and I'm calling you." As the NFL slowly began to adopt neuropsychological testing to diagnose concussions, Pellman brought on Barr to work with the Jets. Occasionally, the two men—along with Casson, another colleague at Long Island Jewish—would appear at coaching clinics to talk about concussions. Barr was struck by how ignorant Pellman seemed of all previous research. By then, Barth, Lovell, and others had been publishing for years. "During these lectures, Pellman's saying things like, 'Nothing has ever been done on concussions or mild brain injury and we're starting from scratch,'" Barr, who had moved on to New York University, said in an interview for this book. "I had been trained in evaluating MTBI, and I knew the literature. But he acted like nothing had ever been published on this before 1995."

Elliot Pellman's views on concussions were perfectly aligned with the NFL doctrine at the time, as articulated by Tagliabue and the NFL's PR machine. When he spoke publicly, he seemed to suggest that they were a routine part of the game and not a major concern. In 1994, the year the MTBI committee was formed, he told *Sports Illustrated* that "concussions are part of the profession, an occupational risk." A football player, he told the magazine, is "like a steelworker who goes up 100 stories, or a soldier." In 1999, by siding with Munsell, the Bears' doctor in the

Hoge case, Pellman—himself an NFL doctor and by then the head of scientific research for the league—had endorsed a treatment model that most leading concussion researchers would have equated with bloodletting and the application of leeches: allowing a severely concussed athlete who had no idea where he was to return to play without even a cursory exam. The same year, Pellman repeated the statistics the league had now floated for a decade—just one concussion every three games—and suggested that injuries to high-profile players such as Toon, Hoge, Aikman, and Steve Young had created a "mirage" that led people to "think the injuries have increased though they've really been there all the time."

Pellman seemed to practice what he preached. Former players described how, as the Jets' doctor, he often allowed concussed athletes back on the field. During a 1999 playoff game against the Jacksonville Jaguars, tight end Kyle Brady reached back for a pass from Vinny Testaverde and was knocked unconscious by a helmet-to-helmet hit. Dazed and nauseous, Brady was helped to the sideline, where Pellman and the medical staff examined him. Suddenly, out of the fog, Brady heard the booming voice of Jets head coach Bill Parcells: "Is he gonna be all right? When's he gonna get back in there?"

"You know, in a classic Parcells kind of way," recalled Brady, chuckling as he described the memory to ESPN's John Barr. "I'm not sure if it was a question. It might have been a command." Brady returned for the next offensive series, still woozy, his teammates telling him where to go. Asked if there was any basis for clearing him, Brady replied: "No. None." But he said he was just as eager as Parcells to see himself back on the field. "At that point, you're kind of like a slobbering dog," Brady said.

Kevin Mawae, who played center for the Jets for eight seasons, said he liked Pellman immensely, respected him "as a man," and even trusted him as his family physician. But he said it was clear in the Jets' locker room that Pellman served multiple masters. Pellman had cofounded a Long Island health care network, ProHEALTH Care Associates, which worked with multiple New York sports teams, including the Jets. The building was filled with memorabilia. "There's definitely some influential weight that goes with being a team doctor, and there's a conflict of interest because they work for the team," said Mawae. As more information about Pellman surfaced—his résumé embellishment, the overlapping relationship between the Jets and his private practice, his brain research for the NFL despite his total lack of qualifications— Mawae began to hear "jokes in the locker room about Pellman's status with the NFL and things like that."

One running joke involved a three-word code—"Red Brick Broadway"—that Pellman had players recite to determine if they were able to play after a concussion. According to Mawae, "The three words were always the same. He would leave you and come back before the next series, and you'd go, 'Red Brick Broadway. I'm ready to go.'" In 2003, Pellman would face pointed questions about his treatment of a wide receiver, Wayne Chrebet, who was allowed to reenter a close game against the Giants after being knocked out for several minutes. "This is very important for your career," Pellman reportedly said before sending him back in. Chrebet was never the same and retired in 2005.

But players such as Mawae and Brady said such incidents were common. On one occasion, Mawae said, he suffered the same injury as Chrebet: He took a knee to the head and blacked out. "Next thing I know I'm laying prostrate on the ground," he said. "The first realization was, 'Wow I just got knocked out.'" After performing a "systems check," Pellman and the Jets' medical staff allowed Mawae to return for the next series, but "my teammates were telling me that I was making calls that weren't even in our playbook."

Reflecting on Pellman's selection as the NFL's top medical adviser and leading expert on concussions, Mawae said: "If you're gonna get a doctor that's a yes man, then it makes it easy for you." He regarded Pellman as a pawn. "Pellman's just a small part in this," Mawae said. "The bigger part is it's a multibillion-dollar industry that cannot afford something such as this."

In North Carolina, Kevin Guskiewicz was beginning to perform his own concussion studies, each with results more ominous than the one that preceded it. He watched the development of the NFL's new concussion committee with incredulity and amazement. Guskiewicz, of course, loved football—the Steelers, after all, had paid his way through grad school while he worked as an assistant trainer—but he felt that the NFL's new committee had willfully excluded the most respected researchers, especially those whose research indicated the potential for long-term problems. "Quite frankly it was comical the way in which that original committee was pulled together; comical is probably the nicest way I could describe it," he said. "It seemed like they were cherry-picking anyone who seemed to be dabbling in this topic who was local in the New York area." Guskiewicz found the choice of Pellman ("a rheumatologist!") "bizarre." He wondered: "Who looked at the résumés of these individuals?"

"I'm trying to think of an analogy here: like in an airport when there's a major breach of security," said Guskiewicz. He thought the NFL's approach to the concussion problem was essentially: "Let's pick these folks, that will be the solution, ignore the problem, and it will all go away."

Lovell was part of the committee, but he too wondered how Pellman, with his limited neurological background, could possibly have landed the job. Pellman offered one explanation when he later wrote about the MTBI committee's formation: "On the basis of my experience with Mr. Toon, I was invited to the Commissioner's office to offer my limited insight into this problem. The Commissioner and I realized that we had more questions than answers. Was this a new problem or just an often misdiagnosed or unrecognized one? Was the premature retirement of these men a statistical anomaly or the beginning of an epidemic? I was asked to mount an effort to answer these questions."

Multiple sources, however, said Pellman had been Tagliabue's personal physician and they believed that was at least part of the reason he was named chairman.

"That's my understanding," said Lovell, a member of the committee from its inception.

In a statement to ESPN, Tagliabue acknowledged he was treated by Pellman but said that the first time he saw him as a patient was October 1997—three years after the formation of the MTBI committee. "No personal medical care had anything to do with Dr. Pellman's appointment to the committee in 1994," Tagliabue wrote, adding that Pellman got the job "based on his experience in sports medicine, his work with the Jets that included Al Toon's concussion-related retirement . . . and recommendations from Jets ownership and management."

The committee didn't publish its first research until October 2003—six years after Tagliabue became one of Pellman's patients. Pellman would continue as one of the commissioner's personal doctors until 2006.

- - -

Pellman, as promised, started from scratch. The MTBI committee began its work by spending months establishing an official NFL definition of a concussion. The lack of a consensus definition "has plagued the study of mild head injury in general and concussive injuries in athletes in particular," the committee wrote in an internal status report circulated in 1996. The new league definition was broad: "any traumatically induced alteration of brain function." That included a long list of symptoms: blackouts, wooziness, amnesia, headaches, vertigo, memory loss, personality change, lethargy, and so on. All constituted an NFL concussion, "or, as we quickly decided, the more academically appropriate term, *mild traumatic brain injury,*" Pellman wrote.

The committee used that definition as the starting point for an epidemiological study it called the NFL Mild Brain Injury Surveillance Study, a system to monitor concussions across the league. The MTBI committee distributed forms to medical personnel from all 30 teams with instructions to keep up-to-date records every week. "A major obstacle to head injury research is the unavailability of willing test subjects," said one memo prepared by a bioengineering firm contracted to participate in the study. "The NFL has graciously sponsored a research program offering its players as those living subjects."

Lovell was put in charge of setting up the NFL's neuropsychological testing program, which he based on the model that he and Maroon had created for the Steelers. A few years later, after Lovell testified on behalf of Hoge—and, by extension, against the Chicago Bears and the league—Lovell thought he'd probably be ousted from the committee and would never work in the NFL again. But Pellman never brought it up, nor did anyone else. Instead, the league gave Lovell $12,000 in seed money to spread the gospel of neuropsychological testing. He traveled from city to city, team to team, armed with a letter of support from Tagliabue, who wrote: "We strongly recommend that all clubs in the NFL implement such a testing program so that neuropsychological data is available to club physicians, or other treating physicians, in the event of player concussions."

The NFL's concussion committee was up and running. Pellman reported directly to Tagliabue. The commissioner was rarely seen at the committee's meetings—Feuer recalled him sitting in on only a couple of sessions, during which he rarely spoke—but his representatives frequently attended. Those representatives included, from the very beginning, NFL attorneys. Two lawyers who supported the early work of the MTBI committee were Jeff Pash, the league's general counsel, and Dorothy C. Mitchell, a young lawyer who served as counsel for policy and litigation. Mitchell's responsibilities included providing legal oversight for the NFL's medical and safety committees. Pellman and his colleagues later wrote that Mitchell "worked tirelessly to initiate the MTBI research."

Dorothy Mitchell's contribution to the MTBI committee wasn't totally clear, but at one point she used information related to the NFL's concussion research to try to discredit an expert witness in Hoge's lawsuit. That witness, John McShane, had been the team doctor for the Philadelphia Eagles and a clinical assistant professor at Thomas Jefferson University in Philadelphia. In 1996, McShane received a $134,000 grant from the NFL to study changes in the brain chemistry of concussed NFL players, a study that included other league-affiliated doctors, including Lovell. But before the study got off the ground, the Eagles sold their medical rights to another provider, and McShane was ousted as team doctor, leaving him without access to the players for his league-commissioned study.

Instead of intervening to keep the study alive, the NFL—first Pellman and then Mitchell—sought to recover the grant money, some of which already had been spent on sophisticated software. The aborted study had long been forgotten until July 2000, when Mitchell FedExed material related to the dispute to the attorney defending John Munsell, the Bears doctor who had treated Hoge. Munsell's attorney walked into court the next day and tried to use the NFL's documents against McShane, a former league physician who was prepared to testify that Munsell and the Bears had negligently sent Hoge back on the field to his doom.

McShane, sitting in the back of the courtroom as he watched the argument unfold, was baffled and angry. He felt he had tried to do research that would help the NFL with its concussion problem, only to be thwarted because the Eagles had changed medical providers. Now he was under attack by the league because he planned to testify on behalf of Hoge. "I couldn't understand why anybody would be mad at me," he said. "I had all good intentions; I wanted to do a study that would provide valuable information. Then this change happened that I had no control over, and they were impugning me. I was just stunned."

The judge ruled that the dispute had nothing to do with the case, and McShane was allowed to testify. But it was an early sign of how the NFL and its ostensibly independent concussion committee were willing to throw their weight around—and for which side. The league was prepared to send Elliot Pellman, in his authority as chairman of the MTBI committee, to testify that Munsell's questionable treatment of Hoge was in fact sound. And the NFL lawyer who helped form that committee was willing to intervene in a concussion lawsuit against an NFL doctor. Before the MTBI committee had published a word of scientific research, it had staked out a position as a defender of the NFL.

The McShane study was just one of a number of early NFL concussion projects. The MTBI committee produced an educational video about how to wear a helmet properly. It looked at special mouthpieces and Kevlar caps that purported to reduce concussions. There seemed to be no end to the parade of gadgetry that passed before the MTBI committee from entrepreneurs seeking the imprimatur of the NFL. Many of the projects were considered and discarded, but Pellman was especially passionate about one initiative: helmet *design*. For various reasons, including the threat of lawsuits and a regulatory process that effectively was run by the helmet companies, there had been little in the way of helmet innovation over the years. With appropriate testing and the right design, Pellman thought, the NFL could use its vast resources to create a concussion-resistant helmet.

This was an attractive but not especially new idea and one that was not nearly as simple as it sounded. From the bloody early beginnings of football, the impulse to create more and better protection had been seen as an antidote to the sport's inherent brutality. Often the solutions were nonsensical or made the violence worse. In 1889, players for Princeton started wearing their hair long in the belief that it would protect them from head injuries, launching a nationwide trend. Around the turn of the century, some players wore "head harnesses"—leather straps that fit snugly around the skull. Others wore hard leather nose protectors that hung from a strap that wrapped around the forehead. None of these devices worked, and some encouraged more head thumping. In 1905, when 18 players died—many from head trauma—several university presidents called for the abolition of football. President Teddy Roosevelt famously stepped in to save the sport, convening an emergency summit at the White House. "Football is on trial," he told representatives of the country's elite college football programs. The summit led to dramatic changes in the way the game was played: The forward pass was legalized, and the yardage needed for a first down went from 5 yards to 10, increasing the emphasis on speed. Football as we know it was saved. But the crisis, in what some would call a setback, also produced the NCAA.

As football evolved through the twentieth century, so did the methods for protecting the head. The head harness morphed into a full leather helmet; by the 1930s, teams were decorating them with colorful logos. But the deficiencies of leather helmets were obvious: They became flimsy and tore, reeked of sweat and mildew, and in the end did not provide much protection. Then, in 1939, Riddell, a Chicago company founded by a high school football coach, patented a helmet with a hard plastic shell. Mass production was delayed by World War II and a propensity of the early plastic helmets to shatter. The designer, Gerry Morgan, later Riddell's first chairman, observed that the human head is "the damnedest thing to fit. It comes in all shapes and sizes—egg heads, square heads, flat heads, and lopsided heads. The head isn't round, it's elongated, especially larger heads." The NFL made helmets mandatory in 1943, and by the mid-1950s, the plastic helmet—ABS thermoplastic, a high-strength polymer—was widely used.

But each technological advance came with a corollary: more destruction. One man's protection was another man's weapon. The face mask is but one example. The need for it was made abundantly clear by players like Hardy Brown, an undersized 49ers linebacker who liked to plunge his shoulder into the face of unsuspecting ball carriers—"the Humper," Brown called his signature tackle—shattering jaws and breaking noses. Brown later bragged that he knocked out 75 to 80 players during his ten-year career. George Halas once stopped a game to check Brown's shoulder pads for steel plates. But no sooner had Riddell started bolting face masks onto its helmets than players figured out they could be used to wrestle men to the ground like steers. One was Dick "Night Train" Lane, a Hall of Fame cornerback for the Los Angeles Rams, Chicago Cardinals, and Detroit Lions whose brutal tackling style became known as the Night Train Necktie. By 1956, the NFL had instituted a penalty for an entirely new term that had entered the English language: *face masking.*

With the advent of the plastic helmet, football significantly cut down on catastrophic head injuries such as skull fractures and hemorrhages, but the flip side was that the human head was suddenly turned into a projectile. That dynamic in the NFL—a step forward for safety, followed by ingenious forms of new mayhem, followed by more rules—continued well into the 1980s and 1990s and was very much alive when Elliot Pellman began his new helmet project in 1995. Shortly after the MTBI committee was formed, Bob Cantu, a neurosurgeon and concussion researcher in Boston, ran into Pellman at a conference sponsored by the American Orthopaedic Society for Sports Medicine. Cantu had never met Pellman, who was still largely unknown among researchers, but he was struck immediately by Pellman's confidence that the NFL had a handle on the problem.

"I still remember Elliot waltzing into those meetings, saying, 'We've got this committee, and the National Football League; we're gonna solve the concussion problem,'" said Cantu. Pellman described how the NFL intended to accomplish this: "He said, 'We're going to build the best helmet imaginable,'" Cantu recalled. "They were going to eliminate this traumatic brain injury problem with a superhelmet. And it didn't matter how much it cost because the National Football League could afford anything."

The creation of a concussion-resistant superhelmet immediately struck Cantu as an idea both appealing and remarkably naive. The appeal was obvious: If the solution to reducing football-related concussions was tied to better equipment, the league could throw money at the problem. There would be no real need to examine how the game was played or the long-term effects on the players. But Cantu felt the solution was simplistic because he did not believe better helmets could prevent concussions, which, of course, were injuries that occurred *inside* the skull. In fact, Cantu thought a new and supposedly improved helmet could make the problem worse as players became emboldened by the illusion of better protection, starting the cycle of mayhem all over again.

Cantu wasn't the only one with doubts. Lovell understood the vagaries of concussion better than any member of the MTBI committee. Over the next several years at his clinic at the University of Pittsburgh, he and his colleague Micky Collins would see dozens of patients a week. Lovell and Collins had been cranking out their own research, and if anything, it continued to reveal how diverse and unpredictable concussions were. They defied easy solutions; Collins called it a "cryptic" injury. Some people recovered quickly; others needed to stay in a dark room for weeks as their brains healed. Some people seemed able to withstand huge amounts of trauma. With others, a slight jostling of the head might trigger an injury. And as Guskiewicz would show, the severity of concussions often grew with each injury.

In the MTBI committee, Lovell said he argued that helmets were fine for protecting the outside of the head. He said he thought research creating more and better protection was an interesting and certainly worthy endeavor. But the goal of engineering a superhelmet to reduce concussions was not a realistic solution, he said.

"I think that was a fantasy," said Lovell. "I've always said it's a fantasy. I never thought that was a realistic thing to do."

In many ways, Lovell thought the idea was understandable, the logical creation of an exuberant rheumatologist who had been put in charge of a brain committee, and of engineers and other MTBI members who didn't spend their lives studying the myriad symptoms of traumatic brain injury.

"It's the fantasy of people who don't spend 50 hours a week seeing patients who are all different," said Lovell.

But Pellman's enthusiasm was undiminished. At the end of 1999, he told the *Philadelphia Daily News*: "Within the next six months to a year, incredible stuff is going to come out. We think we're really going to be able to push the envelope. The helmet manufacturers no longer will have any excuses. We're going to understand the nature of this injury better. We think this is not only going to revolutionize head gear for football players, but across the board. And we definitely think it can have an impact on decreasing the number of concussions."

How does one set out to create a superhelmet? The MTBI committee's idea was to take all NFL concussions between 1996 and 2001 and try to re-create the brain-scrambling hits on anthropomorphic crash-test dummies. (Photos showed the dummies wearing Riddell helmets with odd logos, like the players in *Any Given Sunday*.) The committee examined videotape of each recorded NFL concussion; in 182 cases, there was a clear view of where the point of impact had occurred. From those 182 concussions, the committee gleaned enough information in just a couple of dozen cases to calculate the speed at impact. An Ottawa engineering firm was hired to re-create those hits in the lab, using a weighted pendulum with a curved plastic hammer to simulate a helmet-to-helmet hit. The goal was to establish the amount of force that caused each injury, identify how and where the injuries occurred, and then design a helmet that better protected players against those types of hits.

The initial NFL research elicited some fascinating details about the action taking place on the field. The sheer magnitude of the violence was astonishing. The concussed athletes were being hit by fully armored players moving at speeds between 17 and 25 miles per hour (Usain Bolt reaches a top speed of nearly 28 miles per hour). For 15 milliseconds, their heads were struck with 70 g to 126 g forces. A longer duration, of course, would kill anyone, but the momentum transferred in such collisions is still the equivalent of being hit in the head by a 10-pound cannonball traveling at 30 miles per hour. The numbers alone raised ominous questions about the repetitive nature of football, which, as Vince Lombardi famously noted, "is not a contact sport, it's a collision sport." Everyone experiences elevated g forces from time to time—on roller coasters, stopping short in traffic, even sneezing—but the effects are worse when the elevated g forces are repeated over and over at extremely high levels. Like 25,000 car crashes, as Webster explained it.

By the end of 2001, the MTBI committee had amassed a trove of information about concussions in the NFL. The laboratory experiments alone encompassed not only the videotaped pounding of the crash-test dummies but a film library of hundreds of concussions, not to mention the mathematical calculations on velocity, acceleration, and points of impact. The NFL Mild Brain Injury Surveillance Study had produced an enormous amount of data on the symptoms of concussion, including memory loss, loss of consciousness, concussion rates by position, games missed, and on and on. Lovell's neuropsychological testing program had been up and running for six years: All but three teams—the Vikings, Panthers, and Cowboys—were using some form of the test battery Lovell and Maroon had developed for the Steelers. From the original Group of 27 in 1993, the program had expanded to include thousands of neuropsychological tests on hundreds of NFL players. Pellman's MTBI committee had access to those data, too.

The MTBI committee was now ready to publish its research. But where? There are hundreds, if not thousands, of scientific and medical journals dealing with issues involving the brain, sports, or both, ranging from the *Journal of the American Medical Association* to the *Clinical Journal of Sport Medicine.* But only one had an NFL consultant as its editor in chief. Michael L. J. Apuzzo was a professor of neurosurgery at the University of Southern California. In 1992, he was appointed editor in chief of *Neurosurgery,* the official journal of the Congress of Neurological Surgeons. Apuzzo was a stereotactic neurosurgeon—a highly specialized field that involves the use of three-dimensional mapping to place probes deep inside the brain—and something of a Renaissance man. He had patrolled the Arctic Ocean on a nuclear submarine for NATO; produced a 2,540-page textbook titled *Brain Surgery: Complication Avoidance and Management*; helped design new instruments for microsurgery; and been honored by the queen of Spain. Bob Cantu, who knew Apuzzo well, used words such as *worldly, scholarly, erudite,* and *visionary* to describe him. "And he's also a very prideful person," said Cantu. "He doesn't lack for understanding of his accomplishments, which are significant. And yes, he likes a bit of the stage. . . . But don't most people?" Apuzzo's USC biography spanned nine pages when printed out and described him as "one of the world's best known and respected neurosurgeons."

Some people around the NFL also considered Apuzzo something of a jock sniffer. Among his many endeavors, Apuzzo, a tall, slender man with receding dark hair and plastic-framed glasses, worked the sidelines as a consultant to the New York Giants. Bill Barr, the former neuropsychologist for the Jets, called Apuzzo "a sports guy wannabe. He works in LA, but he shows up at all the Giants games, which is not a convenient thing. That tells me he wants to be in the game so badly that he'll travel all the way across the country for these games. He's a neurosurgeon, but you'd see him on the sideline. Brandon Jacobs goes down with a knee injury and Apuzzo will be down there looking at the knee in his raincoat and golf cap." Apuzzo clearly was thrilled by his association with the NFL. After working the 2001 Super Bowl between the Giants and Ravens, he told an interviewer: "When I was in the military I worked in a nuclear-powered submarine where we'd be submerged for three months doing very dangerous things. We were dependent on each other for life and death, and it was an extremely moving bonding experience. Until this game I'd never experienced anything else like it. Everyone was very aware of what it meant to be a part of this game, to be a part of the team that came so far." Cantu said Apuzzo "really enjoyed the association" with the NFL in general and Tagliabue in particular. Apuzzo frequently worked into his conversations with Cantu that he'd just had lunch with the NFL commissioner in New York, a bit of name-dropping that didn't initially strike Cantu as important but soon would.

As editor in chief, Apuzzo set out to remake *Neurosurgery* in his own image: worldly, eclectic, erudite. He wanted to expand the journal's readership and impact by moving it beyond the narrow world of neurosurgery into what he called "an 'avant-garde' progressive position and internationality." It was the brain science equivalent of Tina Brown's makeover of the *New Yorker*. Apuzzo's avant-garde approach to *Neurosurgery* included transforming some of the journal's covers into abstract art and expanding its sports coverage. He decided to establish a sports section to solicit and publish articles on sports and the brain. Bob Cantu was Apuzzo's pick to edit the section.

Cantu was a logical choice. One researcher called him the "King of Concussions." Cantu had been looking into the relationship between sports and head injuries for perhaps as long as anyone alive. When Apuzzo brought him in, Cantu was in his early fifties, a trim man with short red hair that he combed from left to right. Cantu had grown up in Santa Rosa, California, about an hour north of San Francisco, where his father owned a building supplies company. After pitching for two years at Cal, he blew out his arm, and so he decided to accelerate his entry into medical school at the University of California, San Francisco. Cantu moved to Boston in 1964 to do his residency at Massachusetts General Hospital and never left.

By the mid-1980s, Cantu was chief of neurosurgery service and chairman of the department of surgery at Emerson Hospital in Concord, Massachusetts; for fun, he worked the sidelines at high school football games. At the time, contact sports, especially football, were experiencing a wave of hysteria over something called second impact syndrome. The idea was that a first blow to the head might seem benign, but it primed the brain for the second blow, which killed you. The actual number of cases of second impact syndrome was, in fact, low, but the lack of understanding and the sinister nature of the injury led to a lot of media coverage. Cantu, who was watching teenagers collide every week, decided to start looking into the true nature of those collisions. He didn't want to miss the concussion that preceded the concussion that wound up killing a kid.

Cantu quickly realized there were no guidelines for how long a player should sit out after a concussion, and so he decided to come up with some himself. There wasn't a lot of research to draw on; Cantu admitted the exercise was a bit of a stab in the dark. One of his sources of inspiration was an experiment in which UCLA researchers had bashed rats in the head and then checked their glucose levels, glucose being the chemical that powers the brain. The levels stayed depressed for an average of 5 days but sometimes as long as 10, a possible indication of how long it might take to recover from a concussion. Later, the study's author, David Hovda, ran into Cantu at a meeting and asked him how he had come up with his recommendation that athletes sit out a week after suffering a concussion. Cantu pulled out Hovda's study. "You're making recommendations from rat data?" Hovda asked, grinning.

By the time Apuzzo tapped him as *Neurosurgery*'s sports section editor, Cantu had written dozens of papers on concussions and the criteria for returning to play. He had been named president of the American College of Sports Medicine. He was exactly the type of expert Lovell had expected to see on the NFL's committee. Cantu's concussion guidelines were still somewhat arbitrary, but they gave coaches, trainers, and team doctors something to go on when assessing whether a player should be allowed back on the field. Cantu believed the NFL's research was a perfect candidate for the sports section of *Neurosurgery*; it could help advance the science of an issue that had long been important to him. His doubts about Elliot Pellman notwithstanding, he was curious to see what the NFL, with all its resources, came up with. "I knew the work had been done; I thought the work was important and suggested they submit the first paper to *Neurosurgery*," Cantu said.

The first NFL paper was accepted on May 27, 2003. It was published in the October 2003 issue under the title "Concussion in Professional Football: Reconstruction of Game Impacts and Injuries."

To launch the unprecedented initiative, Tagliabue contributed a bland guest editorial titled "Tackling Concussions in Sports." He wrote that the NFL's research already had "contributed to advancing our understanding of the science of concussions, which is a concern for everyone involved in competitive sports and recreational activities. The accompanying article confirms the groundbreaking character of this research."

Apuzzo was more effusive and colorful in a manner befitting his avant-garde publication. In an editor's note, he compared Elliot Pellman's MTBI committee to Galen of Pergamon, the Greek philosopher and medical researcher who studied the wounds of the Roman gladiators. "Football's participants dwarf Rome's gladiatorial combatants in number, and, in its most sophisticated form, the game's pageantry matches or exceeds the spectacle of Roman-designed events," Apuzzo wrote. "As in the ancient contests, modern football is attended by myriad injuries, the most frequent of which involve the brain."

"As in the past," Apuzzo continued, "the modern arenas of sport offer laboratories for the study of the mechanisms and events attendant to multiple injury end points in athletes, and they offer a substrate of important information for our general comprehension of the problem of human trauma in general."

Apuzzo described the research by "Pellman et al." as "highly responsible NFL-sponsored studies" combining field analysis with lab work and offering "significant new insights" into concussions, including "important data for consideration in the development of new directions in helmet design and testing."

The NFL's era of scientific exploration had begun.

The early reviews were glowing. In its first paper published in *Neurosurgery*, in October 2003, the NFL (Pellman et al.) not only had brought science to the question of why the lights were going out for so many players, it also had addressed an issue on the minds of many researchers who thought deeply about the subject. The paper suggested that the standards used to measure the effectiveness of football helmets in preventing head injuries had to be reassessed. The standards were set by a body known as the National Operating Committee on Standards for Athletic Equipment; everyone called it NOCSAE (pronounced NOC-SEE). It had the ring of a government agency—maybe part of the FTC or the Consumer Protection Agency—but in fact, NOCSAE was a private nonprofit organization funded mostly by the sporting goods manufacturers it regulated, including the helmet companies.

Not surprisingly, NOCSAE hadn't changed the way it tested and certified helmets for years. But now here was the NFL, with all its power and authority, using science as a catalyst for reform. NOCSAE focused primarily on the ability of helmets to withstand blows to the periphery and crown of the helmet, but the NFL's study indicated that many injuries occurred when players got hit in the face mask and the side and back of the helmet. This was progress. Cantu, who served as a consultant to NOCSAE, knew that the standards needed updating. In a review appended to the article, he called the NFL's first paper "the most extensive study to date on the biomechanics of athletic concussion in football" and praised "Pellman and his collaborators for this exciting, innovative and unique study and the NFL for funding this research on a topic very critical to its athletes."

Three months later, the NFL published another study in *Neurosurgery*. This second paper—"Concussion in Professional Football: Location and Direction of Helmet Impacts"—drilled down on where the concussive blows were delivered. Again it was illuminating. Pellman received credit as lead author, but most of the heavy lifting was done by Biokinetics, the Ottawa biomechanics firm brought in by the NFL, and

Dave Viano, a biomechanical engineer at Detroit's Wayne State University who had done crash-test studies for the auto industry. This time the NFL divided the human head into quadrants. The league found that 71 percent of the concussive blows were being struck on the side and back quadrants of the helmet, another repudiation of NOCSAE standards.

Again the reaction was positive. Julian Bailes, the neurosurgeon whose work with Barry Jordan had indicated that alarming numbers of retired football players had signs of dementia, wrote that the NFL had "ushered in a new era in the study and analysis of the many nuances of these high-speed bodily collisions." Alluding to the concussion videos, the NFL, Bailes wrote, was "studying by darkroom analysis an important laboratory for head injury, the football field."

An aura of good feeling settled over the Mild Traumatic Brain Injury Committee. The NFL had revealed itself as a force for good. Yes, the commissioner had appointed a rheumatologist to oversee scientific research into brain injuries, and yes, most of the doctors had ties to the league, but the science was the science. The NFL had resources that no other researchers had at their disposal: a vast library of videotape, an army of willing research assistants, a closed pool of subjects (the players), and, of course, gobs of money. The concussion research community stood by and waited to see what the Mild Traumatic Brain Injury Committee would produce next.

The wait lasted only a month. In the next issue of *Neurosurgery,* the league published NFL Paper Number 3.

This one was different; that much was clear.

The much praised biomechanical studies were over. This time, Pellman et al. had taken the statistics from the NFL Mild Brain Injury Surveillance Study and used them to paint a panorama of concussion in professional football.

It was in many respects a very pretty picture. The NFL didn't have much of a concussion problem, the study concluded. The injury occurred at an extremely low rate—about one every three games—a rate strangely similar to the statistics spouted by Tagliabue and the NFL's PR department for a decade, long before the study had been put in place. When concussions did occur, 92 percent of all players returned to the field in less than seven days—that is, they never missed a game.

Pellman and his fellow authors interpreted this as an indication not that players were being rushed back on the field or hiding their injuries but that concussions were minor events whose symptoms went away quickly with few, if any, long-term consequences. "More than one-half of the players returned to play within 1 day, and symptoms resolved in a short time in the vast majority of cases," they wrote.

The response from the scientific community this time was guarded, even puzzled. Many researchers noted the obvious flaw that blew an enormous hole in the NFL's claims that concussion rates were low: the reluctance of players to report their injuries to coaches and team medical personnel.

Nine months later came yet another NFL study in *Neurosurgery*. This one dealt with *repeat* concussions. Numerous previous studies had shown that one concussion left the brain vulnerable to another concussion if the brain wasn't given time to heal. Guskiewicz had taken it a step further: Repeat concussions, he'd found, appeared to increase the probability of dementia later in life greatly. But that wasn't a problem in the NFL, according to Pellman et al. The league looked at how quickly players went back on the field and concluded that they were at no greater risk than if they had never been concussed at all. The logic was that because players returned to the field so quickly, they must have been okay or the medical staff wouldn't have cleared them. This flew in the face not only of previous research but of widely known realities on an NFL sideline. First, players often didn't report their injuries. Second, they hid their symptoms whenever they could. Third, NFL doctors often deferred to the wishes of coaches and players, just as Pellman had deferred to Parcells. As Steelers doctor Tony Yates had said: "Only a head coach can pull a player off." The entire NFL culture was incentivized toward risk.

For the first time, the NFL also took on the issue of football and brain damage, a growing concern among researchers. The league's scientific opinion? This wasn't a problem in the NFL either. Boxers got brain damage. Football players didn't. It was as simple as that. "This injury has not been observed in professional football," Pellman and his colleagues wrote.

That was technically true: No one had yet cut open the skull of a dead football player to examine his brain for signs of neurodegenerative disease. But after the findings of researchers such as Bailes, Jordan, and Guskiewicz, few doubted that day was coming. Pellman and his colleagues noted that the NFL's study was "admittedly not the best vehicle to search for evidence" of long-term brain damage in football players. Why? Because the league, in fact, hadn't studied the issue. But that didn't stop Pellman and his colleagues from offering an opinion. Yes, there were players who left the game with long-term symptoms after suffering repeated concussions. "They clearly did not have [brain damage] as that seen in boxers," Pellman et al. wrote.

The response to NFL Paper Number 4 was like a cannon going off in the tightly knit concussion research community. Before the paper was published, Cantu, as sports section editor at *Neurosurgery,* sent it around for peer review. Bailes and Guskiewicz were among the reviewers. The two researchers could hardly believe what they were reading. Not only was the NFL dumping on their research, but the league had taken a giant deductive leap by essentially declaring that pro football players were impervious to brain damage, as if they were superhuman. Bailes and Guskiewicz informed *Neurosurgery* that they were rejecting the paper's major findings. They weren't alone. Even Cantu, the editor, had misgivings about the NFL's conclusions and the paper's scientific underpinnings.

In most peer-reviewed journals, rejection by a preponderance of reviewers—particularly the assigning editor—is usually more than enough to prevent a paper from being published. Many scientists feel that's exactly the point of the peer-review process: to prevent science of questionable origin or credibility from making it into the literature— the engine of scientific progress. But *Neurosurgery,* at Apuzzo's direction, used a different process. Reviewers could raise their objections in a comments section appended to the paper, but the paper itself would stand.

Even in the stilted language of science, the comments on NFL Paper Number 4 were scathing. Guskiewicz called the NFL's conclusion that repeat concussions were of no real consequence "potentially dangerous." Bailes stated that the concussion rates calculated by the NFL do "not indicate a true ongoing incidence." In other words: wrong. Cantu wrote: "At first glance, the NFL's experience with single and repeat concussion (no difference) and management (more than 50% of players return to the same game, including 25% of those with loss of consciousness) seems to be at odds with virtually all published guidelines and consensus statements on managing concussion."

The fact that the comments were published provided no solace to the reviewers. "We were like, 'Who reads the commentaries?'" said Guskiewicz. "It's a published paper. It became the gospel."

NFL Paper Number 4 now stood as peer-reviewed science. The NFL's research arm could hardly have staked out a more aggressive position. The league could now claim authority over the questions that soon enough would most threaten its future. It was judge and jury. The NFL was just getting warmed up.

8

ONYEMALUKWUBE

In normal circumstances, Mike Webster's body wouldn't have ended up on the slab. In 2002, there were roughly 17,500 deaths in Allegheny County. Fewer than 1,000 were handled by the coroner's office, which intervenes only when death results from unknown or suspicious causes. Webster had died of a heart attack: Case closed. But for his fame, his very public descent into madness, and the unusual foresight of one man, his body would have been cremated after the funeral.

The man who stepped in was Joe Dominick, the chief deputy coroner. Dominick was a burly Pittsburgh native and die-hard Steelers fan. The son of a carpenter, he had been raised in the milieu of the steel town and then had become part of the new economy when Pittsburgh transitioned into health care. "I watched Mike Webster play football every Sunday, man!" he said. Dominick's 14-year-old son, Alexander, played center on his midget team, and Dominick had raised him on the legend of Iron Mike. Like every Steelers fan, Dominick had heard the stories about Webster's tortured post-football life. When he learned that he had died, Dominick decided to impound the body.

"The first thing I thought was this is a good way to put this issue to rest," he said. "My concern was if Mike died as a result of a drug overdose or he died as a result of injuries sustained that we were able to link to football, it changes the dynamics here. It's no longer a natural death."

The body arrived on a Saturday, and this too was a fortuitous key to the secret inside Mike Webster's head. At the time, the coroner's office had more than a half dozen people qualified to perform an autopsy. The one who happened to be working that day, Dominick thought, was the perfect man for the job. For one thing, Bennet Omalu was a neuropathologist, a specialist in diseases of the central nervous system, although neuropathology was just the latest medical specialty Omalu had picked up. A pathologist by training, he seemed to collect degrees and certificates with the ease of a man picking out produce at the supermarket. Technically, Omalu was a neuropathology *student,* having completed his studies in that discipline at the University of Pittsburgh Medical Center three months earlier. He hadn't yet passed the exams, but he was brimming with curiosity and fresh ideas. "I was intellectually hard," Omalu said. "I had just finished my training."

At this point, it would be hard to conjure up a more unlikely character to wander into the Webster saga than Bennet Omalu. Nigerian by birth, short and stocky, he spoke English with a mesmerizing singsong accent, the pitch of his voice often rising and falling in the same melodic sentence. When Omalu swore, which was often, he made *motherfucker* sound like poetry. His face was equally expressive, conveying a wide range of emotions. Omalu was the ultimate open book: He had no filter, and whatever he was thinking in that moment would be fully expressed, often with no apparent concern for how it might sound to the person on the receiving end. Even his priest, Carmen D'Amico, was sometimes startled by what came out of his mouth: "He'll say things, and it's just like, 'Oh! Bennet, don't say that!'" The more controversial material often focused on his beliefs, a fusion of Roman Catholicism and Igbo tribal mysticism that sometimes became entwined with his medical practice. Omalu believed that the body was a vessel for the soul and that even in death—*especially* in death—the soul had to be honored. He was convinced that spirits inhabited the coroner's office and that the nights belonged to them. Once, while working alone with a dozen or so refrigerated bodies, Omalu thought he saw a figure leaning against the door, staring at him. When he looked again, the figure vanished. He then spotted another shadowy form walking away. Omalu looked at his watch; it was 7:30 P.M. "I said to myself, 'Bennet, you're trespassing. There's usually nobody here at this time; just get the fuck out of here.'

And guess what? What did I do? I quickly stopped what I was doing. I shut off the light. And I got the fuck out of there." On another occasion, Omalu was driving around with a brain in the backseat of his car. The car got a flat tire, and that night the empty dishwasher in Omalu's apartment started without explanation. He attributed these events to the brain's former owner.

Omalu wore impeccably tailored suits and tooled around Pittsburgh in a silver Mercedes-Benz E-Class sedan. He ordered his custom-made shirts without pockets to avoid collecting lint. He later designed his own $6,000 cuff links, which he was planning to sell in Dubai. Omalu sometimes spoke of himself in the third person, especially when provoked to outrage or anger ("He did not even acknowledge there was anybody like Omalu!"). He could seem indiscreet to the point of obliviousness. Once, while conducting an interview for this book, Omalu pulled out his laptop on the patio of a tony restaurant called Wine & Roses and showed images of disemboweled corpses while all around him diners brunched on quiche and eggs Florentine. To people who annoyed him, Omalu would sometimes remark: "I may do your autopsy some day. Remember that."

Omalu's indiscretions and eccentricities sometimes got him written off as a kook. But once you stripped away the mysticism and theatrics, the strange ghost stories and confessions, what was left was an inordinately well-educated immigrant with a razor-sharp mind, soaring ambition, and a keenly honed sense of moral outrage. All this would prepare Omalu well for what was about to occur. Julian Bailes, the neurosurgeon who later would become Omalu's biggest champion, noted that it's often the least conventional people who shake up the world. "Most discoveries of great things are not done by shrinking violets," Bailes said. "They're done by people who want to be noticed or provocative, want to be recognized for discovering things."

Never was Omalu more of an outsider than when it came to pro football. It would have been almost impossible to locate a human being within a 200-mile radius of Pittsburgh who was more ignorant about the sport. Omalu hadn't the slightest clue how football worked. He hadn't watched a game, much less attended one. "I didn't know what a Super Bowl was," he later said. He found the city's fevered obsession with the Steelers baffling and pointless, "part of the American stupidity. You know, in Africa, we believe, yes, the white man is smart but the white man can be foolish." Omalu looked at the game through the lens of a Martian, if that Martian happened to practice neuropathology. Everything about it he found worrisome and dangerous. Why, for example, were the players sheathed in armor? He looked at the helmet and thought: "Why do they have to wear that big casing?"

Omalu was just 32, the junior pathologist on staff. Because of this, he often was scheduled to work weekends. "Guess who was on duty that Saturday?" said Omalu. "Omalu." As he prepared for work, he watched the news accounts of the sad demise of a local football hero, the stories about his Ritalin arrest, the rambling Hall of Fame speech, how Webster had slept in bus and train stations—a man broken mentally and physically. Omalu felt for the poor man. He wondered idly if he might have had some kind of brain disorder. Omalu recently had conducted an autopsy on a woman in her mid-forties. She had died after being beaten into a vegetative state by her husband. Omalu ran tests on the woman's brain and was struck when they revealed an unusual Alzheimer's-like pathology. He didn't do anything with his surprising finding, but the case was still fresh in his mind.

When Omalu arrived at the coroner's office and was told that Mike Webster was his first case, he didn't immediately make the connection.

"Who's Mike Webster?" he said.

"That's the greatest center who ever played," he was told.

"What's a center?" Omalu asked.

Then suddenly he got it: The body on the table belonged to the same broken man they had been talking about on TV.

"Fuck, man!" Omalu recalled thinking. "Thank you, Lord!"

Omalu looked down at Webster's battered corpse—the cracked feet, scarred knees, mangled fingers—and got to work. He always played music during autopsies; it helped calm him and break the monotony of carving up so many bodies. A hopeless romantic, he was going through a Teddy Pendergrass phase of love ballads. Omalu worked with such swiftness and precision that it could seem almost as if he were on autopilot. But with each incision, with each organ he removed, weighed, and sliced, he was looking for clues.

Omalu's belief in spirits extended to his autopsies. He believed he could communicate with the dead and that the dead in turn could tell him how they became dead. Omalu saw himself as their champion, a person who could give them voice. As he worked his way around Webster's body, he conducted an ongoing dialogue, trying to engage Webster's spirit: "Mike, in my heart, I think there's something wrong with you. I can't do this alone, you need to help me. Let's prove them wrong; let's go get them."

The autopsy lasted about an hour, building toward the moment Omalu had been waiting for: the removal of Webster's brain. To understand definitively what had gone wrong with Webster would require months of study. But when he was able to hold the brain in his hands, Omalu felt certain he would see some obvious signs of deterioration. Perhaps it would be shrunken and atrophied like a brain with Alzheimer's disease. But when Omalu removed Webster's brain, he was disappointed. It showed no outward signs of injury or disease. Omalu weighed it: 3½ pounds. It was perfectly normal.

Omalu shrugged.

Sorry, Mike. I couldn't help you after all.

But Omalu found himself thinking back to the case of the battered woman. And so, almost as an afterthought, he ordered his technician to preserve the brain for further study.

He recorded his intentions in the autopsy report: "The brain weighs 1575 grams and has been fixed in formalin for comprehensive neuropathologic examination. A report will be issued on a later date."

Omalu cleaned up and returned to his office. He called his boss, Allegheny County Coroner Cyril Wecht, a Pittsburgh legend. Wecht, among other things, had an uncanny ability to insinuate himself into every major crime and fatality of the day: O. J. Simpson, JonBenét Ramsey, even the Kennedy assassinations. He was an odd breed. People called Wecht a "celebrity pathologist."

"Sir, I've finished the autopsy," Omalu told Wecht. "I've saved the brain and, please, I'm asking for your permission to study it."

"What are you studying the brain for?" Wecht asked.

"Well, they said he had some neuropsychiatric problems. I want to see if he has some evidence of brain damage."

"Do whatever you want to do, Bennet," Wecht told him. "Just make sure you make me fucking famous."

Omalu's full name was Bennet Ifeakandu Onyemalukwube.

His middle name meant: "Life is the greatest gift of all." His parents chose it for a reason: Omalu was born in the middle of a bloody civil war. Nigeria's Igbo tribe, of which his family was part, had annexed the southeastern part of the country to form the state of Biafra. When Omalu's mother went into labor, his father lay in a hospital bed, having nearly been killed when the Nigerian Air Force bombed their village. The two-and-a-half-year civil war ended in 1970, when Biafra was absorbed back into Nigeria. The conflict claimed at least 1 million lives, many from starvation and disease. In the United States, the war would be remembered for its disturbing images of skeletal children. Omalu recalled almost nothing beyond his village receiving rations of dried fish from the World Health Organization.

Omalu's last name, fully realized, meant: "If you know, come forth and speak." This too was fitting, for the Igbo had a reputation for being the most outspoken of Nigeria's three main tribes (the others are the Hausa and the Yoruba). "I'm an Igbo man," said Omalu. "I think we are bold people. That thing that you tell me I can't do is what I want to do." The Igbo are predominantly Christian, with many practicing a mix of Roman Catholicism and native rituals. The Igbo have complicated views on death and burial. Most believe in reincarnation and the interaction between the living and the spirit world. The Igbo are also known as businessmen and traders. Omalu's father, John, was orphaned at three and raised as a house servant by a local parish catechist. When he finished high school, according to Omalu, his "colonial master" paid his father's way to England, where he studied mining engineering and shortened the family name to Omalu. He returned to Nigeria and spent most of his life as a civil servant, eventually retiring as director of the Federal Ministry of Mines and Power.

Omalu was the product of an arranged marriage, the sixth of seven children. He attended the finest schools in Enugu, a city of about half a million people in southeastern Nigeria, living comfortably in a gated community, protected by armed guards, going to school in chauffeur-driven cars. Math and English tutors came by the house twice a week to teach Omalu and his siblings. Bennet was quiet and introverted as a child. He excelled in class but had few friends and was something of a mama's boy. He was tidy and meticulous, voted the "neatest" kid in his class. By his late teens he yearned to break away, dreaming of becoming a jet-setting pilot.

"My childhood dream was to have a girlfriend in every major city of the world," he said. "I fly into Paris. I spend the night with my Paris girlfriend. I fly to Sydney, Australia. I spend the night with my Australian girlfriend. Then I fly to New York. . . ."

His parents nixed that idea and instead sent him to medical school at the University of Nigeria. After getting his degree, he worked four years as an emergency room physician and then, at 26, applied to a one-year visiting scholar program at the University of Washington's School of Public Health. After a year in Seattle, he went to New York to do his residency at Harlem Hospital.

Omalu had no idea what he wanted to do next. Then, one night, he was watching TV and stumbled upon a documentary about the assassination of JFK. There he saw Wecht, pathologist to the stars, making the case that Lee Harvey Oswald could not have acted alone. In his thirties, Wecht had challenged the conclusions of the Warren Commission before Congress; he called the lone gunman theory "an asinine, pseudoscientific sham." His conspiracy theories launched him into the public eye. Omalu was mesmerized. Wecht was a master of the medium: articulate, passionate, compelling—filled with the kinds of juicy details that later would turn forensic pathology into the basis for hit TV shows. Omalu fired off a letter to Wecht, asking if he could come to Pittsburgh for a one-month internship.

The one-month internship became a one-year fellowship, which was followed by two years studying neuropathology at UPMC, which was followed by two years studying for a master's degree in public health at the University of Pittsburgh, which was followed by three more years studying for an MBA at Carnegie Mellon.

Omalu continued to work in the coroner's office; his one-month internship had effectively turned into a full-time job working for Wecht, who seemed to see a younger version of himself in the flamboyant

Nigerian intellectual. "Bennet, you remind me of myself when I was your age," Wecht would tell him. Forensic pathology requires a bit of salesmanship and panache. As Dominick put it: "You gotta have giant balls to be a pathologist, especially a forensic pathologist." In addition to the scientific sleuthing, it requires an ability to get in front of a jury or a phalanx of TV cameras and come off as persuasive. Wecht taught Omalu how to dress and how to talk. The two men often had breakfast together. "He trained me," said Omalu. "He taught me things I wouldn't read in books. For Wecht, how much I respected him, whatever he wanted me to do I would have done."

Omalu went from wearing jeans to wearing $600 suits. Some people in the office referred to him as "Junior Wecht."

"We have a saying in Arabic: 'He knows where to look for the best piece of meat in the pink lamb,'" said Abdulrezak Shakir, a pathologist from Iraq who worked alongside Omalu and saw the relationship with Wecht develop. "What it means is if I go under this guy, that will be better for my future. I wish I have this capability. Not many people have it."

Omalu's close relationship with Wecht drew him into his boss's side business: private medical consultations. The famous forensic pathologist would get requests to perform autopsies and consultations from all over the country. It was a lucrative business. According to Omalu, Wecht charged as much as $10,000 for his services. He paid Omalu $300. "I would do all the work," Omalu said.

When Omalu asked for more money, Wecht told him he was getting "intangible benefits" from the work, Omalu said.

That turned out to be true. One of the private cases Omalu worked on for Wecht was the autopsy of the battered middle-aged woman. It was that case that led Omalu to save Mike Webster's brain.

O malu placed the 3½-pound brain in a bucket of formaldehyde and water. The process, called fixing, hardens the brain, which in its natural state is the consistency of a soft-boiled egg and can be difficult to cut. Webster's brain soaked for two weeks. Omalu then sliced four 2-millimeter sections, each about the width of a dime, from the primary lobes (frontal, parietal, occipital, and temporal). Each of the sections was placed in a small container.

Omalu then drove Webster's brain tissue over to UPMC in his Mercedes. He handed off the tissue to Jonette Werley, a lab technician with more than 20 years of experience working with autopsied brains. Werley bathed the containers in alcohol to flush out the water, then in xylene to flush out the alcohol. She used a microtome—essentially a tiny meat slicer—to shave the 2-millimeter sections into 200 slivers of brain tissue, which were transferred onto glass slides. She stained the tissue with an array of antibodies selected by Omalu, each designed to highlight abnormalities associated with specific types of neurodegenerative disease.

Then Omalu forgot about it. He had a busy life. His decision to save Webster's brain was only a hunch, and he had other things to do. In addition to his work at the coroner's office, he was studying for a master's degree in public health (with a specialization in epidemiology), making regular court appearances, and conducting private autopsies for Wecht. Whatever time he had left he devoted to his girlfriend, Prema Mutiso, a Kenyan whom he later married. The couple had met in church, where Omalu spent most of his time away from work.

Omalu belonged to St. Benedict the Moor, a church founded in 1889 shortly after the National Congress of Black Catholics met in Washington, D.C., to demand greater representation in the Roman Catholic Church. By the time Omalu entered St. Benedict more than a century later, it was almost entirely black, with 80 to 90 percent of the parishioners being African American. The rest were African immigrants—Nigerians, Kenyans, Liberians, Sudanese, Ugandans, Congolese—who had settled in Pittsburgh.

Away from work, where his naked ambition sometimes engendered resentment, Omalu was beloved. He directed his energies into helping others. The church was located in the Hill District, for decades the center of African American life in Pittsburgh, whose rich history includes the Underground Railroad, the glory years of Negro League baseball, and the country's most widely circulated black newspaper, the *Pittsburgh Courier*. The influx of Africans into St. Benedict the Moor had created tensions, but Omalu served as a bridge between cultures. "What was remarkable about Bennet, he was able to, in our church, kind of dispel or dissipate that thinking that some African Americans had about Africans as coming over here as privileged," said Father D'Amico.

Omalu quickly became one of the church's most prominent and valued members. It was obvious to others in the congregation that he had money—from his tailored suits, expensive car, and fine jewelry—but he didn't flaunt it. "He didn't tell anyone his background," said Father D'Amico. "None of us really knew what his work was. We knew he was from Nigeria, but you would never know from meeting him what a brilliant person this man was, the number of degrees he had, and the kind of groundbreaking work that he was doing." Father D'Amico frequently asked him to provide other members with money, clothes, whatever help was needed. Before Mass, rather than having members quietly pray, the priest encouraged them to openly express their gratitude to God about specific blessings in their lives. Omalu became one of the leaders of this "gathering rite," his melodic voice even more spellbinding in prayer.

"It was almost like preaching, you know?" said Father D'Amico. "I said to him, 'Bennet, you're one of the best prayers I know.' It would be so, so beautiful to listen to."

Omalu was so preoccupied by his nonstop life that when slides of Webster's brain came back from the neuropathology research lab, they sat on his desk for weeks. Eventually he brought them home to his apartment, where he kept a microscope on the dining room table. Omalu found that he often did his best work in the middle of the night. He would go to bed early, wake up around 2 A.M., and then work until he had to go to the office.

There, in his apartment, Omalu examined the Webster slides, trying to figure out what they meant. What he was seeing was not normal for a 50-year-old man. But what was it? He was so new to neuropathology that he didn't trust his own eyes. Omalu followed this routine for weeks, waking up at 2 A.M. and examining the slides closely, convinced that they were telling him something extraordinary but wanting to eliminate any doubt before he uttered a word to anyone and risked embarrassing himself.

What Omalu was seeing under the microscope was the buildup of tau, a protein that enables the brain's ability to function but can also strangle it. Without tau, neurons would collapse, cutting off the flow of nutrients and molecules to the cells. But sometimes, especially later in life, tau congeals into clumps called neurofibrillary tangles. These tangles slowly strangle the neurons from the inside. In neuropathology, they are one of the two defining markers in Alzheimer's disease. The other marker is the buildup of beta-amyloid plaques: hardened proteins that surround the cells and poison them.

The staining of the slides is what brings the tau to life; otherwise, you can't see it. Under a microscope, tau appears as tiny brown splotches interspersed among a pattern of normal cells represented as dots, as if someone had dripped dark brown paint on a flecked marble tile. As Omalu examined the slides of Webster's brain, he saw lots of brown splotches. He also saw signs of amyloid plaque, but the pattern didn't look like Alzheimer's as he had been trained to identify it. There was very little beta-amyloid, and it had taken on a slightly different form. Even stranger, the tangles of tau seemed to be distributed haphazardly throughout different parts of the brain, almost without rhyme or reason. In Alzheimer's disease, numerous tangles are present in the hippocampus (an area of the brain involved with memory) before they are seen in the cortex (the outer part of the brain that is critical to cognition). But in Webster's brain it was the opposite: Omalu saw many tangles in the cortex but none in the hippocampus. And besides, Webster was 50: He wouldn't be expected to *have* Alzheimer's disease.

Omalu knew from his training that head trauma could cause tau to form tangles. The presence of a neurodegenerative disease had been chronicled in boxers since 1928, when Harrison Martland, the chief medical examiner for Essex County, New Jersey, published a landmark paper in which he used the expression "punch-drunk" as a medical term. The phrase, he noted, was already part of the vernacular of fight aficionados, who also referred to the condition as "slug-nutty" and "cutting paper dolls." The condition was most pronounced among "poor boxers who take considerable head punishment, seeking only to land a knockout blow," Martland wrote. In severe cases, Punch-Drunk Syndrome was characterized by "marked mental deterioration" that sometimes forced ex-fighters to be sent off to the asylum. Martland estimated that nearly half of all veteran fighters had some form of the syndrome.

Martland has since been lionized for what is now seen as the seminal first study on head trauma and sport. But the reality was that his conclusions were not universally well received, especially by fight fans, who saw them as an unproven denunciation of the sport. It wasn't until 1973 that dementia pugilistica, as it came to be known, was accepted as irrefutable science. A British neuropathologist, J. A. N. "Nick" Corsellis, cut open the skulls of 15 former boxers who had died of natural causes. The autopsies showed cerebral atrophy in 14 of the 15 cases. Corsellis, who put together his own brain bank, the "Corsellis Collection," had shown for the first time that the repetitive head trauma associated with boxing led to the "destruction of cerebral tissue."

However, in Webster's brain, Omalu didn't see one of the hallmarks of dementia pugilistica: an opening in the septum pellucidum, the wall that separates the lateral ventricles in the brain. Plus, from what he had read, Webster didn't seem to have any of the symptoms of Parkinson's disease—slow gait, tremors, and slurred speech—that defined so many old boxers. Omalu's working theory was that Webster may have been suffering from something similar to Punch-Drunk Syndrome, the reason behind his irritability and erratic behavior. Even that would be groundbreaking as there had never been a diagnosed case of brain damage associated with football.

Omalu pressed on, still too reticent to come forward with his findings. He ordered additional stains of Webster's brain tissue, paying for them out of his own pocket. He stacked up every piece of literature he could find on concussions, dementia pugilistica, head trauma, and football on his dining room table and went through it paper by paper. He read Martland, Corsellis, and numerous others on boxing as well as the recent work related to football by researchers such as Jeff Barth, Kevin Guskiewicz, and Micky Collins. He came across papers published by something called the NFL's Mild Traumatic Brain Injury Committee, which was documenting the scientific effects of concussions in pro football.

Finally, in the spring of 2003, Omalu was ready to seek a second opinion. He turned to his mentor, Ronald Hamilton, the neuropathologist who had helped train him during his two-year fellowship at UPMC. Hamilton was renowned as the first neuropathologist to show that Lewy bodies—abnormal masses of protein that develop in nerve cells and are commonly associated with Parkinson's disease—were twice as common in Alzheimer's patients than previously had been known. He had a close and somewhat paternalistic relationship with Omalu. Hamilton viewed his protégé as bright and ambitious but also a bit flamboyant and given to hyperbole. In forensic pathology—particularly Cyril Wecht's brand of forensic pathology—certainty and authority under the bright lights are valued. Not so in neuropathology, in which scientific debates are more measured and deliberate than the fierce advocacy required in the courtroom. Omalu spoke in pronouncements, an attitude that earned him a warning from the head of the neuropathology program that he might not make it in academia if he kept it up. "That's everybody's experience with him. Bennet has a powerful personality, and at first it's just like, *What?*" said Hamilton. "And then you start listening to him more and more—if you have the patience. And you start to realize that he's really right on the mark. It's just that his personality really drives some people nuts."

For his part, Omalu viewed Hamilton not only as a great scientist but as his introduction into a broader world. With characteristic bluntness, he announced one day: "Hamilton is gay. And Hamilton was the one who changed my attitudes toward gay people. I was very homophobic. I thought that gay people are bad people. Hamilton was the first gay person I had met. He was such a good guy; he was so good to me. For the first time in my life I realized that I had been fed lies by the church, by my family and society, that this guy is a good guy with a heart, who cared for me."

One afternoon, Omalu dropped by Hamilton's office at Presbyterian University Hospital and asked if he would look at a special case he had been assigned at the coroner's office.

"What's the case?" Hamilton asked.

"I'm not going to tell you; just look at it," said Omalu.

This was a favorite game among pathologists. You wanted the second opinion to come with a clean slate, not even a suggestion of bias. Omalu's biggest fear was that Hamilton would look at the slides and tell him that what he was seeing was "no big deal," perhaps a variant of Alzheimer's that Hamilton had seen many times before.

Hamilton put a slide under the microscope. Then another. Then another.

This wasn't Alzheimer's disease, not even early Alzheimer's. The game was getting intriguing. Hamilton looked at more slides, keeping his thoughts to himself. This was something he had taught Omalu: Don't muse. Wait until you're ready to make a diagnosis.

"Is this patient a boxer?" he asked finally.

That made the most sense. He figured it would not be unheard of for the body of a boxer to show up at the coroner's office. Maybe he had died in the ring and this was a case of dementia pugilistica.

"No, this guy is not a boxer," Omalu said, a smile coming over his face. "He's an NFL football player. A Pittsburgh Steeler. This is Mike Webster."

Hamilton's jaw dropped, literally.

He knew immediately it was a new discovery, one with profound implications. In some ways Hamilton thought it was obvious; why hadn't it been discovered before? But he had no doubts. The pathology—the haphazardly formed tangles, the scarcity of beta-amyloid—proved it.

"I mean, if I had really felt any kind of hesitation about the diagnosis whatsoever, I would have said no," said Hamilton. "But it was so obvious, so logically beautiful. These are boxers with helmets on that are hitting each other all the time. And Bennet was feeling the same way. So we both came to the same conclusions without being unduly influenced. He didn't say, 'I want you to look at this case. It's a brand new case of something that's gonna be really big.' He just said, 'I want you to take a look at this case and tell me what you think.' "

Hamilton, half in jest, said they should call it "dementia footballistica."

It was a once-in-a-lifetime discovery.

"I knew this was a billion-dollar kind of finding when I saw it," he said.

Hamilton knew he needed more firepower. Omalu would be seen as a nobody—young, eccentric, and Nigerian. He wasn't even officially a neuropathologist. Hamilton didn't want to see him or the findings dismissed out of hand. Hamilton was known and respected, but he knew he needed to go higher.

He called up Steve DeKosky, chairman of UPMC's Department of

Neurology, director of the Alzheimer's Disease Research Center, and an internationally renowned expert in Alzheimer's and related neuro-degenerative diseases. Hamilton knew that if Steve DeKosky concurred that this was a new syndrome and was willing to stake his name and reputation on it, that would stamp it as serious science. DeKosky didn't have time for games, and so Hamilton called him up and told him the story: how Omalu had an interesting case involving a 50-year-old man, how there were tangles of tau throughout the cortex but not in the hip-pocampus and very little beta-amyloid. Hamilton said he originally thought it was a boxer, only to be told by Omalu it was a 17-year veteran of the National Football League.

"Really?" said DeKosky.

DeKosky immediately flashed back to a conversation a few years earlier at a meeting of the Alzheimer's Association. A colleague had recounted speaking with a representative from the NFL Hall of Fame who was concerned about the plight of retired players. Too many were showing up at the annual induction ceremony with serious memory problems. DeKosky had been fascinated. He wondered about the con-nection between all those hits and the problems that were surfacing in Canton. DeKosky did a little research and found that the president of the Hall of Fame Players Association was a lawyer named Ron Mix, a Hall of Famer himself who had played 11 seasons as an offensive tackle, mostly with the Chargers. DeKosky wrote Mix, introducing himself and laying out the design for a longitudinal study that would track Hall of Famers over time. DeKosky never heard back. He hadn't thought about it much until Hamilton's phone call.

Even then, DeKosky was skeptical. He knew Omalu and viewed him the way almost everyone else did: "a wickedly smart guy" but cocky and prone to exaggeration. Hamilton told Omalu to pay DeKosky a visit.

Omalu figured he might get 5 to 10 minutes. Omalu, after all, was little more than a student; DeKosky was the department chair.

Omalu handed over the slides. DeKosky examined them under a microscope.

DeKosky was stunned. Hamilton had been right.

"This will change everything," DeKosky thought to himself. "This will change everything forever."

He felt that Omalu had discovered "a new syndrome. Or, actually, the rediscovery of the physics that says if you beat the hell out of a human brain, this is one of the kinds of degenerative processes that occurs. I knew it was going to change everything, but quite frankly, it was so controversial that I just thought it's going to take a long time before this is accepted."

But that sealed it: If Steve DeKosky agreed, the only other step was to take it public by publishing the research in a medical journal.

That was no small task. It would be another year before the paper was completed. Omalu needed to expand on his research into head trauma and brain injury. DeKosky had to compile a clinical history of Webster by interviewing his family and creating a portrait of how his brain had short-circuited after his retirement. There was also the question of what to call the syndrome. Omalu thought it was critical that he come up with a name already in circulation so that if anyone attacked the findings, he could point to its earlier use in the medical literature. He also wanted something with a good acronym for lay people to remember and understand. In his review of the literature, Omalu saw references to chronic insanity, chronic encephalopathy, traumatic neurosis, traumatic encephalopathy, and occasionally chronic traumatic encephalopathy. Those terms, he thought, were all used generally, not to describe a specific disorder such as dementia pugilistica. He settled on chronic traumatic encephalopathy, or CTE. He thought it was easy to remember, and the language fit: *Chronic* meant long-term, *traumatic* referred to trauma, and *encephalopathy* was a damaged brain.

To a man, the researchers thought they were providing a service to the NFL. DeKosky resurrected his letter to the Hall of Fame, explaining Omalu's findings and expressing the researchers' interest in doing a long-term study.

Omalu titled the paper "Chronic Traumatic Encephalopathy in a National Football League Player." He was the lead author. Hamilton, as the senior neuropathologist, also was listed, along with two of Omalu's colleagues who contributed a section on genetics. In scientific literature, the position of final author is traditionally bestowed as a gesture of respect for the scientist who made the research possible, the "senior author." Omalu initially picked DeKosky, an obvious choice.

He had validated the findings, and his presence gave the paper stature. But Wecht, the coroner, was irate. He was Omalu's mentor, the man who had made him. Webster had been autopsied in his lab. In the end, "Wecht really didn't have anything to do with" the paper, said DeKosky, but he ceded the position, in part because he worried that Omalu might "be fired if he ticked the guy off too much."

The paper laid out the story of Mike Webster's brain, though it didn't name Webster directly, instead describing the subject as a "50-year-old professional football player who died approximately 12 years after retirement from the NFL." Any true football fan who read it—not that any would—could have deduced from the "premortem history" that it was Iron Mike. The authors described the subject as an offensive lineman who was drafted into the NFL at 22 and played 17 seasons, 245 games overall, including 177 consecutive games in a 10-year window and 19 playoff games. Telephone interviews with family members revealed a man suffering from depression, memory loss, and signs of Parkinson's disease.

The first sentence got right to the point: "We present the results of the autopsy of a retired professional football player that revealed neuropathological changes consistent with long-term repetitive concussive brain injury." Translation: This football player got brain damage from the daily pounding of his sport.

The authors described it as a "sentinel case that draws attention to a possibly more prevalent yet unrecognized disease." They recommended additional study to explore this "emergent professional sport hazard."

Omalu first submitted the paper to the prestigious *Journal of the American Medical Association (JAMA)*. Three days later the paper was rejected. Omalu sent out a disappointed e-mail to his collaborators and suggested that they try submitting the paper to a journal called *Neurosurgery*. Reviewing the literature, Omalu had come to believe that *Neurosurgery* was "the official journal of the NFL committee on MTBI," as he wrote to Hamilton and DeKosky.

Submitting the paper to *Neurosurgery* made sense, because Omalu, Hamilton, and DeKosky all believed the NFL would welcome their discovery. Linking football and brain damage wasn't great news, of course, but the league, they thought, would have to confront the implications that football causes brain damage and react accordingly, if only to protect the product.

They were scientists. In the years to come, they would all look back and reflect ruefully on how naive they had been.

"I thought they were gonna call me and embrace me and say, 'Motherfucker, you're such a hero,'" Omalu said. "I thought they were just gonna come and embrace me and give me a kiss on my cheek."

9

THE DISSENTERS

The NFL rolled out Paper Number 5 in *Neurosurgery* in November 2004. By then, the league's Mild Traumatic Brain Injury Committee had moved well beyond concussion videos and crash-test dummies. With each new study, the NFL was mounting a scientific argument. In essence, that argument amounted to this: Don't worry, be happy. Concussion rates in the NFL are extraordinarily low. The number of concussions is a meaningless predictor of future injuries; theoretically, one can have an infinite number of concussions and still be fine. There is no link between football and brain damage because football players don't get brain damage. To those on the other side of the argument, there was a kind of ham-fisted logic about this science of denial. NFL Commissioner Paul Tagliabue had created a research arm that exactly mirrored his skepticism about the so-called concussion crisis.

NFL Paper Number 5 dealt with the modest 8 percent of players who had missed at least one game because of a concussion, described by Pellman and his colleagues as "the most severely injured of the NFL concussion cases." Who were these players, and what happened to them? To start with, they were mostly quarterbacks, defensive backs, wide receivers, and kick returners "injured in high-speed, high-acceleration collisions." Although this observation ignored the violence taking place in the Pit, it made some sense. The players on the perimeter were being hit with extraordinary force. It stood to reason that the most spectacular collisions were likely to result in the most severe injuries. Quarterbacks, who were often exposed and used their brains more than any other players, were perhaps most sensitive to the effects of concussions, as seen in the cases of Aikman, Young, and many others. Not surprisingly, these players had more acute symptoms: lingering memory loss, disorientation, sensitivity to light, lethargy, and so on.

From there, Pellman and his colleagues went on to draw a number of conclusions that left some of the nation's leading concussion researchers shaking their heads in wonderment. One finding was that even these severely injured players recovered very quickly and, when they returned, were not at greater risk for further injury. This conclusion ran counter to nearly all previous research, which held that one concussion left you predisposed to another. But the NFL's logic was the same as in the previous studies: The fact that players went back on the field was an indication that they were fine; otherwise team medical personnel wouldn't have cleared them. It is perhaps germane to note again that nearly half of the NFL's concussion committee was made up of team doctors. Pellman, who was one, commended them for their superb diagnostic skills. He noted that only a small percentage of these players had been allowed back on the field the same day they suffered their injuries, an indication that "NFL team physicians and athletic trainers are extremely effective in screening out the most severely injured players on the sidelines within a short period of time after injury." NFL doctors might actually be "overly conservative and cautious," Pellman and his colleagues posited, in light of how quickly the players recovered and the risk of long-term brain damage—a risk that Pellman and his colleagues calculated was exactly zero:

"This 6-year study indicates that no NFL player experienced . . . cumulative chronic encephalopathy [brain damage] from repeat concussions. While the study did not follow players who left the NFL, the experience of the authors is that no NFL player has experienced these injuries."

The NFL hadn't actually *studied* retired players, but that didn't stop the league's experts from concluding that none had sustained long-term brain damage. Pellman and his colleagues would repeat this statement, in some form, over and over and over.

Except that not even the NFL believed it to be true.

The MTBI committee's controversial assertion that football didn't cause brain damage, which would create so much trouble for the NFL, was undermined by the league's quiet dealings with Webster and other injured veterans. At the same time the MTBI committee was publishing its research, Bob Fitzsimmons, Webster's lawyer, and a Baltimore attorney, Cy Smith, had taken the Bert Bell/Pete Rozelle NFL Player Retirement Plan to court to try to get more money for Pam Webster and the kids. The retirement board, of course, had determined in October 1999, while Webster was still alive, that he had had irreparable brain damage from repeat concussions related to his career. Webster's cognitive difficulties, the board wrote, were "the result of head injuries [he] suffered as a football player with the Pittsburgh Steelers and Kansas City Chiefs," a statement Fitzsimmons would describe as "the proverbial smoking gun." Now, over four years later, Pellman's committee—a separate entity but also under Tagliabue's control—was denying in a prestigious medical journal that such injuries were possible.

As Fitzsimmons and Smith pressed their lawsuit, they obtained confidential documents that showed, among other things, that it wasn't just Webster. The NFL retirement board had granted benefits to several other players with long-term brain damage. One was Gerry Sullivan, a contemporary and friend of Webster's who played guard and center for the Cleveland Browns from 1974 to 1981. Sullivan had the usual litany of NFL horror stories. On one occasion, during a punt return, he recalled plodding down the field to try to catch Oilers return man Billy "White Shoes" Johnson, which he equated with "trying to catch a rabbit." Sullivan was applauding himself for getting anywhere near White Shoes Johnson when another Oiler ear-holed him. "The first thing to hit the floor of the Astrodome was my head," Sullivan said. "Back then, they just had about a half inch of Grass-Tex—some kind of poly product that looked like grass—and then a slab of concrete. They peeled me off the field." The next thing Sullivan knew he was sitting on the bench, "vomiting on my jersey. Thankfully the Oilers had Earl Campbell. They had a really long sustained drive, and they were able to get me to where I was, you know, semi-functional." Sullivan sucked on an oxygen mask while a trainer asked him how many fingers he was holding up. "We were really kind of thin on the offensive line; that might have been the reason I went back in," he said.

When his career ended, Sullivan became chief operating officer of a company that leased automatic ice makers. A witty, self-deprecating man, he had been highly respected by his colleagues until, for no apparent reason, his moods began to vacillate between "manic hilarity and extreme anger," according to a letter the company's president wrote to the NFL retirement board. Sullivan threatened employees and punched holes in ice machines and walls. In 2005, based on the evaluations of several doctors, the retirement board awarded Sullivan "total and permanent" benefits related to his chronic brain injury.

Yet another document produced by the league showed that the same board had awarded permanent benefits to at least two other players whose doctors concluded they had gotten brain damage from playing pro football. The board redacted the names of those players, and the documents were stamped "confidential."

The longer the Webster lawsuit went on, the more evidence surfaced that the NFL had been handing out benefits to brain-damaged former players for years. To win, Fitzsimmons and Smith needed to prove that Webster's brain damage had left him disabled at the end of his career and not six years later, as the board had determined. This wasn't hard, because all five doctors who examined Webster—including Edward Westbrook, the neurologist brought in by the NFL—had attested to this. Still, the retirement board fought it all the way to the appellate court, which awarded $1.8 million in benefits and damages to Webster's family. The ruling stated flatly: "Mike Webster, the Hall of Fame center best known for anchoring the offensive line of the Pittsburgh Steelers professional football team from 1974 to 1988, developed brain damage as a result of the multiple head injuries he suffered as a player." The ruling noted caustically that the NFL retirement board had asked the court "to do two things: first, to disregard the testimony of the Board's own medical expert (in addition to *all* the others) . . . and, second, to hold that the *absence* of contemporaneous evidence is itself 'substantial evidence.'"

But perhaps most interesting about the 35-page ruling was a footnote on page 28 in which the court referred to "eight other cases of . . . disability due to brain damage." It was unclear who the players were—

the names were never disclosed—but the United States Court of Appeals for the Fourth Circuit clearly was aware of them. Of course, so was the NFL.

This was indeed a curious situation: two NFL committees, both involved in health matters, with completely opposite views on the subject of football and brain damage. The NFL retirement board, charged with dispensing disability benefits to deserving former players, was headed by the NFL commissioner (a nonvoting member served on his behalf) and was made up of three owners' and three players' reps. That board, which consulted with neurological experts around the country to render its decisions, had accepted long-term brain damage as a fact of NFL life for some players. Pellman's Mild Traumatic Brain Injury Committee, the NFL's research arm, had been formed by the same commissioner and reported directly to him. That committee stated unequivocally and repeatedly that NFL players didn't get brain damage. The MTBI committee went so far as to declare: "Professional football players do not sustain frequent repetitive blows to the brain on a regular basis."

At first, opposition to the MTBI committee was limited to a few scientists who tried to prevent this assertion and its dubious corollaries from appearing in the pages of *Neurosurgery*. They were, not coincidentally, the same neuroscientists whose research had warned that the league was facing a catastrophic health crisis.

One was Kevin Guskiewicz, the earnest young researcher studying retired NFL players at the University of North Carolina. Guskiewicz was respected as a thorough researcher and an honest broker even when concussion experts began to split into warring factions over the NFL. But Guskiewicz could hardly believe what was happening to him. From his earliest memories—riding a bike to watch the Steelers from a hill in Latrobe to taping Merril Hoge's ankles as an apprentice Steelers trainer—football was in Guskiewicz's blood. His three kids were playing Pop Warner. Guskiewicz had hoped his research on depression and dementia would help make the sport he loved safer. Instead, he found himself under attack. When Guskiewicz published his seminal depression study, which showed that players who sustained at least three concussions were far more likely to be clinically depressed later in life, Hank Feuer, the Colts' neurosurgeon and a member of the MTBI committee, dismissed it as "virtually worthless." The fact that it was merely a survey—the most comprehensive one of its kind in the history of the NFL—made it worthless, according to the league's doctors. "They didn't have information from the doctors confirming it," Ira Casson, the MTBI committee's neurologist, told the *New York Times*. "They didn't have tests, they didn't have examinations. They didn't have anything. They just kind of took people's words for it." (A decade later, Feuer would still describe Guskiewicz's study as "the worst type of research that you can publish.")

The crux of the NFL's argument was that players were more likely to come clean with their coaches and team doctors than with independent researchers. But the reverse, in fact, was true. Young and Hoge, after all, had pleaded with their coaches and team doctors to let them back on the field—even after the concussions that destroyed their careers. Hoge was so desperate that even after he was forced to retire, he called Joe Maroon at 2 A.M. to insist he could play. Numerous studies had shown that when athletes were asked directly by independent researchers, the incidence of concussions skyrocketed. Annual concussion rates in college were over 70 percent, and rates in the Canadian Football League were nearly 50 percent. Were NFL players' brains really that different?

Guskiewicz thought that what was going on was obvious: The NFL wasn't promulgating science; it was trying to protect its business. Later, when he was asked to deliver the commencement address at his alma mater, West Chester University, Guskiewicz described his stunning realization that rather than helping his favorite sport, his research had been perceived as "incriminating toward arguably one of the most popular and profitable industries in America." His findings were "the last thing the NFL wanted to hear," Guskiewicz told the graduates. The league went into "damage control mode," using its own scientists to try to "put out the fire" and discredit him. He dismissed the work of the NFL's committee as "industry-funded research at its best."

As the papers continued to roll out in *Neurosurgery*, Guskiewicz, who was one of the peer reviewers, savaged them. "Very suspect," he called the latest. But seemingly there was no stopping them. Bob Cantu, the Boston neurosurgeon who was serving as sports section editor of the journal, said he was equally opposed to the papers and tried to get them killed. Like Guskiewicz, he had come to believe that the NFL's research arm had set itself up as protector of the league. "The feelings that we had from the articles were that the authors were being self-serving to the NFL and that's what the NFL wanted," Cantu said, "and that they would ingratiate themselves to the NFL if they essentially produced data that would make the NFL look good and, in the process, maybe solidify their positions with the NFL."

"The flaws were too great," Cantu said. "We didn't think they should be published."

But when Cantu went to Mike Apuzzo—the editor in chief and neurological consultant to the New York Giants—the response was always the same, he said. Apuzzo told him: "This is important information that readership wants to hear. I will give you and the other reviewers the opportunity at the end of the paper in the comments section to comment about the weaknesses of the paper and your negative feelings about it." But Cantu, like Guskiewicz, felt that was inadequate. "Nobody really seriously reads the comments at the end of the paper," he said. "And the person, no matter how bad the comments are, can simply say, 'Well, I got cited in a peer-reviewed journal that's very respected and prestigious.' The damage is done."

Cantu was 74 and had authored more than 350 scientific publications over 45 years by the time he was interviewed for this book. He said he had never seen another "instance where essentially the editor stepped in and went against what the reviewers' comments were."

Cantu felt Apuzzo's close relationship with Tagliabue and the NFL had influenced his judgment. "I know that Michael discussed meeting with the commissioner and how he enjoyed it, and I think that's totally appropriate," Cantu said. "But at the time he first mentioned that, it didn't dawn on me just how enamored with the whole thing maybe he was. Because as time would roll on there was one article after another of questionable accuracy."

But Cantu felt that wasn't all of what was going on. "I don't want to give the impression that [Apuzzo] was cherry-picking what went into the journal based on just his view of the NFL," he said. "I think he was letting NFL things in because he thought they were hot. They sizzled and would sell the journal, and the journal would have a greater readership, a greater interest and drive because of it."

Under Apuzzo's editorial retrofit, *Neurosurgery* had effectively doubled in size. Total submissions rose 285 percent. Ad revenue increased dramatically. In his USC bio, Apuzzo wrote that reader penetration under his leadership "increased astronomically, from 6,000 in 1992 to 13 million in 2005," because the journal was bundled on a data platform with elite publications such as *JAMA* and the *New England Journal of Medicine*. Asked if he thought the NFL papers contributed to *Neurosurgery*'s success, Cantu replied: "I'm probably not in a position to know with certainty, but if I were to take a calculated guess, *immensely*." One reviewer described the NFL papers as "an irresistible read."

A USC spokeswoman initially offered to set up an interview with Apuzzo for this book, which, she wrote, "sounds like a great project." But when she contacted him, Apuzzo declined and said he did not believe his participation would "benefit him or the university," the spokeswoman wrote. Apuzzo did not respond to numerous e-mails and calls.

Cantu valued his position at Apuzzo's prestigious publication. For that reason, he said, he never threatened to resign when Apuzzo published the NFL's research over his objections. "I didn't go to the mat with the editor, in all honesty, because I felt that he would just strip me of being section editor," he said. "I liked being in that role, and I didn't really want to lose it. And I believed I would have lost it if I simply said, 'It's me or these articles.'"

"Oh, for God . . . Jesus," responded one former member of the MTBI committee when Cantu's remarks were read to him. "I mean, think about what you're saying here. He's the *section editor*. He's putting his name out there as a section editor. Right? And he's telling me that the general editor told him, 'You have to do this,' and he didn't make a ruckus? He didn't walk away? He's the man of great ethics, the man on the white horse?"

Others also felt Cantu was trying to have it both ways, trying to disavow science that he in fact commissioned and presided over. Another former MTBI member, interviewed during the 2012 election cycle, called Cantu "the Mitt Romney of doctors. You can never pin the guy down. He flaps in the wind."

But there were distinct sides now to the NFL's concussion crisis. On one side was the National Football League, promoting the worldview that everything was fine. On the other side were neuroscientists such as Guskiewicz and Cantu and Bailes. That side was small but growing. Collectively, the researchers who stood up to the NFL became known as the Dissenters.

Up to that point, Mark Lovell had managed to steer clear of the controversy building around the NFL's committee. Armed with Tagliabue's letter of endorsement, he continued to travel the country, selling teams on his concussion test. By the mid-2000s, most had embraced it in some fashion. Lovell was the director of what had become known as the NFL Neuropsychology Program, a lofty title that he never bothered putting on business cards. He considered his presence on the MTBI committee a sideline, a perk on top of his main job running the sports concussion program at the University of Pittsburgh Medical Center. One of Lovell's favorite spots in the world was a retreat in Pennsylvania's Amish country where he'd often get away to write and reflect. The hideaway fit how he perceived himself: low key, with an innate desire to lie low.

That was all about to end.

Now Pellman and the MTBI committee wanted to gather the results of the NFL Neuropsychology Program and see what they said about the ability of pro football players to withstand concussions. Pellman, of course, had no background or expertise in neuropsychological testing. No matter. As head of the NFL's concussion committee, he again appointed himself lead author on the study. At this point, the conclusions of NFL Paper Number 6 would have surprised no one. It was all part of the same narrative. Pellman and his colleagues wrote that the results "corroborated" the league's earlier findings that NFL players "demonstrated a rapid recovery." NFL players also "did not demonstrate evidence of neurocognitive decline after multiple concussions," they wrote. The findings, finally, "support the authors' previous work, which indicated that there was no evidence of worsening injury or chronic cumulative effects of multiple MTBIs in NFL players." The response to the paper also was predictable: Guskiewicz, Cantu, and Bailes recommended killing it. Without that option, they spiced their appended comments with words like "unfortunate," "preliminary," and "premature."

But the criticism was about to take a more serious turn. Lovell, who signed off on the paper as a coauthor, would take a major hit. The league had gathered the data for the study from the network of neuropsychologists Lovell had spent years assembling. One was Bill Barr, the team neuropsychologist for the New York Jets. Barr by then had moved his practice to NYU Medical Center, where he was chief neuropsychologist at the Comprehensive Epilepsy Center. Barr viewed the Jets gig as something of a lark and a career builder. Each Sunday, he watched the game on TV. Whenever his wife tried to pry him off the couch, he'd respond: "Hey, I'm working here!" Most of the "psycho neurologists" around the country knew one another, so it wasn't surprising that Lovell also was acquainted with Barr. Their history wasn't totally amicable. In the 1990s, when Micky Collins was an up-and-coming researcher, Lovell and Barr both had recruited him as a research fellow. Collins had picked Lovell, to whom he remained devoted. "I never thought Bill forgave me or Micky for that," Lovell said. But Lovell and Barr had stayed on good terms, even publishing together. In 2004, the same year the NFL's treatise on neuropsychology came out, Lovell and Barr coauthored a chapter on American football in a textbook on brain injury in sports.

Barr worked as the Jets' neuropsychologist for nearly 10 years, at which point he ran afoul of Pellman and the NFL's concussion committee. On December 11, 2004, he appeared at a sports concussion conference at Madison Square Garden. He spoke about his own research, including his role in a two-part series he had recently coauthored with Guskiewicz and others in *JAMA*. One of the major findings was that one concussion increased the risk of another—the exact finding the NFL was trying to refute. Barr told the audience he was preparing another study on the optimal time to administer neuropsychological testing, which he concluded was 5 to 10 days after an injury. That, too, diverged from NFL policy, which under Pellman and Lovell was 24 to 48 hours.

A week later, Barr said he got a call from Pellman, who had not attended the conference. Pellman, as the NFL's medical director and

Jets doctor, oversaw Barr's work as the neuropsychologist for the team. Pellman said he heard that Barr had been "bad-mouthing" the NFL, according to Barr.

Barr told Pellman that he had merely described his own research. Pellman, according to Barr, responded by advising him that he'd have to clear all future concussion research through him, regardless of whether it was related to the NFL. Barr refused. He told Pellman that would compromise his integrity as a scientist and a faculty member at NYU.

"Then your time with the Jets is over," Pellman informed him, according to Barr. Pellman later would vehemently deny Barr's account to Peter Keating of ESPN, calling it "ridiculous."

Barr was still fuming a few months later when he heard that the NFL was about to release a paper based on data from the NFL neuropsychology program. His first thought was: "Are you kidding me? You're doing *what*? I haven't heard anybody talking about this data for years and now you're almost done with the paper?" Barr had accumulated hundreds of baseline tests while working for the Jets. He said neither Pellman nor Lovell asked him for the data. Barr said he contacted Pellman, who told him he excluded the Jets because of Pellman's role as team doctor. That made no sense, Barr protested, telling Pellman that leaving out the data would bias the study. "He kind of blew me off," said Barr. "He was like, 'No, no, no, I don't need the data. We're okay, we're gonna do it.'" Pellman later denied this conversation to ESPN's Keating, the first journalist to explore the NFL's adventures in concussion research. "Bill Barr was a consultant for the Jets who tested individual players to help us make decisions," Pellman told Keating. "I did not discuss the committee's research with him."

When Paper Number 6 came out, Barr thought something stank, particularly the statistics that Pellman and Lovell used to support the conclusion that everything was right with the NFL's world. The study reported that only 22 percent of concussed players—143 athletes—had submitted to neuropsychological testing. For a five-year study, that was an extremely low number. Why? Part of it was that the tests were voluntary; not all players were participating. But Barr knew that his own data for several years weren't included. Then, three months later, the *New York Times* published its report that Pellman had attended medical school in Guadalajara, not New York, as he had told Congress. The *Times* hadn't connected Paper Number 6 and the credentials flap, but when Barr saw the story, he decided to dig deeper into the mystery of what had happened to his data. His central question was whether Pellman, with Lovell's assistance, was embroidering the NFL's science in the same way he had embroidered his résumé.

Barr began to contact other neuropsychologists from Lovell's network to see if he could find out whether their data had been excluded from the study.

On March 30, 2005, the day the *Times* published the Pellman piece, Barr wrote an e-mail to Rick Naugle, the neuropsychologist for the Cleveland Browns. "You might have seen this story in today's news," Barr began, attaching the link. He continued: "I have actually had some questions about the NFL study on neuropsychological testing that was published by Pellman and his colleagues last year in *Neurosurgery*. The number of reported baselines and injured players doesn't match up with what I would expect for the five year study period from 1996 to 2001."

Naugle replied that he sent Lovell data on "2 or 3 players." He added: "I have a few hundred baselines. Mark does not have those data."

Barr also wrote to Chris Randolph, a neuropsychologist for the Chicago Bears. Randolph said he had collected baselines for 287 players. No one from the committee had requested his data.

He wrote to John Woodard, the neuropsychologist for the Atlanta Falcons. Woodard had collected baseline tests for 173 players. He too was never asked for his data.

By the time Barr was done canvassing neuropsychologists from Lovell's network, he calculated that at least 850 baseline tests—and perhaps thousands more—had been excluded from the NFL's results. Barr was concerned that Pellman and Lovell had cherry-picked the data to reinforce the league's argument that the impact of concussions was negligible and players recovered quickly. Barr said Pellman called him one year before the paper came out looking for information on three former Jets: Kyle Brady, Fred Baxter, and Keyshawn Johnson. None had been with the team in years, but they had come back quickly from their concussions, and that fit the profile of the players who were reported on in the NFL's study. "I think they had an agenda on what they wanted to find in the research before they conducted the research," said Barr. Pell-man later told Keating this was false: "Team doctors talk to specialists and ask them for results all the time," he said. "It's part of their job."

Lovell denied that data were purposely excluded. He said that Nau-gle and Randolph had refused to provide data and that a "miscommu-nication" prevented Woodard from providing his. Barr, he said, later privately told the NFL that "we had all of his data on multiple occa-sions. So do we have it or do we not? I don't know. He's the only one who knows the answer to that." Lovell believed that Barr had launched his attack to get back at Pellman for firing him and that Lovell wound up as collateral damage.

Lovell's role in the controversy was bewildering. His pioneering research had helped expose the NFL's concussion problem. Leigh Stein-berg had featured him in his seminars to convince the NFL the world was round. He had taken the witness stand to accuse the Chicago Bears of ruining Merril Hoge's career by failing to take his concussion seri-ously. Yet now many of his fellow neuroscientists suspected that Lovell was involved in the NFL's effort to cover up its concussion problem.

Lovell denied that was the case. "I don't think the NFL ever wanted to have a concussion problem. I don't think anybody ever does," he said. "But, I mean, the suggestion that there was some kind of grand con-spiracy, I don't think, honestly, knowing the people on the committee—that never happened. Or none of us would have been involved with it."

Yet much of what the NFL believed about concussions was there in black and white, with Lovell's name attached to it. Beyond the allega-tions about the missing data, Lovell had put his name to research that concluded, among other things, that (1) concussions are minor injuries and nearly all NFL players recover quickly and completely and (2) pro football doesn't cause brain damage, *ever*. Oddly, Paper Number 6 even suggested that neuropsychological testing was at best of limited use in assessing football-related concussions and at worst useless. Was Lovell really bashing his own profession, the research that had come to define him? Even his partner Maroon seemed taken aback, noting in his review that "the authors seem to suggest that the role of neuropsychological testing is 'minor.' Such a strong statement does not seem to be justified."

Lovell, backpedaling years later, argued that he was a victim of the inner workings of Pellman's committee, which he said produced the more inflammatory assertions without his knowledge. When the MTBI committee wrote up its findings, he said, it was a collaborative effort. Each author wrote a section related to his work. The sections were then compiled by the lead author, which in nearly all cases was Pellman. Lovell claimed that he contributed sections on the history of neuropsychology and football, the evolution of the NFL Neuropsychology Program, and the methodology of the study. His name was on the paper as a coauthor, but he claimed he didn't write the passages that produced the most controversy and, later, legal action.

Neuropsychology was of limited use in diagnosing concussions?

"Obviously I didn't write that," Lovell said.

Multiple concussions do not increase the risk of further injury?

"I didn't write that."

NFL players don't get brain damage?

"I didn't write that," Lovell said again. He acknowledged he could have protested to the committee to try to get the passages changed. But there was already a lot of back-and-forth between the authors, he said, and he didn't pay atttention to sections he didn't write. Lovell said the language was "actually softened a great deal."

"Could I have said, you know, 'God dammit!'" said Lovell. "Probably. Didn't."

One former committee member said it was essentially revisionist history for Lovell to try to disavow responsibility for a paper that, after all, had his name on it. Versions of the papers were indeed passed around among all the authors, the committee member said, and changes were made constantly upon request. "I wouldn't have any argument with someone saying, 'Gee, looking back on it, I wish I hadn't agreed to that,'" the former MTBI committee member said. "But to say, 'They put something in there that I didn't agree with'? Everyone had the opportunity to look at everything and had the chance to say, 'I don't agree with that, and I don't want to be an author on it, let's change it.' And it probably would have been changed."

It was an eventful four months for Elliot Pellman and his MTBI committee. Pellman had fired a neuroscientist who disagreed with the NFL's concussion policies; his own credentials had been exposed as inaccurate and inflated; and he had published a controversial study that was based on questionable data.

In April 2005, Barr sent a letter to his dean at NYU "to clarify the nature of [the] professional relationship I have had with Dr. Pellman since the early 1990s and to review the series of events that ultimately led to the abrupt termination of this relationship."

He described how Pellman, after Barr refused to clear all research through the NFL, not only fired him but "threatened me with a lawsuit" if Barr ever tried to publish research related to his work with the Jets.

"The idea that someone would attempt to restrict my academic activity and prevent the communication of my research findings, as a precondition for continued employment, was most disturbing," Barr wrote. "I would appreciate it if you could keep this letter on file in the event that I have any further encounters with Dr. Pellman."

Barr would have future encounters with the NFL; that was certain.

Despite the work of the Dissenters, the NFL's concussion research machine was unstoppable. During one prolific stretch in 2004 and 2005, the league churned out five papers in as many months; the first four listed Pellman as lead author. The committee ultimately pumped out 16 papers on concussions, an extraordinary number for a single group of researchers publishing in one journal. Cantu, who commissioned the first paper for *Neurosurgery,* thought that it was overkill, that one or two studies would have sufficed: "For the life of me, to this day I don't understand how it turned into that many papers." But Apuzzo insisted on taking them all, he said. In February 2005, Maroon, one of the reviewers, wrote: "This article represents the seventh and final contribution by the NFL Committee on MTBI on the various aspects of head injury in professional football." Yet a month later, without explanation, there it was: Part 8! Some concussion researchers began to mock *Neurosurgery* as the "Official Medical Journal of the National Football League" or the "Journal of No NFL Concussions." No sooner would Guskiewicz review one paper than another would arrive in his in-box. Guskiewicz, of course, was rejecting the work. But oddly, Apuzzo would still call him, asking where his review was so that the paper could be published. "He'd say, 'You know, I'd really like to get this paper out, because we're delayed and we're waiting on your commentary,'" said Guskiewicz. "And I'm like, 'Mike, you just sent it to me 10 days ago. You know, I've got a life.'"

"We all talked about this often: Who was driving this?" said Guskiewicz. "Who was pushing him? We never knew. It was just odd. And very questionable."

Whether it was Pellman who actually wrote the papers—9 out of 16 would list him as the lead author—also was unclear. Two former committee members insisted that none of the studies was ghostwritten, a not uncommon practice in the research community, but the idea that a rheumatologist with no experience in neuroscience could write that many papers on the subject struck many as unlikely. Pellman, after all, had never authored a paper on the topic before taking over as head of the MTBI committee, according to a search of PubMed, a database of scientific literature. Some seasoned researchers felt lucky to publish a paper or two a year. But the reassuring treatises kept coming. Pellman and the NFL now were saying that concussions were so minor that players were generally safe to return to the same game even if they had lost consciousness. Not only that, although the league had studied only NFL players, they wrote, "It might be safe for college/high school football players to be cleared to return to play on the same day as their injury." The authors suggested that "rather than blindly adhering to arbitrary, rigid guidelines, physicians keep an open mind to the possibility that the present analysis of professional football players may have relevance to college and high school players."

After a while, the Dissenters threw in the towel. If any assertion could be published unchallenged as peer-reviewed science in *Neurosurgery*, they reasoned, what was the point of peer reviewing the studies? "Quite frankly, people like Kevin and myself just quit reviewing these papers," said Cantu. "We just said, 'These are poorly written, you can't use this data to make the claims they're making, and we won't even bother to write comments anymore because it's just so flawed and so bad. We won't be a part of this.'"

"We were like, 'I'm outta here,'" said Guskiewicz. When Apuzzo sent him papers to review, Guskiewicz refused. Soon Apuzzo stopped asking. Cantu said Apuzzo's solution to the peer review uprising was not to shut down the NFL's research but to find other reviewers who were willing to chime in.

Lovell continued to argue that he was on the outside of this unruly debate and that except for the three papers that had his name on them, he barely paid attention to the literature the MTBI committee was churning out every month. "I probably only read five of the papers," Lovell said. "Other than that I had absolutely nothing to do with the papers." That argument avoided one important fact: As a body of work, the papers were an expression of NFL dogma. Over and over, they repeated the same essential themes, making it nearly impossible to disassociate oneself from the overall message. Lovell was a coauthor on NFL Papers 3, 6, and 12; all asserted that NFL players didn't get brain damage from playing football and/or seemed to have superhuman qualities that limited their susceptibility to concussions. Paper Number 12 included the observation: "In our opinion, it is unlikely that athletes who rise to the level of the NFL are concussion prone."

"That's just kind of a stupid statement," Lovell said when it was read back to him. "What do you mean by 'concussion prone'? What does that mean? I didn't write it, but it's stupid either way."

"Well, your name's on it," it was pointed out.

"No, no, no," he said. "I mean, is my name on that sentence?"

The researchers associated with the NFL's work would all take a hit to their reputations, but Lovell in many ways had the farthest to fall. By the time he arrived on the committee, he had spent years helping athletes understand the seriousness of head trauma. He had helped bring concrete measurements to an injury that team trainers and doctors had only guessed at. Now Lovell found himself accused of carrying water for the NFL. Whether Lovell was a passive or an active participant in this stunning transformation was subject to interpretation. Lovell argued that he was merely swept up in the politics of the committee but played a very minor role. "I'm not a, you know, NFL company man," he said. "Do I regret some of the things that were said that had my name on it? Yes. Would I say them again? No." But others portrayed Lovell as a scientist caught in a web of conflicts that proved too lucrative, seductive, or both for him to disengage, if in fact he wanted to.

Lovell had come a long way. Back in 1993, when he and Maroon had come up with the idea to measure the Steelers' brain functions, Lovell had started with just pencil and paper and 27 reluctant subjects. He had since refined that test and developed it for the computer. With financial backing from UPMC, the test was now being mass-marketed under the brand name ImPACT. Many brain scientists didn't consider ImPACT much different from the alphabet soup of neuropsych tests that were out there, such as ANAM, which was used by the Army, and NEPSY, which was designed for kids. But ImPACT, through its association with the NFL, had come to be known as the football concussion test, an impression that Maroon, Lovell, and Collins constantly encouraged.

By the mid-2000s, ImPACT had taken off. When the company was founded, Lovell's overlapping roles didn't draw much attention. But as the torrent of NFL papers continued, many researchers saw an obvious conflict. Lovell was overseeing the NFL Neuropsychology Program at the same time he was pushing ImPACT to NFL teams. The league's research helped him promote his company. Paper Number 12 read almost like an advertisement: "Many studies using the ImPACT have indicated that it is reliable and valid." Lovell's financial stake was disclosed in small print at the end of the paper. Soon, nearly every NFL team was using ImPACT. So was most of the NHL, which adopted mandatory neuropsychological testing in 1997. As concerns about concussions grew, the association with the NFL proved a gold mine for the company's marketers, who turned ImPACT into a Kleenex-like synonym for concussion assessment. Micky Collins, Lovell's brash protégé, became an ambassador and indefatigable marketer, hitting the road to promote both the research and the test behind it. "I've given a thousand lectures, two thousand lectures," he said, emphasizing that his primary focus was on concussion awareness and management. "I mean, I've been spending time away from my family because of it, educating and really promoting the data." By the end of the decade, with the national hysteria over traumatic head injuries peaking, over 90 percent of the high school trainers who used computerized testing to assess concussions were using ImPACT, according to the company. The test, which sold in kits for $350 to $750, had been translated into 17 languages.

Collins, like Lovell, went to great lengths to try to distance himself from the NFL committee. Within minutes of sitting down for an interview in Pittsburgh, he declared: "First of all let's make this on the record: I wasn't involved in any of the NFL research, none. I just want to make sure you're clear on that. I'm not on any papers. I'm not on an NFL committee. I've never been on an NFL committee."

That was technically true. Collins had never had a direct role with the committee. But after a while it became hard, if not impossible, to figure out where the NFL ended and ImPACT began. A case in point was Pellman's pet project: the concussion-resistant superhelmet. After the early tests involving the crash-test dummies, the idea had been forgotten, buried under the avalanche of disputed research the NFL was cranking out. But the idea was very much alive. After the first biomechanical studies, Riddell, the NFL's official helmet maker, got to work designing the concussion-resistant helmet, which was based on specs that had come out of the NFL's research. For $500,000, Riddell even hired the Ottawa biomechanics firm, Biokinetics, that had performed the crash-test studies for the league.

Early on, the helmet project suffered a setback. In November 2000, Biokinetics sent a confidential report to Riddell warning that no football helmet—no matter how new and improved—could prevent concussions. That assessment confirmed what researchers such as Cantu and others had believed all along and essentially torpedoed Pellman's grand vision. The report, unearthed years later by *Frontline*'s Sabrina Shankman, went so far as to state that even if Riddell created a helmet that surpassed industry safety standards, there was still a 95 percent likelihood that a player would sustain a concussion from a strong enough blow. "No helmet can prevent a concussion. Full stop," Chris Withnall, the Biokinetics senior engineer who wrote the report, told Shankman.

Riddell built the helmet anyway, with Withnall's name on the patent. The company called it, ambitiously, the Revolution. Its principal defining features were flaps that extended over the lower jaw and additional protection around the ear hole. The NFL's video reconstructions had found that most concussions resulted from blows to the face mask, jaw, and side of the head. The Revolution's main selling point was that its design was based on research aimed at reducing concussions.

But how could Riddell make that claim after Biokinetics had privately warned that no helmet could prevent concussions? The answer came in summer 2002, a few months after the Revolution was released. Collins got together with Thad Ide, Riddell's senior vice president for research and development. "For the record, I don't know who approached whom," said Collins. Together, they came up with an idea for a research project involving ImPACT, Riddell, and the University of Pittsburgh Medical Center. "Both Thad and I reciprocally thought it was a really good idea to do a study," Collins said. "Riddell was coming out with this new helmet technology. I'm not an engineer. All I know is that we could create a methodology that could study it."

The idea was to compare high school football players, some wearing the Revolution and others wearing their old helmets. The study would use ImPACT to determine recovery time after a concussion was diagnosed. Riddell provided the helmets and paid $75,000 to UPMC to subsidize the salaries of Lovell and Collins while they worked on the study.

The potential for conflict was obvious. Lovell was a member of the NFL's influential concussion committee. He was on record as saying the creation of a concussion-resistant helmet was "a fantasy," yet he had taken money from the NFL's official helmet maker to produce a study examining whether its new helmet reduced concussions.

Collins, who led the study, suggested that he was motivated in part by the need to bring in research dollars to justify his position at UPMC. "I needed money to fund my salary," he said. "I was going to get my ass fired, you know? So I'm looking for any kind of funding to do this research. Any struggling academic is looking for that. So that was part of it." He said he understood that Riddell probably was shopping for research that would support its claim that the Revolution reduced concussions. "I'm not an idiot; I know Riddell wanted the results to look good, okay?" he said. "I mean, obviously. I understand that. But I am one of the leading experts in concussion; I've done as much research as anyone. I can be trusted as an academic to do a good research project."

Lovell, Maroon, and Riddell's Ide were listed as coauthors. Although this paper would be published in *Neurosurgery*, the study was not technically part of the NFL series.

Not surprisingly, the study concluded that wearing the Revolution helmet reduced the "relative risk" of concussion by 31 percent and the "absolute risk" by 2.3 percent. The change in helmet design that grew out of the NFL's research, Collins and his colleagues wrote, "appears to have beneficial effects in reducing the incidence of cerebral concussion in high school football players."

Riddell rushed out a press release:

RESEARCH SHOWS RIDDELL REVOLUTION FOOTBALL HELMET PROVIDES BETTER PROTECTION AGAINST CONCUSSIONS

The study, which will be published in February's edition of Neurosurgery, *found that athletes who wore the Riddell Revolution helmet were 31 percent less likely to suffer a concussion compared to athletes who wore traditional football helmets. The authors of this study estimate that the Revolution's patented technology could translate to 18,000 to 46,000 fewer concussions among the 1.5 million high school players who participate in football each season.*

Later, a UPMC spokeswoman provided e-mails that she said showed how the university had tried to prevent Riddell from misrepresenting and exploiting the research. The e-mails included Riddell's press release with proposed corrections. Riddell made a few changes, including striking the sentence, "There is now proof that one football helmet provides better protection against concussions." But most of the press release, including the banner headline, stood.

Cantu was still the section editor at *Neurosurgery* when the Riddell-funded Revolution study came across the transom. It seemed that his worst fears had been realized. Years earlier, Pellman had announced to the world that the NFL planned to create a concussion-resistant super-helmet. And now here was the result: a helmet that couldn't prevent concussions any more than any other helmet, created with the NFL's stamp of approval and peer-reviewed research that was funded and even coauthored by the company that planned to sell it to kids.

Cantu attached a blistering commentary to the study, suggesting that it failed to pass the "sniff test" and writing: "This article, in my opinion, suffers from a serious, if not fatal, methodological flaw."

That flaw was that the new Riddell helmets had been compared with random older models of indeterminate age.

Collins conceded that the varying ages of the helmets was "a major flaw" that skewed the results.

Years later, when asked about Cantu's criticism, Collins launched into a tirade that was very much of its time. "For him to criticize this study is a bunch of fucking bullshit," Collins said. "The flaws in this study were outlined. Everything was fair and balanced in that paper. And Cantu, he was part of the editorial staff! If he didn't want to publish it, why was it published? I have no problem with Bob wanting to reject the paper. There were serious flaws with the study, okay? I understand that. But when I picked up the paper for the first time and read the comments, I was like, 'Holy shit. Bob is ripping the shit out of me.' I'm like, 'Are you kidding me? Didn't pass the sniff test?' "

Micky Collins was a headstrong young researcher who once had admired Cantu as a giant in the field. "I was a young kid, and I respected the shit out of Bob Cantu," he said. But tests like ImPACT, which revealed an endless variety of concussions, had made Cantu's grading scales obsolete, Collins thought. "And guess what Bob did? Bob defended them until he looked like an idiot," said Collins. "Basically it was like an ugly death."

For his part, Cantu was still the King of Concussions. He had spent more time studying the injury than any researcher in the country. His voice carried a lot of weight.

But there was a larger issue beyond the debate over the Revolution helmet and the conflicts of interest and the competition between an older researcher and a younger researcher.

Collins, whether he acknowledged it or not, had aligned himself with the NFL, like Lovell, his mentor.

Cantu was a Dissenter.

That epic battle was building.

10

"THE LADY DOTH PROTEST TOO MUCH"

Not long after Omalu and Co. submitted their paper on Mike Webster to *Neurosurgery*, two things became clear. One was that the widely held view in some circles that *Neurosurgery* had been converted into a house organ of the NFL—the Official Journal of No NFL Concussions—was not entirely true. Apuzzo continued to rubber-stamp the NFL's research despite the mounting protests that it was flawed and self-serving. But now, in February 2005, he agreed to publish Omalu's paper as well. The publication of the Webster study set up competing narratives in the same medical journal: One said NFL players didn't get brain damage from football, and the other said they did. This development seemed to support Cantu's theory that Apuzzo more than anything was interested in topics that "sizzled" and boosted his readership. Whether Apuzzo had totally thought this through was unclear. The Webster paper would prove so hot that it ended up scorching almost everything it touched, especially the NFL.

That was the second thing: The big wet kiss Omalu had been expecting from the league would not be forthcoming. Instead, the NFL's doctors took out their scalpels and long knives. Omalu had gotten a hint of how controversial his study would be during the torturous review process, as he was asked to cleanse the paper of any suggestion that the

NFL's MTBI committee should have confronted the issue of long-term brain damage years earlier. An original version of the manuscript included a preamble detailing the history of the MTBI committee. It gave a summary of the retirements of Al Toon and Merril Hoge and stated that after Hoge's premature retirement, for the first time "NFL executives and medical personnel took notice of the possible neurodegenerative sequelae of professional football." None of that made the final draft.

The paper was published as a "Special Report" in the July 2005 issue of *Neurosurgery*. After a brief period of deceptive calm, Omalu received a call from a man who identified himself as Donald Marion, a member of *Neurosurgery*'s editorial board. Marion told Omalu that doctors from the NFL's MTBI committee were calling for his paper to be retracted.

"You know what that means, what that would mean to your career?" Marion said.

Omalu knew. He sat down and wept. He knew that in the world of scientific research, a demand for a retraction was the nuclear option. It generally was reserved for allegations of fraud, plagiarism, or cheating.

"But I haven't done anything wrong," Omalu pleaded.

Marion said that he had been asked by Apuzzo to mediate the dispute. He told Omalu that he would receive a copy of the NFL's demand and that he should confer with his coauthors to put together a response. That evening, Omalu e-mailed DeKosky and Hamilton, summarizing the conversation.

Omalu indicated that he had the impression Marion believed the demand was without merit and might have been directed by the league office. "Interestingly he thinks their paper is laughable and politically motivated," Omalu wrote to his colleagues. "He has asked me, however, to write up a very simple scientific explanation without becoming political. He said they all know that it was the NFL that may have instructed Dr. Pellman and his group to pen the commentary."

Despite Marion's reassurances, Omalu was terrified. As he prepared to read the NFL's letter at his Pittsburgh apartment, he poured himself a shot of Johnnie Walker Red and gulped it down. The letter was signed by the three leading members of the MTBI committee: Elliot Pellman, Ira Casson, and Dave Viano.

"We disagree with the assertion that Omalu et al.'s recent article actually reports a case of chronic traumatic encephalopathy in a National Football League (NFL) player," the letter began. "We base our opinion on two serious flaws in Omalu et al.'s article, namely a serious misinterpretation of their neuropathological findings in relation to the tetrad characteristics of chronic traumatic encephalopathy and a failure to provide an adequate clinical history.

"These statements are based on a complete misunderstanding of the relevant medical literature on chronic traumatic encephalopathy of boxers (dementia pugilistica). A review of the relevant medical literature, including that cited by Omalu et al., in the chronological order in which it was published demonstrates the flaws in Omalu et al.'s assertions."

As Omalu read on, he began to relax. "By the time I got to the third paragraph I smiled," he recalled. "I even laughed. I knew that Pellman, Casson, and Viano did not know the subject and that their letter was embarrassing and shameful. I said to myself, 'Isn't it un-American?' I respect this country, I'm a foreigner, but I came here to chase my dreams, that the three doctors who are the heads of the NFL Brain Injury Committee don't even know the basic science of brain damage. I became angry."

The letter was six pages long, longer even than the original paper, much of it a scientific overview of the history of CTE in boxers. Pellman, Casson, and Viano used phrases such as "complete misunderstanding," "completely wrong," and "completely lacking." They made two primary arguments: that Omalu et al. had a case that didn't meet the criteria for CTE and that there wasn't enough clinical evidence showing Webster was mentally impaired. They insisted Omalu's findings met only one of the four standards necessary to call this CTE even though Omalu and his colleagues had never claimed this was identical to what was found in boxers. The NFL doctors suggested that the clinical history on Webster was essentially useless because it had been limited to a few phone calls with family members. They pointed out that Webster had no history of concussions or any indications that he had ever left a game because of a blow to the head.

"Omalu et al. go on to state that 'there was no known history of brain trauma outside professional football.' In fact, there was no known history of brain trauma *inside* professional football," they wrote, suggesting that during his 17-year career in the NFL there was no evidence that Webster's brain was so much as jostled.

Casson, Pellman, and Viano suggested alternative theories for what might have happened to Webster's brain, theories that the league would continue to cite for years: alcohol, steroids, possible drug abuse. Ironically, the theories were reminiscent of those proposed by defenders of boxing after Martland, like Omalu a medical examiner, described Punch-Drunk Syndrome in boxers in 1928.

"We have demonstrated that Omalu et al.'s case does not meet the clinical or neuropathological criteria of chronic traumatic encephalopathy," they wrote. "We, therefore, urge the authors to retract their paper or sufficiently revise it and its title after more detailed investigation of this case."

It was signed:

IRA R. CASSON
ELLIOT J. PELLMAN
DAVID C. VIANO
New York, New York

The doctors didn't identify their connection to the NFL, as if they were merely independent physicians who had banded together in their outrage.

Omalu wondered about their backgrounds. He did some quick research and had to laugh: Pellman, the committee chairman and now one of Omalu's main critics, was a rheumatologist. The head of the NFL's brain committee was an arthritis expert?

When he finished, Omalu e-mailed Hamilton and DeKosky. "To say the least, it is a laughable commentary," he wrote.

Hamilton wasn't at all amused. "I read over their critique and I do not think it is laughable. . . . It is very serious indeed," he responded. Hamilton was more confident than ever about the validity of their research; the criticism was baseless, he felt. What concerned him was the NFL's attempt to erase their work from the record. He thought it was the work of a self-interested corporation trying to censor his independent research. "I like to think of them as being honorable scientists who are simply stating an alternative hypothesis, but the fact that they wanted me to trash the paper and say that it was bad science, that cued me in to that they were kind of, oh, setting up walls," he said. "Trying to set up a barrier. To shut it off. To try to make sure that everybody knew that these Hamilton and DeKosky, Wecht, Omalu characters were just insane."

Over the next couple of weeks, the men exchanged e-mails discussing the main points of their defense: Webster's brain had widespread neurofibrillary tangles in several areas that "for a 50-year-old, are very very 'unnatural'"; that although Webster suffered other ailments, none was consistent with the presence of these tangles; that the boxing papers the NFL cited—in particular Corsellis's seminal research—also lacked detailed clinical histories; that the pattern of the tangles—throughout the cortex but nowhere in the hippocampus—is significant in that it signaled neurodegenerative disease inconsistent with Alzheimer's or other known disorders.

Hamilton wrote in one e-mail to his colleagues: "Without any clinical history, most neuropathologists familiar with dementing disorders would ask: did this patient engage in boxing? So when told that he played football, I think most would say, 'Yeah, OK.'"

Of course, there were no neuropathologists on the NFL committee.

Omalu, Hamilton, and DeKosky also dug further into the history of Webster's life after football. The NFL had blistered them for the limited clinical information documenting his mental illness, describing it as "completely lacking." Omalu and his colleagues discovered that just a few months earlier a federal judge had awarded Webster's family $1.8 million in a lawsuit against the NFL's disability board, which had compiled testimony from five doctors who concluded that Webster had brain damage.

"Their comments about us not having the detailed clinical history is stunning in its hypocrisy," DeKosky wrote in an e-mail to Hamilton.

As the group prepared its response to the NFL, Omalu knew he had another secret weapon that he thought would blow the NFL's protestations out of the water: He had discovered another case of CTE in a dead football player.

- - -

On June 7, 2005, Terry Long killed himself by drinking antifreeze. Long had played eight seasons in the NFL for the Pittsburgh Steelers, lining up alongside Mike Webster for five of those seasons in the mid-1980s. In some ways, Long was like Webster: an undersized hulk who bulked up through weight training and steroids. Long was 5-feet-11, at least 280 pounds, "half-crazy," as one former Steelers employee described him. At the same time, Long had a bighearted personality that drew him close with the Rooney family and his coach, Chuck Noll, whom Long viewed as a father figure.

After graduating from high school, Long enlisted in the military and served two years with the Special Forces Unit of the Army's 82nd Airborne Division. He played football at Fort Bragg—"I hated the military but loved playing football," he later said—and earned a scholarship to play at East Carolina. There he was designated "Strongest College Football Player in the Nation" after squatting, bench-pressing, and dead lifting a combined 2,203 pounds at the North Carolina State AAU Powerlifting Championships. He had a 40-inch waist, a 54-inch chest, 21-inch arms, a 20-inch neck, and 30-inch thighs. He ran the 40-yard dash in 4.8 seconds.

Long was an All-American at East Carolina and was selected by the Steelers in the fourth round of the 1984 draft. He played in 105 NFL regular-season games and 4 playoff games. In his final season, 1991, he tested positive for steroids at the beginning of training camp. When Noll told him, Long wept. The next day, he tried to commit suicide, first by sitting in a running car inside a closed garage and then, when that attempt was foiled by his girlfriend, by eating rat poison.

Like Webster's, Long's life after football was a dramatic downward spiral marked by bouts of depression and mood swings as well as a series of bad business decisions that led to financial problems. In 2003, a chicken- and vegetable-processing plant he owned was destroyed by fire. Two years later, on March 29, 2005, he was charged with setting the fire to collect $1.1 million in insurance, and he filed for bankruptcy that same day. Long also was accused of defrauding the state of $1.2 million in a separate business scheme. Soon afterward, he again tried unsuccessfully to kill himself, this time by drinking a bottle of Drano.

A little over two months later, Long's body lay in the Allegheny

County coroner's office—another dead Pittsburgh Steelers offensive lineman who had essentially lost his mind.

In the years to come, Pittsburgh brain researchers would sit back in wonder at the string of events that turned their city into "Ground Zero" for the NFL's concussion crisis, as the *Post-Gazette*'s Chuck Finder put it. First, Noll's offhand remarks to Maroon in 1991 about the lack of quantifiable evidence for a concussion, which led to the development of ImPACT and one of the most successful concussion research institutions in the country at UPMC. Then Webster, his condition diagnosed by the young Nigerian pathologist who happened to be working that day. This time, Omalu wasn't on call. The autopsy was performed by Abdulrezak Shakir, Omalu's Iraqi colleague, who had worked in the coroner's office for 17 years. It is not common practice to save the brain during a forensic autopsy; after being weighed and examined, the vital organs usually are sewn into the body cavity. But Shakir, thinking about Omalu's research, preserved Long's brain for his colleague.

Omalu repeated the process he had followed with Webster. When the tests came back, he had "Chronic Traumatic Encephalopathy in a National Football League Player: Part II." Omalu sent the slides to Hamilton, who responded with an e-mail: "I have looked over your new NFL case. Fantastic! It is classic 'dementia pugilistica,' at least according to the entire chapter in Esiri and Morris (I will copy for you)."

This time, Wecht, the celebrity pathologist, wasn't interested in waiting for a medical journal to publish the findings. He went straight to the media with the news: Terry Long had sustained brain damage from playing football.

Shakir's autopsy report left no room for doubt: Long's brain damage had been caused by "repeated mild traumatic injury while playing football." The brain, Wecht said, showed signs of meningitis—inflammation—that stemmed in part from all the blows Long had taken playing football.

"A football helmet gives you an awful lot of protection," Wecht said. "But you don't have to be a doctor or an engineer or even a football player to realize that the helmet does not block out all the measured force produced when some 300-pound player with a hand the size of a

Christmas ham whacks you in the head dozens of times a game, season after season."

The NFL responded swiftly. This time the league's defender was Maroon, who had been the Steelers' neurological consultant during Long's career. "I think the conclusions drawn here are preposterous and a misinterpretation of facts," he told the *Post-Gazette*. "To say he was killed by football, it's just not right, it's not appropriate. I think it's not appropriate science when you have a history of no significant head injuries."

Maroon said Long's only recorded head trauma was from a 1990 car accident when he swerved to avoid hitting a deer. "I was the team neurosurgeon during his entire tenure with the Steelers," Maroon said. "I rechecked my records; there was not one cerebral concussion documented in him during those entire seven years. Not one."

Maroon cited Long's previous suicide attempts and his steroid use as other possible causes. "The bottom line is, in a patient who has not had truly documented head injury, no evidence of concussions—I would have seen him if he had—who has had a history of substance abuse, a history of suicide attempts with extremely neurotoxic materials, and then to conclude that this brain was damaged from football is more than a long stretch," he said.

Wecht knew Maroon well—his son Danny was a neurosurgeon in Maroon's practice and often worked the sidelines with the Steelers—and he became concerned by the aggressive denials. Wecht called Omalu at home.

"Bennet, are you sure?" Wecht asked.

"Cyril, if Terry Long did not have CTE, may I drop dead tonight," said Omalu.

Wecht ordered Omalu to speak to the media. Omalu, as it turned out, had Long's medical records, including those from the Steelers. They included a 1987 letter written by Maroon describing a concussion Long had suffered after colliding not with a deer but with an opposing player. Maroon wrote that Long was light-headed, had difficulty concentrating, and walked unsteadily. He recommended that Long sit out a week. Omalu told the *Post-Gazette* those symptoms were consistent with "massive concussive injuries."

One day earlier, Maroon had insisted that Long had not had a single concussion from playing football. Now he had to admit that he had "overlooked" the letter. But he said a concussion like Long's "happens in the NFL on a weekly basis." He said it was still a stretch to link Long's death to football. Pellman rushed to Maroon's defense, calling Omalu's conclusions "speculative and unscientific."

The Long case became even more confusing when a toxicology report came back and revealed that the swelling in Long's brain had been caused by the antifreeze he had ingested and not by football, as Wecht had told the media. When the toxicology report came back, Wecht had quietly changed the cause of death on the autopsy report to "suicide." Omalu was unfazed. The presence of neurofibrillary tangles was consistent with CTE, which, he said, could only have been caused by football. "People with chronic encephalopathy suffer from depression," Omalu said. "The major depressive disorder may manifest as suicide attempts. Terry Long committed suicide due to chronic traumatic encephalopathy due to his long-term play." Omalu added, "The NFL has been in denial."

"I think it's fallacious reasoning," Maroon shot back, "and I don't think it's plausible at all."

While the Long dispute played out, Omalu, Hamilton, and DeKosky put the finishing touches on their response to the NFL's demand for a retraction of the Webster paper. Not surprisingly, Omalu's initial response had been emotional. He called the NFL's reasoning "archaic" and "naive" and accused the MTBI committee of "ignoring possible long-term neurodegenerative outcomes of play in the NFL" for over a decade. Omalu described his reaction as "a typical manifestation of an Igbo man: 'Who do you think you are? Who do you think you are fucking with? C'mon, bring it on!' "

DeKosky wanted something more measured. "Ron, I don't want anything to do with this preachy polemic," he wrote in an e-mail to Hamilton. "The only way to respond to THEIR polemic is with a short, fact-based response."

Hamilton agreed to play editor and dial it back from the original Igbo. He stripped out Omalu's indignation and reduced the letter to two pages, although he did allow himself one bit of amusement, beginning the response to the NFL with a quote: "The lady doth protest too much, methinks" (Shakespeare, *Hamlet* III, ii).

That, too, was cut out of the final version, which was published in the May 2006 issue of *Neurosurgery,* alongside the NFL's demand for a retraction. Omalu, Hamilton, and DeKosky wrote that they had not suggested that Webster's brain was identical to that of a punch-drunk boxer. Boxers endure more severe head trauma, they wrote, largely because they don't wear helmets. "We doubt Casson et al. really feel that NFL offensive linemen do not experience repeated episodes of head trauma," the letter said. "It is far more likely that the majority of the head trauma in the NFL, as well as in American football in general, is underreported by the players and the team staff, who accept the occasionally 'dazed' recovery during the game and postgame headaches simply as part of the sport, not unlike bruises and sprains." They reminded the NFL's concussion committee that Webster's brain damage was well known in the league. "Of course, the NFL, at least the Disability Plan, acknowledged the cognitive impairment and its relationship to his profession," they wrote.

In conclusion, they wrote, "Our case is important primarily because it indicates there may be brain damage in NFL players that is currently under-reported." They said the NFL needed to begin a long-term study and they would be "happy to collaborate."

Left unsaid was the self-evident fact that the NFL's demand for a retraction had been denied. The Webster paper stood.

When Apuzzo and *Neurosurgery* published the Long study six months later, the NFL kept up its attack. The diagnosis of CTE was still wrong. Football players didn't get brain damage.

The public brawl was taking a toll on Omalu. The young Nigerian immigrant who had barely heard of the NFL suddenly found himself the target of some of the most powerful doctors in the country, who had the full weight of a rich and powerful corporation behind them.

One afternoon, the phone rang at Omalu's desk at the coroner's office. Omalu thought twice about answering. He was never sure who might be calling these days and what might happen next. But he picked up.

"Hello, is this Bennet?" said a baritone voice with a slight drawl.

"Yeah."

"This is Julian Bailes. I'm the chairman of the Department of Neurosurgery at West Virginia University."

"What can I do for you?"

"Bennet," said Bailes. "I believe you."

I n Omalu, the Dissenters had found an ally. In many ways, his discovery was a validation of their own work. Bailes and Guskiewicz
had found a large number of players with signs of dementia. Omalu
and his colleagues had taken it a step further, confirming neuropathological changes in the brains of two players who were mentally impaired at
the time of their deaths. Yet the NFL had dismissed Omalu, Hamilton, DeKosky, and Wecht in the same way the league's doctors had dismissed Bailes and Guskiewicz. The Dissenters found it appalling. Their
concern was no longer whether this was a problem; it was how many
players like Mike Webster and Terry Long were out there: walking time
bombs who were a danger to themselves and a nightmare to the people
who cared about them.

Bailes told Omalu he wanted to help any way he could. Cantu also
threw his support behind him. One day, Omalu received an e-mail from
a man who identified himself as one of Cantu's former patients. His
name was Chris Nowinski, and he told Omalu he wanted to interview
him about his work for a book he was writing about the concussion
crisis. They arranged a time to chat, and during the 45-minute conversation, Omalu educated Nowinski on CTE and his certainty about
its significance. He also talked about the NFL's hostile reaction to his
research.

Nowinski soaked it up. He was a new breed of Dissenter: not a
research scientist but a concussion activist, for lack of a better term.
He was trying to create public awareness of the underreported problem. Nowinski was tall, blond, and preppy, a former Harvard lineman
and pro wrestler who became interested in concussions as a result of
his own painful fieldwork. At the time, Nowinski was just 27, but he
had been bashed in the head for years. Nowinski had played football at
John Hersey High School in Arlington Heights, near Chicago, starting
out as a spindly 6-foot-3, 160-pound middle linebacker. He loved the
sanctioned violence and macho culture. Nowinski played with a broken hand, gulped down ibuprofen to fight through an injured shoulder,
lived for the big hit. In one game, he sprinted down the field on punt

coverage and knocked out the returner with a helmet-to-helmet hit. Nowinski stood over his opponent and played to the crowd. He lifted weights constantly. By the time he graduated, Nowinski was a 6-foot-5, 230-pound defensive end. He also was an excellent student—in junior high, he was the Illinois champion in the Scientific Olympiad in the map-reading category—and a budding actor, performing in *West Side Story* in high school.

Nowinski's successful career at Harvard was marred by at least a couple of concussions, though they weren't diagnosed at the time and he didn't miss any action. Once, during an intrasquad game, he collided so hard with a teammate that they both fell down sideways, toppling like bowling pins. "That was the first time I remembered the sky turning orange," he said.

By his senior year, Nowinski was 6-5 and 295 pounds and harbored dreams of playing in the NFL. He worked out for a handful of teams, but when it became clear he wasn't going to make it, Nowinski began to focus on life after football. Although he had majored in sociology, Nowinski landed an internship at Trinity Partners, a Boston-area consulting firm. One of his bosses, John Corcoran, was a pro wrestling fan. He knew Nowinski had a background in sports and theater and also loved the spectacle of pro wrestling. Corcoran suggested that he try it. It turned out to be a perfect fit, a chance for Nowinski to combine his athletic skills with his acting bug.

After work, Nowinski spent his evenings training at Killer Kowalski's Pro Wrestling School in Malden, Massachusetts, founded by the fabled wrestler who mentored some of the sport's future stars, including Triple H, Big John Studd, and Chyna. Nowinski made $20 in his first match, wrestling under the name Jake Champski in front of 150 people at an armory in Portland, Maine. He then put together a video application that earned him a spot on an MTV wrestling reality show, *Tough Enough*. The writers dubbed him Chris Harvard, creating a character fans would love to hate: the snobbish Harvard graduate who taunted his opponents with his superior intellect. Nowinski repurposed a chant he recalled hearing from the fans of an opposing high school back in Illinois: "Five, ten, fifteen bucks, we own the company, you drive the trucks!" In 2002, he was signed by the WWE and made his debut on

Monday Night Raw, with 5 million people watching. He was a rising star.

"I played the hateable character very well," he recalled. "I had, you know, they liked to use the term 'natural heat.' People just liked to dislike me."

Chris Harvard wore tight crimson trunks with the school logo on his butt. Sometimes he recited poetry to incite the crowd. At one match in Moncton, New Brunswick, he shouted:

> *Roses are red,*
> *Violets are blue,*
> *The reason I'm talking so slowly*
> *Is because no one in Moncton has passed grade two.*

Nowinski, of course, knew that the sport was staged, that the moves and the results were choreographed. But there was no way to comprehend the true violence of pro wrestling until he was in it. "You don't appreciate how the sausage is made," he said.

Nowinski got kneed, elbowed, drop-kicked, punched, and otherwise smashed in the head. That was all very real. The concussions began with a kick to the chin from Bubba Ray Dudley's boot. Nowinski sucked it up and kept going. When more concussions followed, he never gave himself time to recover. Soon he was experiencing pounding headaches and blurred vision; sometimes he forgot how his matches were supposed to play out, like an actor forgetting his lines. He began sleepwalking. One night his girlfriend woke up at a hotel in Indianapolis and saw Nowinski standing on the bed, trying to climb the wall. She tried unsuccessfully to wake him by shouting his name, only to watch him leap off the bed and slam headfirst into the wall.

After that, Nowinski set out on a journey to try to figure out what was going on inside his head. He visited a series of head trauma experts, including Lovell at UPMC, but never felt that he truly understood. Finally, he was referred by a friend to one of the world's leading concussion experts, a doctor right in his own backyard. It was Cantu, one of the original Dissenters. Nowinski had found his savior, a man who took the time not only to define concussions for him but to explain how poorly understood they were and the dangers of not allowing them to heal. The two met many times over the coming months, and Cantu became more than Nowinski's doctor; he became his mentor, his teacher, his friend, and his champion. It was Cantu ultimately who encouraged Nowinski to write the story of his concussions, to help educate the world. Cantu saw "a dynamic individual, a very brilliant mind, whose background is 180 degrees from mine. He had lived reality TV life. He had lived the star athlete life. And he knew how to use the media to get across ideas in a way that, duh, never occurred to me in 30 years of writing papers. Reminds me of the monk in the monastery approach, as compared with what can happen instantaneously if you get that message out."

"Medical guys write books all the time, but no one reads them," Cantu told Nowinski. "You have a platform from wrestling."

As Nowinski began his work on the book, Cantu directed him to other research scientists and some of his other patients. Nowinski also reviewed the literature on concussions. That was how he came upon Omalu. Nowinski's book, *Head Games: Football's Concussion Crisis,* was published several months later, with an introduction by former professional wrestler turned governor Jesse "the Body" Ventura. Nowinski's dedication read: "To the players, young and old, whose lives have been changed forever by head injuries."

On November 20, 2006, Nowinski was checking SI.com when he read that the 44-year-old Andre Waters, a former Philadelphia Eagles safety, had committed suicide by shooting himself in the head. Nowinski remembered that Waters, nicknamed "Dirty Waters," had a reputation as one of the hardest hitters in the game. Waters had spent 12 seasons in the NFL. In 1994—the NFL's Year of the Concussion—he had told the *Philadelphia Inquirer* that he had tried to count how many concussions he sustained during his career and lost count at 15. His treatment? "I just wouldn't say anything," he said. "I'd sniff some smelling salts, then go back out there."

Reflecting on Omalu's work, Nowinski played a hunch. He contacted Dr. Leszek Chrostowski, the associate medical examiner in Tampa, where Waters had killed himself. Nowinski explained who he was and asked Chrostowski if he was aware of the literature connecting concussions and depression. He then politely made an unusual request: Could he please obtain what remained of Andre Waters's brain for further study?

"He said, 'There's no evidence that there's any connection,'" Nowinski recalled. "He kind of implied that I was crazy to think so."

Nowinski sent the medical examiner Omalu's paper as well as the studies done by Bailes and Guskiewicz for the Center for the Study of Retired Athletes. He then called Omalu to tell him about Waters.

"If I can get you another brain, would you study it?" Nowinski asked.

"Absolutely," said Omalu.

Omalu called Chrostowski to support Nowinski's efforts. The medical examiner agreed to give them the tissue if they could get permission from Waters's family. Omalu told Nowinski he wanted no part of calling the family, and so Nowinski's career as a brain chaser was launched. It was the hardest assignment imaginable. He would have to cold-call the family members of somebody he didn't know who had just put a gun in his mouth and pulled the trigger. Nowinski wrote up a script, closed the door to his room, and practiced for half an hour.

"The most difficult cold call I've ever been part of," he said.

Nowinski spoke with one of Waters's sisters, describing his own experiences with concussions and the cases of Mike Webster and Terry Long, raising the possibility that her brother might have had the same terrible disease. The family agreed. Despite the bullet wound, enough tissue had been recovered from Waters's brain for Omalu to examine it. The medical examiner sent the tissue to Omalu in Pittsburgh.

Nowinski began to prepare for the possibility that Waters might have CTE. He thought it would be huge news, a third documented case of a former NFL player diagnosed with brain damage after dying tragically. He didn't want to wait for the slow wheels of science to turn—the publication of yet another peer-reviewed paper—before word got out. He wanted people to know. "There were people that were going to kill themselves between now and then because they didn't know what was happening to them," Nowinski said. "And there were kids who were going to play through concussions because they didn't know that it mattered. And to have something with this sort of public health implication sitting on a shelf for a year when you know it's true, and it's the third case of three, was to me impossible."

While trying to get his book published, Nowinski had been introduced to a New York–based freelance journalist named Alan Schwarz. Schwarz had been encouraging: He told Nowinski that his book was well written and thoroughly researched. Schwarz then pointed him to a literary agent and a couple of prospective publishers. Schwarz had no particular expertise in concussions; he was primarily a baseball writer, an expert on statistics who had graduated from the University of Pennsylvania with a mathematics degree. Schwarz described himself as "an accidental journalist." He had decided to become a sportswriter only after learning that he needed a master's degree to teach high school math, his longtime ambition. Schwarz had recently published his own book: *The Numbers Game: Baseball's Lifelong Fascination with Statistics.* Now Nowinski called Schwarz again, thinking perhaps he could help with the Waters story.

"I think I have something good," Nowinski told Schwarz. "I think I have something important. But I'm not sure what to do with it. And you're the only one who ever took me seriously."

Schwarz, then 38, had a developing relationship with the *New York Times.* He had written some baseball stats columns and a few front-page stories, including a profile of a 111-year-old former Negro League player who was living in St. Petersburg, Florida. Schwarz told Nowinski he would try to set up a meeting with Tom Jolly, the *Times'* sports editor. Nowinski traveled to New York for the meeting and explained the story and how he was awaiting the results of the analysis on Waters's brain. Schwarz thought he was there as the go-between, but Jolly told him as he was leaving that he would write the story on the Waters results.

Schwarz was excited, but he didn't immediately recognize it as big news. "I didn't necessarily have the keenest nose for news," he said.

Then, in January, the slides came back: Waters had brain damage. Omalu told Nowinski, who relayed the news to Schwarz. Schwarz contacted several experts for comment: Cantu, Bailes, Guskiewicz—most of the Dissenters—and members of the NFL's concussion committee. Guskiewicz told him: "I think that some of the folks within the NFL have chosen to ignore some of these earlier findings, and I question how many more, be it a large study like ours, or single-case studies like Terry Long, Mike Webster, whomever it may be, it will take for them to wake up." Schwarz didn't know what he was getting into. He figured he would write the story and move on. "I thought it was going to be one story and that was it," he said. "You know, you do a story on this thing, and then you get back to writing about baseball."

When he drafted the piece, Schwarz focused on Nowinski's compelling life story and how he'd gotten possession of Andre Waters's brain. It was basically a human interest story about a concussed former wrestler turned activist. Late in the day, after the story had passed through the news desk, Schwarz was told to rewrite the top to get straight to the heart of the matter: "Since the former National Football League player Andre Waters killed himself in November, an explanation for his suicide has remained a mystery. But after examining remains of Mr. Waters's brain, a neuropathologist in Pittsburgh is claiming that Mr. Waters had sustained brain damage from playing football and he says that led to his depression and ultimate death."

"The beginning was restructured at the last second because the *Times* had a better idea of what news was," Schwarz said. "I knew what a feature was, and I could do a pretty good feature. But they recognized what this could be."

The story ran on page 1 of the *New York Times* on January 18, 2007. That was the day the NFL's concussion problem hit the mainstream. The story had been percolating for over a decade, from Greg Garber's ESPN piece on players such as Toon and Hoge back in 1994, to Peter Keating's powerful *ESPN The Magazine* story in 2006 about Pellman's dubious reign as head of the concussion committee ("Dr. Yes"), to Wecht's public announcement in Pittsburgh that Terry Long had brain damage.

But the *New York Times* had elevated the story by virtue of being the *New York Times*.

"Without the *Times,* it never moves," Nowinski said. "It cannot be overstated how important it was."

- - -

When Bailes contacted Omalu—"Bennet, I believe you"—he explained that he had been asked by the American Association of Neurological Surgeons to see if he could examine Omalu's research. Omalu readily agreed. Bailes thought the meeting also presented a huge opportunity to bring the NFL into the fold. The denials could go on for only so long before the league had to act, he thought. Bailes decided to invite his former boss, Maroon, to the session. Despite Maroon's harsh criticism of Omalu, Bailes thought he was a serious, reasonable man and would respond to evidence.

By that time, Omalu and Maroon had struck a truce. Omalu had gone to visit the distinguished neurosurgeon in his office at UPMC, and the two had talked it out after Maroon's "fallacious reasoning" comment in the *Post-Gazette*. Omalu, in fact, had proposed making Maroon director of a longitudinal study of CTE in retired players that he, Hamilton, and DeKosky were planning to propose to the NFL. Omalu, like Bailes, felt the NFL would eventually have to come around. In an e-mail to Hamilton and Hamilton's boss, Clayton Wiley, Omalu attached a copy of the proposal and wrote: "I intentionally suggested that Dr. Maroon should be the Director of the project since the NFL will be more likely to fund the study if they know that their own man is at the helm of affairs and will be less likely to undermine them."

Omalu, Bailes, Maroon, Hamilton, and DeKosky gathered in Hamilton's office on the fifth floor of the A Wing at UPMC Presbyterian. Nearby was a conference room with a multiheaded microscope that would allow Bailes and Maroon to look at the slides while Omalu walked them through the material.

Omalu was nervous. It was one thing to write a paper, but the young Nigerian was about to present his findings to two of the top neurosurgeons in the country, Bailes and Maroon; an internationally recognized Alzheimer's expert, DeKosky; and Omalu's widely respected mentor, Hamilton. Bailes took pages of notes. He was struck by the magnitude of the moment, the potential significance to the game he had played and continued to love.

"To realize the implications and that we were on the very cutting edge of it, it's a very striking realization," Bailes recalled. "It was not going to be a fun journey."

Maroon hadn't said much throughout the meeting, but finally he asked Omalu: "Where do you think this is going?"

"To be honest, I don't know," Omalu said quietly. "But I think many, many more players have this disease than we have acknowledged."

"Do you understand the impact of what you're doing?" Maroon asked.

"Yes," Omalu said.

Maroon seemed to be coming to his own moment of reckoning. He had been with the Steelers for two decades. He had helped launch ImPACT, the neurocognitive test that raised awareness within football about the serious effects of concussions. But in recent years, as the debate grew, more often than not he had sided with the NFL, praising the committee's research and casting doubt on Omalu's findings.

Maroon asked Omalu again: "Do you really understand the impact of what you're doing?"

"Yes," Omalu answered.

The conversation continued, and Maroon asked Omalu one more time: "Bennet, do you *really* understand the impact of what you're doing?"

"Okay, what is the impact?" said Omalu.

Maroon tilted his head back.

"If only 10 percent of mothers in America begin to conceive of football as a dangerous game," Maroon said, "that is the end of football."

11

A MAN OF SCIENCE

Do you really understand? Suddenly, there were a lot of interested parties posing the exact same question. For years, really, the battle over the NFL's concussion policies had been confined largely to the pages of a medical journal and the few researchers who cared. People later forgot that the original Dissenters were a vociferous Gang of Four: Bob Cantu, Kevin Guskiewicz, Julian Bailes, and Bill Barr. (The superagent Leigh Steinberg was an honorary member, by virtue of his awareness campaign.) Within those circles, the NFL's scientific transgressions were certainly a big deal, a source of constant discussion and indignation. But very little of the dispute had seeped out into the real world. Now the number of people openly challenging the NFL was growing by the day. They included reporters from powerful media organizations, especially Alan Schwarz of the *New York Times* and Peter Keating of ESPN; Omalu and Nowinski; and a growing number of prominent former players.

Harry Carson, the New York Giants linebacker of 13 years, had been profoundly affected by Webster's death. He had flown to Pittsburgh to attend the funeral out of respect for his former opponent and had spent time talking to Garrett, who described in detail his father's horrific final years. Later, when Carson learned that Omalu had diagnosed Webster with brain damage, he was heartbroken. He partly blamed himself. Carson flashed back to the brutal tactics he had employed to try to neutralize Webster's incredible strength—how he gathered "all of my power from my big rear end and my thighs into my forearm," which he unleashed on Webster's head. "I'm the guy that he would fire off the ball to hit, and I would hit him in the face with my forearm, you know?" Carson said. "And so I was distributing the damage."

Carson was well positioned as a spokesman for the cause of former players, a distinguished, imposing man still built like granite. He combined the sensitivity of a Manhattan psychoanalyst with the naked violence of the Pit. "I wasn't known for getting my hands on the ball," he wrote in his autobiography, *Captain for Life*, "but I was known for knocking a player's dick in the dirt if he came my way and I got a good shot on him." When O. J. Simpson told Carson that no player had hit him harder, "that made my year," Carson wrote. Carson was so respected by his peers that coach Bill Parcells sent him out alone for the coin toss before the 1987 Super Bowl against the Broncos.

After his retirement in 1988, Carson had been open about his own struggles with depression. He confessed that he once considered driving his car off the Tappan Zee Bridge into the Hudson River. "I'd seen where there were people who would stop their car on the bridge and then jump off the bridge," he said in an interview for this book. "If you're on the Tarrytown side, there's a curve. And I was thinking, 'What if I accelerated, hit the guardrail, and go through?'" Carson found that there seemed to be no rhyme or reason to his moods; they simply came over him like squalls. Only after he went to a neuropsychologist and described his symptoms—migraines, mysterious twitching in his arms and legs, sensitivity to bright lights—did it begin to make sense. The neuropsychologist diagnosed him with postconcussion syndrome related to his career.

The diagnosis seemed to liberate Carson. It also awakened him to the devastation he recognized among many of his peers. Carson held a dark view about NFL-style capitalism, how it chewed up and spit out players. "When someone gets hurt, you just find another part," he said. "The reality is nobody gives a shit about those guys. I mean, their time is over. They don't bring anything of value to the table. Some people feel like they need to just shut up, go away and enjoy your retirement and that's it." Webster's death, he felt, had been a moment of shame for the

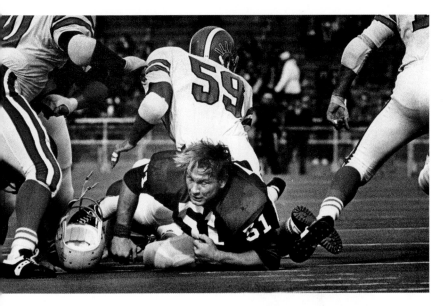

At the University of Wisconsin, Mike Webster began his transformation into "Iron Mike," obsessively driven by fear that he would never escape his tormented childhood.

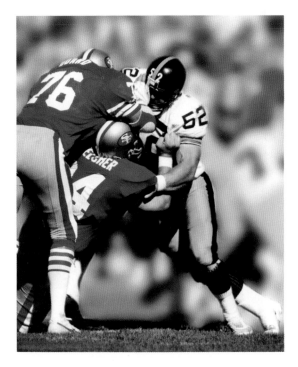

Webster played 17 seasons, winning four Super Bowls, becoming the strongest man in the NFL, and going six years without missing a single offensive play. But his struggles with mental illness would define his legacy as much as his Hall of Fame career.

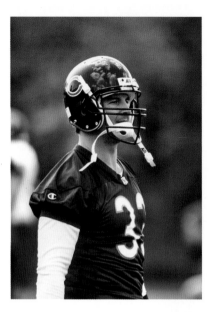

Merril Hoge retired at 29 after a concussion that left him unable to recall his daughter's name and briefly caused him to go blind. He sued the Chicago Bears doctor for negligence.

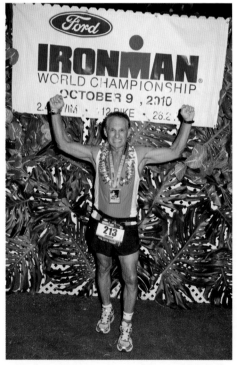

When confronted with the first cases of football-related brain damage, Joe Maroon, longtime neurological consultant to the Pittsburgh Steelers and a competitive triathlete, said, "If only 10 percent of mothers in America begin to conceive of football as dangerous, that is the end of football."

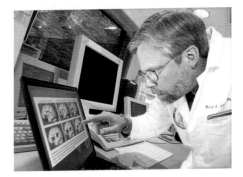

Mark Lovell, a neuropsychologist, cofounded ImPACT, a hugely popular concussion test, and was a charter member of the NFL's Mild Traumatic Brain Injury Committee. He later disavowed the committee's major findings.

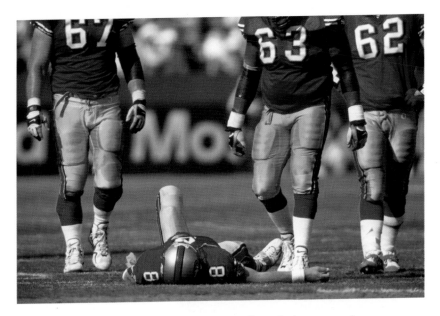

Steve Young insisted he was the "vanilla guy" whose concussions were routine, but his retirement after numerous head injuries forced the NFL to confront the growing crisis.

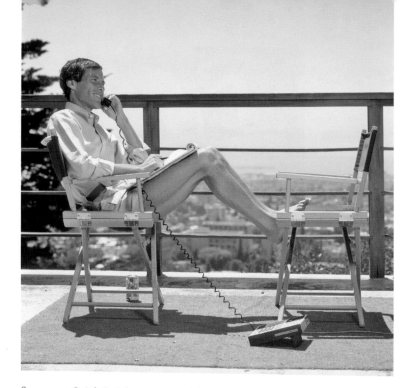

Superagent Leigh Steinberg represented practically every starting quarterback in the NFL; he ultimately became concerned that football might destroy the men who helped build his empire.

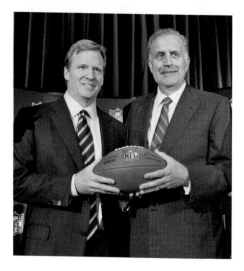

When he retired as NFL commissioner in 2006, Paul Tagliabue (right) dumped a health crisis and a public relations disaster in the lap of his former right-hand man, Roger Goodell (left).

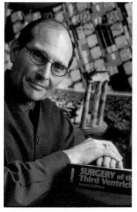

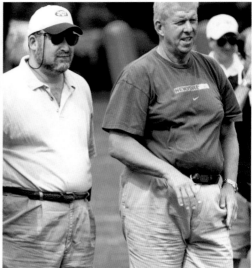

As head of the journal *Neurosurgery,* USC professor and New York Giants consultant Michael Apuzzo rubber-stamped the NFL's concussion research over the objections of peer reviewers, according to one of his editors.

As Jets team doctor, Elliot Pellman (left), who also headed the NFL's research arm, sent severely concussed players back into games, sometimes under pressure from head coach Bill Parcells (right), according to former players.

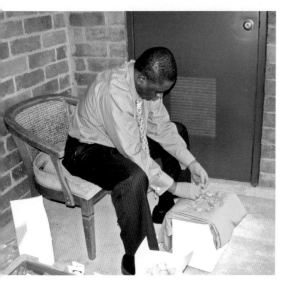

Bennet Omalu, the Nigerian pathologist who documented the first case of football-related brain damage, often conducted research on the porch or dining-room table of his Pittsburgh condominium.

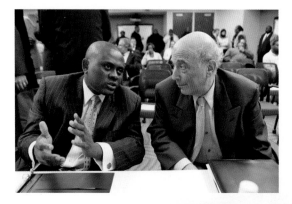

Five years after Ira Casson (right) and his colleagues sought to discredit Bennet Omalu and his research on football and neurodegenerative disease, the two men met for the first time at a 2010 congressional hearing in Detroit.

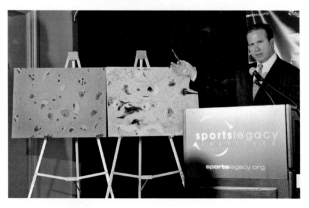

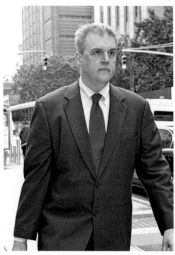

Above: Former Pittsburgh Steelers doctor Julian Bailes presented evidence linking football and brain disease to NFL officials, including Commissioner Roger Goodell, only to face mocking skepticism from the cochair of the league's concussion committee.

Left: Former New York Jets neuropsychologist Bill Barr accused the NFL of cherry-picking data to support its assertion that pro football players recovered quickly and completely from concussions.

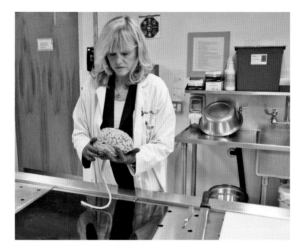

Ann McKee, a Packers fan and charismatic neuropathologist, became the unofficial spokeswoman for CTE. She came to believe that "most NFL players are going to get this. It's just a question of degree."

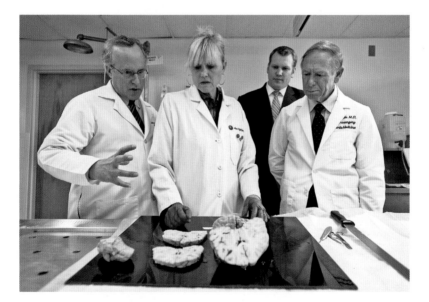

The BU Group (left to right): Bob Stern, Ann McKee, Chris Nowinski, and Bob Cantu. After splitting with Omalu, Nowinski assembled a team that gained international recognition as the leading researchers on football-related brain damage.

Kevin Guskiewicz, a University of North Carolina neuroscientist and former Steelers trainer, found dramatically higher rates of depression and dementia in NFL players. He compared the formation of the NFL's MTBI committee to an airport security breach.

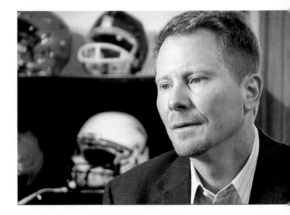

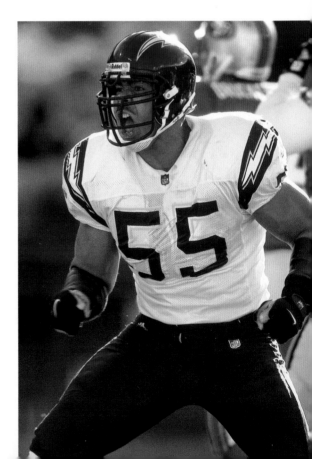

Junior Seau, one of the greatest linebackers in NFL history, was a San Diego icon. When he killed himself in 2012, several prominent research institutions engaged in an ugly battle over his brain.

NFL, one of the lowest points in the history of the league. The NFL had abandoned Webster to the streets and fought him in court even after he was dead. "I felt like Mike lost his dignity," said Carson. "That's the thing with me that is important."

In 2006, after years of being passed over, Carson was elected to the Pro Football Hall of Fame. He delivered his speech without notes. Standing in the same spot in Canton, Ohio, where Webster, a decade earlier, his mind already riddled with disease, had struggled to gather his thoughts, Carson used the occasion to call out the NFL:

> When I was elected to the Pro Football Hall of Fame, some people asked me, "Why aren't you happy about being elected?" Well, I can't be happy about it until I get one or two things off of my chest, and please indulge me.
>
> As a Hall of Famer, I want to implore the NFL and its union to look at the product that you have up on this stage. These are great individuals. The honor of making it into the Hall of Fame is great, but it was even greater to have the opportunity to play in a league with 18,000 individuals. These are some of the best individuals I've ever encountered. We'd get on the field and we'd fight tooth and nail, we'd try to knock each other out, then we'd walk off the field, pat each other on the rear end, and say, "Congratulations, hang in there," whatever. Those individuals I am extremely proud of participating in a game, and it is just a game, I'm extremely proud to have participated in that game with those 18,000 individuals.
>
> I would hope that the leaders of the NFL, the future commissioner, and the players association do a much better job of looking out for those individuals. You got to look out for 'em. If we made the league what it is, you have to take better care of your own.

Carson's speech, coming as the first documented cases linking football and brain damage were revealed, added his powerful voice to the growing list of people calling for the NFL to take action. The setting was symbolic. It had been just a few years earlier that Steve DeKosky, the Alzheimer's expert, had been ignored when he asked the Hall of Fame if he could study players for signs of neurological disease. Webster himself had viewed the Hall as a sick ward for discarded legends. And now here was Carson, one of its newest members, using his induction speech as a platform to "implore" the NFL and the union to do the right thing. As more and more Hall of Famers became mentally ill, their brains and bodies destroyed, the Canton shrine took on a completely different meaning.

Tagliabue had created the NFL's Mild Traumatic Brain Injury Committee under pressure in 1994. Now, in 2007, the committee's body of work—a veritable fortress of denial—was beginning to crumble. Schwarz, who was brought on full-time by the *Times* shortly after the Andre Waters story was published, was helping to accelerate the process by writing stories that chipped away at the committee's tortured logic. Schwarz and his editors realized that it was far more than one story: The entire sport was in crisis. Schwarz began to look at it from other angles. In one story, he went back to one of the NFL's most controversial pieces of research, NFL Paper Number 7, which concluded that returning to play in the same game posed no significant risk and suggested that "it might be safe for college/high school football players to be cleared to return to play on the same day as their injury." It was an extraordinary statement: The NFL seemed to be prescribing the same aggressive approach for college and high school players, without actually studying them.

Two and a half years later, Schwarz interviewed the authors. Two of the five, Colts neurological consultant Hank Feuer and Cynthia Arfken, an associate professor in Wayne State University's department of psychiatry and behavioral neurosciences who was brought on to conduct the statistical analysis, described the paper's conclusions as unfounded and inappropriate. They hadn't studied high school or college players, and so there was no basis for those claims. Arfken told Schwarz that the controversial "it might be safe" passage had been written into a final draft without her knowledge. Two other authors, Ira Casson and Dave Viano, the same scientists who had attacked Omalu, acknowledged putting in the provocative statement at the last minute to address, they said, comments by peer reviewers who had asked for analysis of the implications for high school and college players. Viano and Casson said both Arfken and Feuer had had a chance to review the final draft.

Feuer, a charter member of the MTBI committee, told the *Times* he "would change that sentence; I'd eliminate it." Years later, in an interview for this book, Feuer offered the same explanation as Lovell about why information he didn't believe had made it into the paper: He hadn't read it, only the material that was relevant to him.

Arfken had ended up on the paper entirely by chance. She got a call from Viano one day out of the blue; though they were colleagues at Wayne State, they didn't know each other. "He called me because my name started with *A*," Arfken said in an interview for this book. "He just went down the alphabet."

Schwarz accurately described this internal split as "the first crack in a united front long presented by the NFL's concussion committee." Among other things, the story revealed one of the more insidious aspects of the NFL's work: its influence over the national feeder system that funneled elite players into the league. The NFL's science hadn't taken place in a vacuum. Three million kids between 6 and 14 years old played tackle football. There were 1.1 million high school players and 68,000 college players. The NFL's research had been followed by medical personnel who were making decisions involving those kids.

"That was a major disservice, and it continues to be an ongoing one in conversations I have with parents and coaches and players," Gerard Malanga, a New Jersey team doctor for several high schools and colleges, told Schwarz. "They will reference back to that article. It creates confusion when there's increasing clarity on the subject. They say what I tell them about it not being safe to go back in the same game is totally wrong, and they're backed by the NFL. So they go to a doctor who tells them what they want to hear. It's happened. Sure it's happened. And we remain the guys holding our breath that the kid doesn't get hurt again."

The MTBI committee's helmet studies were another example of this trickle-down phenomenon from the NFL's research. The NFL's designs on creating a concussion-resistant helmet had been shot down by the biomechanics firm involved in the project. Lovell and Collins both believed the idea was a fantasy. Yet armed with the flawed UPMC study (coauthored by Lovell and Collins), Riddell, the NFL's official helmet maker, sold about 2 million Revolution helmets, mostly to high school and college players. The company employed an aggressive national advertising campaign that emphasized the Revolution's concussion-reducing properties, using numbers lifted straight from the Riddell-funded UPMC study—numbers that were both misleading and derived from the flawed NFL research.

Riddell developed PowerPoint presentations to educate its sales representatives on how best to market the Revolution to teams, school districts, and leagues. That material underscored the helmet's "Concussion Reduction Technology," which purportedly reduced concussions by 31 to 41 percent, the sales reps were told. At one point, the company sent out a rush mailer making the concussion-resistant claim for its youth line of helmets. The UPMC study had not examined that line. Realizing that the mailer was false, not just misleading, Riddell's director of marketing modified it by striking one word: "Ground-breaking research shows that athletes who wear Riddell Revolution ~~Youth~~ helmets were 31% less likely to suffer a concussion than athletes who wore traditional football helmets."

The claims had a major impact on the helmet industry. Riddell was able to sell the Revolution at a $50 premium, which it attributed to the cost of creating the Concussion Reduction Technology and underwriting the UPMC study. One Southern California sporting goods dealer who sold football helmets made by Schutt—Riddell's main competitor—and other brands said the market for non-Riddell helmets in his region had all but dried up. "We just didn't sell many helmets at that point," he said in an interview for this book, asking that his name not be used because he was still in the business. "I think more than anything else, the end user, the dads, were believing what Riddell was saying. And that had a big effect. We were trying to sell the helmets, but if a coach or a dad believes this to be true, they're going to purchase that product."

Schutt modified its helmets to stay competitive. Riddell sued Schutt for patent infringement. Schutt countersued for false advertising and deceptive trade practices. A Wisconsin judge ruled in Riddell's favor. Schutt, the judge wrote, had failed to prove that Riddell's concussion claims were "literally false."

"Although the presentations and internal discussions may suggest that sales representatives were trained to mislead, they fail to suggest that representatives were trained to make literally false statements," the judge wrote.

- - -

Do *you really understand?*

Ted Johnson was a hard-hitting New England Patriots linebacker for 10 years, winning three Super Bowls before his retirement in 2005. When he saw that Andre Waters had been diagnosed with brain damage by Omalu after shooting himself in the head, he decided to tell his own dark story. It was a story both unique to Ted Johnson and now familiar, with echoes of Webster, Hoge, and countless others. Johnson, like Webster, found that he couldn't function without gulping down huge quantities of stimulants, in his case Adderall. His addiction, depression, and self-loathing frequently confined him to his bed, where he lay in the dark for days. He had migraines and memory loss and felt certain he was losing his mind.

Johnson first told his story in 2006 to the *Boston Globe*'s Jackie MacMullan, who was about to publish it until Johnson was arrested for assault and battery for pushing his wife into a bookcase. After the incident, Johnson begged MacMullan to delay the piece; she reluctantly agreed, not wanting to take advantage of a man she thought was clearly unstable. What happened next revealed a lot about not only Johnson but also Nowinski, who was intent on exploiting his budding relationship with the *New York Times* to the fullest. With MacMullan still sitting on her exclusive, she received word that Johnson had given his story to Alan Schwarz and the *Times*. MacMullan was furious at Johnson, who later told her that Nowinski had advised him to spurn her because the *Times* would bring "the best bang for the buck." The betrayal was so audacious that Nowinski's embarrassed colleagues and *Times* editors alerted MacMullan, who, after screaming at Nowinski, scrambled to get her own story published.

The two pieces ran on the same Sunday: February 2, 2007. They were devastating. Johnson traced his problems to a concussion he had sustained in a 2002 preseason game against the New York Giants. Four days after the injury, still groggy, he took the practice field wearing a noncontact red jersey. Before a set of running drills, however, an assistant trainer handed him a blue jersey—essentially an order to get out and hit. Johnson knew right away the switch had been made not by the team's medical staff but by the Patriots' head coach, Bill Belichick. He feared that if he refused, he'd lose his job and his $1.1 million salary. "I'm sitting there going, 'God, do I put this thing on?'" he said. He added that such intimidation is common in the NFL. "That day it was Bill Belichick and Ted Johnson," he said. "But it happens all the time."

Johnson got hit in the head on the first play, leaving him dazed. When he reported the second concussion to a trainer after practice, the Pats sent him to Massachusetts General Hospital.

"You played God with my health," Johnson said he later told Belichick. "You knew I shouldn't have been cleared to play, and you gave me that blue jersey anyway."

MacMullan got hold of Belichick. The coach told her that he and Johnson apologized to each other during the air-clearing meeting. He never denied ordering Johnson to wear the blue jersey. "If Ted felt so strongly that he didn't feel he was ready to practice with us, he should have told me," Belichick said.

Rendered in painful detail—Johnson also revealed that he nearly underwent electroshock therapy—the Ted Johnson story read like another real-world counterargument to years of NFL denials. Johnson hadn't returned to play because the Pats' astute medical staff had cleared him; his head coach had ordered him to go out and hit. His first concussion wasn't unconnected to the second; his brain had been primed for further injury. Johnson estimated he'd had as many 30 concussions during his career. Cantu, his doctor, concluded that he had post-concussion syndrome and incipient dementia.

As the voices challenging the NFL proliferated, the league began to respond. It was a little like the scene in *Titanic* when the ocean liner struggles to avoid the iceberg. The league rushed out a series of new policies. The "88 Plan" was established in honor of John Mackey, the legendary Colts tight end, who was experiencing advanced dementia. Mackey, the former head of the players union, sometimes spooned his coffee, thinking it was soup; was unable to recognize people he had just met; and flew into illogical rages distantly connected to his illustrious career. Mackey wore two rings—one from Super Bowl V, when the Colts scored 10 points in the fourth quarter to beat the Cowboys, and one from his induction into the Hall of Fame. In 2006, when airport security asked him to remove the rings, he became enraged, ran toward the gate, and had to be wrestled to the ground by armed guards, screaming and mumbling: "I got in the end zone!" The 88 Plan, named after Mackey's old number, provided up to $88,000 a year for players with dementia, Alzheimer's, amyotrophic lateral sclerosis (ALS), or Parkinson's. It originated with a wrenching three-page letter that Mackey's wife, Sylvia, had sent to Tagliabue, describing her husband's condition as "a slow, deteriorating, ugly, caregiver-killing, degenerative, brain-destroying tragic horror." Dozens of applications soon poured in.

The NFL also adopted mandatory neuropsychological testing—providing more business to Lovell, Collins, and ImPACT—and established a hot line for players to report improper concussion treatment by their coaches or trainers. The policy immediately became known as the Ted Johnson Rule.

The league also reconfigured its concussion committee. Pellman, whose résumé embellishment had been exposed two years earlier, was removed as chairman, although he was allowed to stay on as a committee member. Casson and Viano replaced him as cochairs. It wasn't exactly a major shake-up: The triumvirate that had steered the NFL's science for the past 13 years remained intact, just rearranged slightly. The committee added three new members, including Joe Maroon, whom the NFL originally described as a "non-affiliated" doctor. That was quickly amended after it was pointed out that Maroon had worked for the Pittsburgh Steelers for two decades.

There was an odd schizophrenia to the policy changes. The league and the union had created a special fund for players with brain damage while at the same time vehemently denying that football caused brain damage. When Schwarz pointed out this apparent contradiction to Greg Aiello, the league spokesman replied that dementia was a disease that "affects many elderly people." The NFL's criticism of Omalu continued. Casson told the *Washington Post* that Omalu's work was riddled with "glaring deficiencies" and suggested that he had exaggerated his findings.

Casson, the new cochair, baffled researchers and laypersons alike. Even more than Pellman, he would become associated with the NFL's refusal to admit it had a problem—the league's true disbeliever. A bald, combative man, Casson was emphatic: He didn't believe the evidence.

His denials were all the more confounding because of his experience with boxers. Casson's 1982 study in the British *Journal of Neurology, Neurosurgery, and Psychiatry* was regarded as a breakthrough and had been particularly well timed, coming the same year that Duk Koo Kim, a South Korean lightweight, died of a brain hemorrhage after fighting Ray Mancini outside Caesars Palace. Casson and his colleagues performed CT scans on 10 boxers shortly after routine knockouts. Five showed signs of cerebral atrophy. Experience appeared to be a predictor: the more bouts, the more brain damage. Among the five boxers with 20 or more fights, four had cerebral atrophy. Of the five with fewer than 12 fights, only one had it. Rather than a single punch, Casson and his colleagues wrote that "a cumulative effect of multiple subconcussive head blows is the most likely culprit," a fact that, when applied to football, had dramatic implications for the men in the Pit.

The year after his study came out, *Sports Illustrated* brought in Casson as a consultant to examine a CT scan of Muhammad Ali's brain. The scan had been taken in July 1981, before Ali was cleared for his last fight, against Trevor Berbick. "They read this as normal?" said Casson, poring over the scan. "I wouldn't have read this as normal." At *SI*'s request, Casson also performed neurological exams on three other living fighters: the heavyweights Jerry Quarry and Randall (Tex) Cobb and a bantamweight named Mark Pacheco. Quarry and Pacheco had abnormal CT scans and signs of cavum septum pellucidum, a shearing of the ventricles. The exercise foreshadowed the debate about football 30 years later. Casson had become part of a long line of researchers to reveal the devastating effects of the sweet science on the brain. But on the question of whether boxing should be banned, Casson replied no. "A boxer ought to know what he's getting into if he wants to go on and be a champion," he said. "He should know what he may be sacrificing. A doctor has to tell the boxer if he thinks the fighter should stop, but in the end it's not really a medical decision. Society has to decide what we're going to do about boxing."

Casson had studied boxers for decades and had come away with no doubts that the sport caused brain damage. But when it came to football, he wasn't buying it. He later told Congress: "My position is that there is not enough valid, reliable or objective scientific evidence at present to determine whether or not repeat head impacts in professional football result in long term brain damage." In a 2010 article for *Neurology Today*, Casson quoted Charles Darwin: "False facts are highly injurious to the progress of science for they often endure long." He wrote that Guskiewicz's dementia and depression studies at North Carolina suffered from "inherent methodological limitations," especially a possible bias in how players self-reported their injuries. He wrote that the buildup of tau protein seen in the brains of "a few retired NFL players" was not "exclusive to head trauma." NFL doctors had been treating concussed players "in a cautious and conservative manner for many years," he asserted. Casson concluded: "The public has been led to believe that dementia and depression are a frequent and inevitable consequence of a career in professional football. This 'false fact' is belied by the presence of a large number of retired players who, despite experiencing multiple concussions, have gone on to have brilliant careers in broadcasting and other endeavors."

Cantu, while tearing into the NFL one afternoon at a conference in Las Vegas, described Casson to the audience of 100 researchers as "a neurologist that had studied boxers and should have known better." Guskiewicz came to believe that Casson was the single most destructive force for the NFL during the entire era of denial, worse even than Pellman. "Whoever picked Ira Casson should have been fired before *he* was fired," said Guskiewicz. Casson, in fact, had been selected personally by Tagliabue, he told Congress and others.

Even people who liked and admired Ira Casson felt that he was his own worst enemy. "Ira is a good man; he just can't keep out of his own way," said Lovell. "So dogmatic. He became a lightning rod. Presentation matters. I think everybody has a reasonable point of view. But when you dogmatically say this is all just like a scam, everybody writes you off. And Ira got kind of written off as a nut. His presentation is such that if you're looking for a villain, you know, he became it."

That April, as the NFL ocean liner was making its groaning pivot, Casson sat down for an interview with Bernard Goldberg, the writer and Emmy-winning TV correspondent. Goldberg, the author of works such as *Bias* and *100 People Who Are Screwing Up America (And Al Franken is #37)*, was also a correspondent on HBO's *Real Sports*. Goldberg was trying to sort out the growing controversy around football and brain damage. He interviewed Casson, the new cochair of the MTBI committee, to get the NFL's views.

"Is there any evidence, as far as you're concerned, that links multiple head injuries among football players with depression?" Goldberg began.

Casson cocked his head slightly.

"No," he replied emphatically.

"With dementia?" asked Goldberg.

"No."

"With early onset of Alzheimer's?"

"No."

The interview was taking place nearly two years after Omalu's report on Webster and months after the studies on Long and Waters had been published. By then, the NFL had established the 88 Plan in John Mackey's honor. The drumbeat of accounts of mentally disabled players like Ted Johnson kept growing louder.

"Is there any evidence as of today that links multiple head injuries with *any* long-term problem?" Goldberg asked finally.

"In NFL players?" said Casson. "No."

Goldberg said he walked away thinking: "Well, he's pretty sure of himself."

The NFL had replaced Elliot Pellman with a man who from that point forward became known to critics as Dr. No.

The rumors began to circulate that spring of 2007, when so much change seemed to be in the air. The NFL was planning a Concussion Summit, it was said, and even the Dissenters might be invited. "And then sure enough the invitation came by e-mail," Guskiewicz said. "I think we all sort of thought, 'Okay, maybe this is a good sign.' I'll be honest with you. I was a little nervous. You didn't know what to expect."

The NFL had undergone one other major change. Paul Tagliabue had retired after nearly 17 years as commissioner. He was replaced by his right-hand man, Roger Goodell, the league's chief operating officer.

It was hard to ignore how Tagliabue, as he walked out the door, had dumped a mushrooming health crisis in Goodell's lap. "Commissioner Goodell inherited a nightmare, truly inherited a nightmare," said Bob Stern, a Boston University neuropsychologist who soon would become involved in the crisis. "He inherited a cover-up." Tagliabue, of course, had long shared the MTBI committee's skepticism about the magnitude of the concussion problem. There was no indication that his views had changed. But if anyone was equipped to grasp the huge potential ramifications for the NFL—and the need to change course fast—it was Roger Goodell. After taking office at age 47, Goodell adopted an expression for what he believed was one of his main responsibilities as commissioner: "Protect the shield," he called it, safeguarding the integrity of the game. By then, Goodell had spent more than half his life in the league. He had dreamed of being NFL commissioner since his teens. Goodell's idol was his late father, Charles, a Republican senator from New York who lost his party's support and then his seat after sponsoring a bill to end the Vietnam War. When Goodell graduated from Washington & Jefferson College in 1981, he wrote to his dad: "If there is one thing I want to accomplish in my life besides becoming commissioner of the NFL, it is to make you proud of me." Goodell started his quest to become NFL commissioner from the bottom. He personally wrote letters to Tagliabue's predecessor, Pete Rozelle, and all 28 teams, asking for an opportunity to serve. He landed an internship in the NFL's secretarial pool, where he clipped newspaper articles and fetched coffee for the league's PR department. Goodell was now the most powerful man in American sports.

When Goodell took over the previous September, the concussion issue was not at the top of his agenda. At the time, the primary concern was how to divide the league's expanding riches, which would soon approach $10 billion a year, and the possibility of an impending work stoppage. The focus had changed quickly with the publicity surrounding players such as Waters and Johnson and the obvious disconnect between their personal stories and the attitude of the league's doctors, articulated most forcefully by Ira Casson.

The Concussion Summit was designed to get the new commissioner up to speed. There had been nothing like it in the history of the NFL. The league would gather all medical personnel—doctors, trainers, neurological consultants—in one room and debate the science of concussions. All the original Dissenters—Guskiewicz, Cantu, Barr, and Bailes—were invited to make presentations. Apuzzo was the keynote speaker. The attendees were greeted with a large packet of material emblazoned with the NFL's red, white, and blue logo. It included all the MTBI committee's *Neurosurgery* papers on a compact disc, a laminated sheet of "Concussion Information for NFL Players and Family"—Point 1: What is a concussion?—six pages of references to peer-reviewed studies on ImPACT, and even the Guskiewicz and Bailes depression study that the league had shredded.

Omalu—the man who had started it all—was conspicuously left off the invitation list. No one could say why. Bailes was asked to present Omalu's research.

"Why did they ask you? Why didn't they ask me?" Omalu said to Bailes when he first heard about the summit. Here was his opportunity to try to persuade the NFL that he was right, that he wasn't evil.

"I don't know, Bennet," Bailes said.

"He felt like he was being ostracized," said Bailes, who agreed. "It was pretty shocking that Bennet wasn't called. If it was real scientific discourse, they would want to have him there and they would want to pick his brain. You'd want to have *the* source there. Why would you want somebody else? Get him there, put him on the spotlight, like the witness stand, scientifically. Why wouldn't you want to do that? It's the truth."

The daylong meeting took place in a 218-seat amphitheater at Chicago's Westin O'Hare. The audience was composed mostly of white men in coats and ties. Goodell made the opening remarks at 9:15 A.M., emphasizing the NFL's commitment to the concussion issue and thanking the MTBI committee for its work. Apuzzo spoke next. Barr, who by then had developed perhaps the least charitable view of the proceedings, described the presence of the *Neurosurgery* editor–New York Giants consultant as "very strange. To me, it was like whatever pact they signed with the devil about having him publish their findings, he probably said, 'You guys owe me. I want to talk at the conference.' It's kind of embarrassing to have your grandfather get up there when you don't want him to, but that's what it was. He basically said, 'I do this for the Giants and I'll be happy to help any team that needs help with it.' He really conveyed to me he was really just interested in being part of the game in a pathetic way."

Apuzzo gave way to a series of 10- to 40-minute discussions on the topics of the day. Casson and Viano summarized the NFL's research. Cantu spoke about guidelines for returning to play. Guskiewicz gave a presentation on the risks of returning to the same game. They were all touchy subjects, the source of much of the hostility between the Dissenters and the league, but the atmosphere was civil, even collegial. It could have been any dry medical conference.

Then Bill Barr took the stage. His topic was ostensibly the "Role of Neuropsychological Testing in Return to Play Decisions." But really he had shown up to firebomb the NFL's research. As Goodell looked on, Barr repeated his allegations that Pellman and Lovell had left out thousands of baseline tests in NFL Paper Number 6, the paper that supposedly had shown that players recover quickly from concussions.

"I said that the data collection is all biased," Barr said. "And I showed slides of that. Basically I pointed out that we had been obtaining baselines on players for 10 years, and when you look at the study it only included a small amount of data. My calculations were that their published studies only included 15 percent of the available data. Let's put it this way: There were nearly 5,000 baseline studies that had been obtained in that 10-year period. And only 655 were published in the study."

Barr hadn't come right out and said it, but essentially he was accusing the NFL's researchers of fraud. The implication was that Pellman and Lovell had purposely excluded data that didn't support their findings. Those NFL researchers were in the room. Pellman, after his demotion from committee chairman, had been left off the program but was still on the committee and was seated in the audience. Lovell was still director of the NFL Neuropsychology Program and in fact had also been asked to make a presentation to the group.

Lovell already felt sick—literally. At four that morning, he had woken up vomiting, the result of a seafood allergy that had flared up after he'd gorged himself on crab legs and shrimp at a banquet the night before. "I was vomiting for like five hours," he said. "Then I had to give two presentations in front of two hundred people in this highly charged [atmosphere]. You literally had people sitting on one side of the room and the other." Lovell thought he might not make it. "I was deathly ill," he said. "I didn't think I'd be able to present, and I knew how that would look." Steelers doctor Tony Yates, who was also Lovell's physician, bailed him out by giving him Zofran, a medication used to treat nausea after chemotherapy.

Lovell recovered enough to present but now found himself under attack in front of the new NFL commissioner. Cantu watched from the audience, cringing. He'd had his own scientific disagreements with Lovell, of course, but he felt Barr's attack was inappropriate. "I really felt badly for Mark because I didn't feel that was the setting to be exposed to all this," Cantu said. Lovell tried to rebut the allegations. He told the audience that he had used all available data at the time of the study and that it was unclear why he might not have received all of the information.

The next scheduled speaker was Joe Waeckerle, a Kansas City Chiefs doctor and member of the NFL committee. Waeckerle was scheduled to present a 10-minute "Editor's View of the MTBI Research," but according to Cantu, Waeckerle instead announced to the audience: "Well, we now have these ethics issues to assess."

The NFL's Concussion Summit had suddenly turned into an informal ethics inquiry, with Lovell as defendant.

At one point, according to Lovell, Barr was asked about the missing data: Did the NFL have them or not?

"Yes," Barr replied, according to Lovell.

Barr said he did provide data to Lovell, but only up to 2000, four years before the paper was published. After that, he said, he was never asked for the information. As a result, the league had only part of his data. He said Lovell and Pellman never set up an organized system to collect all the data that were being compiled by the individual teams. But when the NFL wrote up the study, it implied that the data were comprehensive.

The NFL debated the ethical questions surrounding NFL Paper Number 6 before deciding that Lovell hadn't done anything wrong. "It came down in favor of Mark," said Cantu, who was still uncomfortable with what had just unfolded. "The net effect was he got exonerated in the open forum. But there was enough said before that it just was awkward, to say the least." Barr agreed that the consensus was that Lovell "didn't do anything intentional to not put data in there, but I don't think anybody concluded he did a great job on that research."

As the session broke up, Barr left the stage and made a beeline for the bathroom. "I had to take a wicked pee," he said. As he walked out of the amphitheater, Micky Collins, Lovell's protégé and partner in ImPACT, followed him outside, fuming.

Collins chased down Barr before he could make it to the men's room.

"What are you doing!" Collins screamed, according to Barr. "You're ruining everything! You're an idiot! Everybody hates you!"

"He got his nose right up in my face, like managers in baseball when they get in the face of the umpire and they want everybody to know they're arguing," Barr said. "I'd never had anything like that before—where somebody is just right in my face."

"Calm down, man," Barr said he told Collins. "Micky, I feel like you're going to hit me or something."

Barr looked down the hallway. Television cameras were hovering nearby. Collins began to calm down, he said.

"You don't understand what we're trying to do," Collins told him. "We're trying to do good."

"Micky, I don't believe in the science you're doing," said Barr.

Collins suggested that he come to Pittsburgh to see how ImPACT really worked.

"Micky, you're talking to me like you're trying to convert me in a religion," Barr said.

"You know what? It *is* kind of a religion," said Collins, according to Barr.

Collins acknowledged that he had confronted Barr but said he never raised his voice. He said he was upset about Barr's shabby treatment of Lovell.

"Bill, Mark Lovell is the most ethical human being I've ever met," Collins said he told Barr. "For you to attack him is wrong. You look like a buffoon."

He said he never compared ImPACT to a religion. "I would never use that language. That makes it sound like a cult; it's creepy." He said he merely told Barr that people gravitated to ImPACT "because it works."

In many ways, the confrontation had been building for years. It was a product of jealousy over ImPACT's wild success; the tension over the perceived conflicts involving Lovell, Collins, the NFL, and Riddell; and, of course, the allegations over the missing data first aired the year before by ESPN's Keating. Lovell even believed that his long-ago victory over Barr in the recruiting battle over Collins was a factor.

Regardless, the NFL's Concussion Summit already had featured an ethics probe and a near brawl involving two neuroscientists.

And it was only lunch.

Bailes presented in the afternoon, standing in for Omalu. The topic was "Does Concussion Lead to Pugilistic Dementia and Alzheimer's?" Also presenting were Maroon and Casson. They made quite a trio: Bailes, the genteel and brawny southerner; Maroon, the diminutive triathlete (and Bailes's former boss); and Casson, brimming with certitude.

The presentation was unusual in that Bailes was effectively describing someone else's work. This, too, provided a stark contrast. Omalu—a graduate of the Cyril Wecht School of Theatrical Pathology—was every bit the showman; love him or hate him, you couldn't take your eyes off him. Bailes, by comparison, was a plodding presenter.

It was nonetheless an extraordinary moment. As the NFL commissioner and the league's medical hierarchy looked on, microscopic images taken from dead football players appeared on the screen. Bailes explained that the brown splotches represented brain cells strangled by the tau protein. The almost certain cause, Bailes said, was repetitive head trauma related to football.

As Bailes went through one slide after another, he described the devastating symptoms produced by the disease: depression, dementia, even suicide. It was hard to imagine—the images seemed so benign, like flecks of paint on white marble. It was hard to connect the images to a man drinking antifreeze or knocking himself unconscious with a stun gun. Bailes didn't talk about that. He showed the slides and described what he thought was the cause. "The facts spoke for themselves," he said. "There wasn't really very much editorialization that I had to do. I tried to stay narrow and focus on just what the findings were. Having taken care of brain-injury patients for the previous two decades or more, I knew that the only cause that was known in medical science was this exposure" to head trauma.

As he spoke, Bailes scanned the audience for a reaction. He was feeling the weight of the moment. The conclusions he was delivering to the NFL and its new commissioner, he felt, were "extremely profound": Their game was causing brain damage. How much wasn't clear. But the results, combined with his own studies on depression and dementia in living players, were ominous. Bailes's gaze fell upon a man seated in the first few rows. As sobering as the news was, he seemed to be . . . *smirking*. Bailes looked more closely. The smirker wasn't looking at him but at Casson, who was standing off to the side.

Bailes turned to look at Casson. "I saw him rolling his eyes," said Bailes. He was stunned. As Bailes delivered his sobering presentation, the cochair of the NFL's Mild Traumatic Brain Injury Committee was mocking him! Bailes had presented dozens of papers and had never witnessed anything like it. Struggling to describe what he felt in that moment, he called Casson's reaction "unprecedented, totally unprofessional, egregious. . . . What other word can I say? It was unbelievable, inappropriate, unbelievable."

Bailes kept going. When he got to the end, he was met with silence. "There were maybe one or two questions," he said. "It was a lack of interest, a lack of intellectual scientific medical curiosity. And absolutely no line to, 'What's the next step?' "

Casson was now questioning Bailes's conclusions, which, of course, were Omalu's. Casson brought up his own experience with boxers and said these cases were definitively not dementia pugilistica as he understood it. The buildup of tau protein could have been caused by many factors, he said, including substance abuse and steroids. "He was really digging in and just totally unwilling to budge, and that was really their view on everything," said Barr, who was back in the audience. "They were like, 'Okay, I'll listen to you, but you're wrong. We gave you a chance to talk today, but you're wrong.' "

"I'm a man of science," Casson declared.

Years later, that was the line that stuck with everyone. Casson repeated it throughout the afternoon as a response to conclusions with which he seemed to disagree.

"I'm a man of science."

The clear implication was that what Bailes had just presented was not science.

Even Collins, who thought Omalu's research was over-the-top, was stupefied by Casson's performance. "I just sat there thinking, 'Why is Ira Casson such an asshole?' " he said.

Guskiewicz was apoplectic. It wasn't that long before that he and Bailes were standing together on the Pittsburgh Steelers sideline—Bailes a young neurosurgeon, Guskiewicz an apprentice trainer. As much as anyone, Bailes had helped launch Guskiewicz's career as a neuroscientist. Together, they had started the Center for the Study of Retired Athletes at a prestigious institution, the University of North Carolina, with the explicit goal of assisting and conducting research on former NFL players. Since then, they had surveyed and examined thousands. Many of the players were fine, Guskiewicz knew. Many were not. Now here was Ira Casson essentially heckling his partner and dismissing all of their work.

Guskiewicz thought the NFL's Concussion Summit had the makings of a *Saturday Night Live* skit, with Casson as the parody of a man in denial.

"Oh, my gosh, as long as I live I'll never forget that day," Guskiewicz said. "I use that as a teaching point with my students. I'm like, 'The day that you have to stand up in front of a group and tell them that you're a man or woman of science, your credibility is shot, especially when you have nothing to put in front of people to convince them.' That was a bad, ugly, ugly day for the NFL."

When the doors flew open, the league tried to put a positive spin on it. A dialogue had been opened. Further research was needed. The league was planning its own study on retired players, which it predicted would bring clarity. "You're looking for an answer," Pellman told Schwarz. "And the answer is there is no answer."

Apuzzo, speaking to a motley collection of football writers and broadcasters, described a concussion as a little-understood "ephemeral kind of event" traceable to prehistoric times, "when people would have a concussion, appear to be dead, and then rise. And what this did was to lead our ancestors in medicine 12,000 years ago to begin to bore holes in dead people's bodies thinking they were going to bring them back to life. So it's a very dramatic thing when that happens." As the editor of *Neurosurgery,* Apuzzo told the sports media, "I really am privileged to feel that I'm a journalist and a part of your family." But he was also the "principal neurosurgical consultant" to the New York Giants: "I triage the Giant players," he explained.

The NFL seemed to draw a distinction between Bailes and Omalu. Bailes was a reasonable man, the league said. He was at least open to dialogue and debate. Omalu was "out there stating things unequivocally," said Pellman. Goodell also weighed in on Omalu's assertions that the players had brain damage. "I'm not a doctor," he said, "but you have to look at their entire medical history. To look at something that is isolated without looking at their entire medical history, I think is irresponsible."

To Bailes, there was no distinction. He and Omalu were delivering the exact same message: Football causes brain damage. The NFL establishment appeared to have a problem not just with the message but with the messenger, too.

When Schwarz said he heard that the behind-closed-doors exchange got a bit heated, Pellman replied: "I wouldn't even use the word 'heated.' I would use the word 'lukewarm.' "

In fact, the rancor spilled into the ensuing days. Dave Viano, the new cochair of the committee with Casson, tried to get Guskiewicz to sign on to a statement that doubts remained about the effect of repeat concussions. Guskiewicz said the statement was similar to one contained in a pamphlet released to NFL players that fall:

> *Current research with professional athletes has not shown that having more than one or two concussions leads to permanent problems if each injury is managed properly. It is important to understand that there is no magic number for how many concussions is too many. Research is currently underway to determine if there are any long-term effects of concussions in NFL athletes.*

"How can you put out this statement? Do you really think you're going to pull the wool over the eyes of these people?" Guskiewicz said he wrote Viano, referring to league medical personnel who had attended the summit. "And he spouted back to me something like, 'That's insulting to me and to our committee that you would suggest that we're trying to pull the wool over anybody's eyes.' "

"Really???" Guskiewicz said he wrote.

"I was just like, 'Come on, get real. Who do you think you're talking to?'" said Guskiewicz. "That was when I realized that he was all about protecting the company, its name, and not about his own integrity. And that's where I lost respect for him. I thought he was one of the few true scientists on that committee."

Guskiewicz detected a faint glimmer of hope right after he left the meeting. He ran into Jeff Pash, the league's general counsel and the number two executive at the NFL. Pash, much to his surprise, was complimentary. "Keep doing what you're doing," he told Guskiewicz.

Guskiewicz came to believe the Concussion Summit was "the game changer, the turning point," but not for the reasons the NFL would cite in the statement he had refused to sign. Guskiewicz realized that Goodell and Pash "were in the back of that room saying, 'I've got a freaking train wreck on my hands here.'"

12

THE BRAIN HUNTERS

Although neither was invited to Chicago, Omalu and Nowinski had loomed large over the Concussion Summit. It was Omalu's findings, after all, that Bailes had presented. By then, Omalu had linked football to neurodegenerative disease in three dead NFL players: Webster, Long, and Waters. Nowinski had helped put the issue on the national agenda by feeding the Waters story to the *New York Times*. With the league scrambling to regain control over the crisis, Nowinski and Omalu moved to formalize their partnership.

The plan had begun to take shape in January 2007, shortly after the Waters story was published in the *Times*. When things settled down, Omalu wanted to travel to Florida to meet with Waters's family to compile a complete clinical history for his next paper. Nowinski set up the meeting and made plans to join him. Amazingly, the two men still hadn't met face-to-face. They decided to link up at the airport in West Palm Beach and then make the 45-minute drive to Belle Glade to see Waters's family.

Nowinski had seen a picture of Omalu that had run with the story, but the photo was taken from the waist up, Omalu wearing a white lab coat over a tailored light blue dress shirt and a striped tie. He was posed in the middle of a long hallway at the coroner's office in Pittsburgh, staring seriously at the camera. He easily could have passed for 50. When Nowinski saw him in person for the first time, he was taken aback.

"You look much younger than I thought," Nowinski told him. "You look smaller. You look like a college kid."

As they strode through the airport, they made quite a pair: the 28-year-old former Chris Harvard from suburban Chicago, tall, blond, and muscular, and a short, loquacious 38-year-old Nigerian doctor who had earned three degrees and five medical certificates and believed he could talk to the dead.

Nowinski found he enjoyed Omalu's energy and youthful personality. Omalu referred to his faith several times and seemed at ease with his new friend. He discussed a book he was beginning to write about his own experiences with the concussion issue and his battle with the NFL. He asked Nowinski if he would be willing to write the introduction.

As they drove west on U.S. 98, Nowinski broached the idea of forming a partnership with Omalu. He imagined a nonprofit organization based at a research institution that would seek to acquire the brains of dead athletes—primarily football players—and determine if they had CTE. Nowinski, like Omalu, believed the prevalence of the disease was extensive. He had become disgusted by what he viewed as the NFL's pattern of denial. In researching his own book, he had read all the *Neurosurgery* papers and, channeling his mentor Cantu, ridiculed "the NFL's tobacco industry–like refusal to acknowledge the depths of the problem."

Nowinski wanted to fight back against what he saw as a dangerous message. "I knew that if people trusted the NFL implicitly and the NFL leads the sports culture and the NFL didn't take concussions seriously, no one could take concussions seriously," he said.

He wanted to be an advocate for the athletes. He needed someone to carry the science. That would be Omalu's role. Nowinski thought that he and Omalu, along with respected older colleagues such as Cantu and Bailes, could compel the NFL to confront a reality it had spent years dodging. Omalu thought it was a good plan. He, too, liked the idea of directly challenging the NFL, which had tried to discredit him, but he thought the work also was consistent with his faith and a chance to bring some degree of peace and hope to former players and their families.

A few weeks after returning from Florida, Nowinski e-mailed a two-page document to Omalu. It was titled:

PROPOSAL TO INSTITUTIONALIZE NEUROPATHOLOGICAL INVESTIGATIONS ON PROFESSIONAL ATHLETES BY AFFILIATING WITH A UNIVERSITY RESEARCH CENTER

The proposal began with a summary of the current state of the research: three cases of former NFL players diagnosed with the "first indisputable evidence" of brain damage caused by football. "This has created a media storm, and may provide the needed momentum to force multiple sports to increase safety measures for athletes, especially at the youth level."

The primary goal outlined by Nowinski was to acquire more brains. He laid out a list of "Current Problems," including no formal process for gathering specimens. In the first two cases, the brains had essentially fallen into Omalu's lap, he noted. The third was acquired "solely on the efforts of one curious researcher"—himself. Nowinski also identified the potential for competition: "This is cutting-edge, groundbreaking, and controversial with real financial consequences for many parties. With the recent media attention surrounding the issue (NY Times, Wash Post), there will likely be new entrants to the field without pure research intentions."

Aligning with a university would give them credibility, Nowinski wrote, which would help as they cold-called families and medical examiners who wondered if they were "credible or crackpots."

Nowinski's two potential candidates to house the institute, both based in Boston, were the Massachusetts Alzheimer's Disease Research Center at Massachusetts General Hospital, which already had a brain bank with 1,000 specimens, and the Harvard Brain Tissue Resource Center at McLean Hospital, which held 6,000 brains. Nowinski noted that separate funding would be needed to pay for a "primary investigator" to find brains and develop an "automated program."

Nowinski and Omalu tossed around names for the organization before settling on the nonthreatening Sports Legacy Institute. They also wanted to come up with a catchier name for the disease itself. CTE was fine as an acronym, but Nowinski and Omalu wanted a name the media and players would embrace. Nowinski e-mailed Omalu some suggestions, trying to work the initials NFL into the disease: necrotic football linked dementia, neurofibrillar football linked dementia. But Omalu responded: "These names seem too long and do not have that sting to them." Nowinski tried again: (1) Football-induced CTE (FI-CTE), (2) Neurofibrillary Football Linked Dementia, (3) Footballer's Dementia (FD), and (4) Mike Webster's Disease. Later, Omalu sometimes referred to the disease as gridiron dementia.

To give their team additional firepower, Nowinski brought in Cantu, the man who had inspired his activism. "Remember, of anyone that you speak with in this entire business, he can be trusted most of all not to share confidential information or take ideas. He's already The Man," Nowinski wrote Omalu. For his part, Omalu brought in his own champion, Bailes. For legal advice, they added Bob Fitzsimmons, the head coach of Team Webster, who had taken the NFL disability board for $1.8 million. Barbara Jones, an attorney who had been Nowinski's agent on his book *Head Games,* also briefly came on board.

After the Waters story, Nowinski and Omalu had become sought after, in demand for media interviews and conferences. In late April, two months before the NFL meeting in Chicago, Leigh Steinberg, the agent, had resurrected his own concussion summits from the mid-1990s, aware that his earlier efforts had generated a lot of discussion but little change. The concussion crisis had come full circle. Nowinski and Omalu were invited to make a presentation, as were Cantu, Bailes, and Guskiewicz. Lovell was the only member of the NFL committee to attend. Invitations were sent to the commissioner's office, the NFL Players Association, and owners and trainers from every team. None accepted.

Steinberg excavated some of his material from a decade earlier, describing concussions as "a health epidemic, the consequences of which are a ticking time bomb that may not be seen in their totality for 10, 15 or 20 years." He continued: "What are the stakes? It's one thing to go out and play football and understand that when you turn 40, you can bend over to pick up your child and have aches and pains. It's another thing to bend down and not be able to identify that child."

But it was Omalu who had a far more disturbing story to tell. He put together a PowerPoint slide show for the scientists, players, and media to complement his presentation, "The Neuropathology and Delayed Sequelae of Concussion in NFL Players." If people thought they were in for a jargon-filled description of neurofibrillary tangles and beta-amyloid plaques, they were mistaken. Omalu opened with a series of autopsy photos. First came Webster, naked from the waist up, right eye open, left eye closed, and Frankenstein-like sutures along each of his arms. Next was Terry Long, also naked from the waist up, eyes slightly open, his tongue drooping out of his mouth. Omalu didn't show Waters only because Waters had blasted a hole in his head.

The pictures shocked many people in the audience, even the scientists who had examined their share of dead bodies. Many felt Omalu had crossed the line. "Some of us knew it was in poor taste," Nowinski said. But Omalu felt this was the nature of his business and an effective way to convey his message. It would not be the last time he showed pictures of dead players in a public setting.

When Nowinski gave his presentation, he used the name for football-induced brain damage that he and Omalu had settled on for the time being: neurofibrillary football linked dementia—NFL dementia.

By then, the newly formed Sports Legacy Institute had its sights on the brain of another player: Justin Strzelczyk (pronounced STREL-zik), yet another former Steelers offensive lineman. Strzelczyk had died two and a half years earlier at age 36 after leading police on a 37-mile chase on Interstate 90 through central New York. The chase concluded with Strzelczyk driving his pickup truck across a median at 100 miles per hour and colliding head-on with an oil tanker. He was killed instantly in the explosion. Strzelczyk had experienced a Webster-like transformation. He had played 133 games over nine seasons in Pittsburgh, retiring in 1998, but by the time of his death had become nothing like the free-spirited, goofy, intelligent man who had been beloved by family, friends, and teammates. Instead, he was paranoid and delusional, devastated by financial troubles and a failed marriage.

Bailes had been with the Steelers when Strzelczyk played; his death, like Webster's, had stunned him. He remembered Strzelczyk as a "fun-loving guy" who would tool around on a Harley, play the banjo, and carry around a bag of candy to distribute to kids "like some modern Santa Claus."

"His death really troubled me," Bailes said.

Now, as the Sports Legacy Institute sought brains, Bailes had a

hunch. He wondered if any of Strzelczyk's brain tissue had been preserved during his autopsy. That led to a call to the medical examiner,
who confirmed that he had kept some of the tissue.

Two months later, Schwarz had another story, this one on the front
page of the *Times'* sports section announcing that Strzelczyk had signs
of "brain damage that experts said was most likely caused by the persistent head trauma of life in football's trenches." Among the experts
quoted were Omalu, Bailes, and Ron Hamilton, Omalu's mentor, who
had played such a critical role in the validation of Omalu's original
work. Hamilton, the story said, had confirmed Omalu's findings on
Strzelczyk. He told the newspaper: "This is extremely abnormal in a
36-year-old. If I didn't know anything about this case and I looked at
the slides, I would have asked, 'Was this patient a boxer?' "

That story also became the forum for Nowinski, Bailes, and Omalu
to formally announce the creation of the Sports Legacy Institute. They
couldn't have done it better with a press release. Nowinski described his
plan for a nonprofit organization based at a still-unidentified university.

"We want to get an idea of risks of concussions and how widespread
chronic traumatic encephalopathy is in former football players," Nowinski told the *Times*. "We are confident there are more cases out there in
more sports."

To date, the NFL's efforts to shoot down the theory that football
caused brain damage had not gone well. Those efforts included—
but were not limited to—demanding a retraction from leading experts
in neurodegenerative disease, making public statements in an attempt to
discredit independent researchers, and convening a Concussion Summit
in which the cochair of the NFL's concussion committee mocked one of
the nation's top neurosurgeons in front of the new NFL commissioner
as he showed slides of diseased former players.

The NFL needed a new strategy. Ira Casson and his colleagues on
the league's concussion committee decided to bring in their own independent expert to examine Omalu's work—if, of course, he was willing
to subject it to further scrutiny. The cases already had been validated by
numerous researchers, including Bailes, who had been dispatched by the
American Association of Neurological Surgeons. Bailes continued to be

shaken by what he had seen. These weren't just case studies that Omalu was presenting; they were human beings Bailes had known personally during his days with the Steelers, people who had spent time with him and his family.

The night of the memorable meeting with Maroon—"Bennet, do you really understand what this means?"—Bailes's wife, Colleen, found him in his basement office, still staring at the slides of Webster's brain.

"This is a sad day for the NFL," Bailes told her.

Bailes had met Colleen in Pittsburgh when he was working for Maroon and she was working as a cardiothoracic nurse in the intensive care unit at Allegheny General Hospital. He knew she would understand. As they sat in the basement, Bailes first showed his wife a slide of a normal brain, then one of Webster's, splotched with the tau protein that had caused him so much pain.

"Here's Mike, our dear friend. Here's his brain," Bailes told Colleen.

She, too, was crestfallen. "For me, it was just really sad to have it come down to a slide of somebody who I knew," she said. "There it was: on a slide. It was just sad. And then he was the first. Little did we know others would follow."

But the NFL still wanted its own opinion. Casson set out to find an independent expert. He didn't have to look far. Casson had an affiliation with Long Island Jewish Medical Center, part of the North Shore–Long Island Jewish Health System. He was aware that North Shore–LIJ recently had opened an Alzheimer's Center. Its director was Peter Davies, a leader in Alzheimer's research. Davies was also recognized as an expert in tau, the protein at the heart of the CTE debate.

Casson contacted Davies and asked if he would assess Omalu's research and report back to the NFL committee. Davies agreed and soon afterward met with the committee at the NFL's headquarters on Park Avenue. Davies told the doctors he couldn't tell much from Omalu's papers in *Neurosurgery*; they showed just one picture from one slide that revealed one neurofibrillary tangle. Davies was baffled and annoyed; he never would have published a paper with so little evidence. He needed to see multiple regions with multiple stains of brain. Davies was skeptical of the finding, and it was clear to him that he wasn't alone.

"I think there was a really high level of skepticism" on the committee,

Davies said. "And in fact, you know, the thought of real exaggeration that [Omalu] was making a mountain out of one picture of a tangle."

"I need to see the tissue that Omalu took the pictures from," Davies told the committee.

Maroon, who had been added to the committee amid the turmoil, volunteered to serve as a liaison. That made sense: He lived in Pittsburgh, knew all the players, and had seen the slides.

Casson offered to pay Davies, but Davies declined. He wanted to avoid even the appearance of a conflict. "If you want my opinion, you'll get what I think, not what you pay for," he told Casson.

A few weeks later, Davies found himself seated in a large conference room at West Virginia University with Maroon, Bailes, and Omalu. By that point, Omalu had obtained brain tissue from six NFL players and two professional wrestlers. Omalu was wary. He saw Davies as a researcher, not a real-world forensic pathologist. He was a scholar, not a doctor. At that point, Omalu wouldn't have trusted anyone sent by the NFL. For his part, Davies saw Omalu as an overzealous coroner slightly out of his depth. The role of a medical examiner was to determine cause of death, not identify new diseases. He thought Omalu's research and staining were crude, not up to his standards. Later, he noted that Omalu, of course, wasn't a neuropathologist. When informed that in fact Omalu was, Davies exclaimed: "Wow, that's surprising! I didn't know that." It wasn't necessarily a recipe for agreement.

Yet the more Davies analyzed the slides, the more astonished he became. It was clear that Omalu was on to something big. Davies confirmed that what Omalu had found was definitely not Alzheimer's or any other disorder he had seen. The pattern of tau was unique, the tangles everywhere.

"It was obvious there was something there," he said. "I knew there was something going on."

Davies wanted to take the tissue back to his lab. He told Omalu that his lab could provide a more exacting level of staining. Omalu panicked. Should he really give up tissue to someone who had been hired by the NFL? But he agreed, telling Davies he would get him whatever he needed.

"I knew if they destroyed my slides, that was a good opportunity for me to sue them and become a multimillionaire," Omalu said.

A few days after the meeting, Maroon, now seemingly a convert, sent Omalu an e-mail of thanks: "The personal effort you made to meet with us is deeply appreciated. Like Socrates, you have been a major 'gad-fly' (in a complementary sense) in stimulating and provoking a more detailed examination in the underlying pathophysiology of TBI in sports." One day later, Davies wrote to Omalu: "I remain convinced that you have discovered something, a new phenomenon. . . . This discovery could prove of great importance to the field of neurodegenerative disease research."

Davies kept the NFL committee informed of his progress, forwarding his correspondence with Omalu to Casson and Maroon. At one point, Omalu suggested that he and Davies pursue research together, a suggestion that Davies encouraged. Casson tried to warn him off: "I would suggest great caution regarding Dr. Omalu's proposed paper."

Once back in New York, Davies received the tissue from Omalu. His lab began to process it. The NFL and Casson were eager to hear the conclusions of Davies's study. "Do you have any information regarding your staining of Dr. Omalu's material yet?" Casson wrote. "We are all very anxious to hear about your findings." A few weeks later Casson checked in again: "How is your analysis of the slides going? I am very interested in hearing about your findings." And then, a few days after that: "Dear Peter, I am really looking forward to your report." Omalu, too, was on pins and needles. The early signs had been positive, but he wasn't sure what would come back now that Davies had the material to himself. "Should we expect the results soon?" he wrote.

As Davies peered into his microscope, he couldn't believe what he was seeing.

"I remember that day, you know, it's one of those days where you're just so blown away by what you see: *What on earth am I looking at?*" Davies said. "I've never seen anything like it. With the best stains around, we're seeing far too many tangles. Way too many. More than I've ever seen in anything else before."

The results were so off the charts, Davies thought his technicians had botched the staining. He had them do it again. That was part of the reason for the delay. When the slides came back, the results were the same.

On January 28, 2009, Davies sent an e-mail to Omalu, beginning to lay out his findings. He was perplexed by one thing. There seemed to be two distinct groups: one with unprecedented widespread disease and the other also with numerous tangles, but not nearly as prevalent. He wondered if there might be a reason other than head trauma for the differences. He began to speculate that perhaps steroids were a factor. Nevertheless, Davies was convinced. The following day he wrote Omalu: "This is amazing stuff: you really have opened a major can of worms!"

Two days later Maroon, still acting as a liaison between Omalu and the NFL, wrote Davies: "I have been asked to comment on this and wondered if you could coach me a little on just where we stand on this. ANY input is appreciated."

Davies wrote back 38 minutes later:

> *I am forced to consider at least three different scenarios:*
>
> *1. That Bennet is right, and that repeated head injury produces this pathology, in certain (genetically distinct?) individuals resulting in a very aggressive disease.*
>
> *2. That some systemic factor (steroid abuse?) causes the pathology.*
>
> *3. That the two factors interact such that those abusing steroids become much more sensitive to head injury. Steroids may "prime" neurons for tau pathology following head injury, and render vulnerable whole populations of neurons that otherwise would not show signs of damage.*

When Maroon informed Casson, the cochair of the NFL committee indicated that he thought the findings still didn't implicate football: "WOW!!! Amazing," he wrote Davies. "This seems to raise more questions than it answers. Is it fair to say that something is going on here but it is not clear exactly what that something is?" He again cautioned Davies against collaborating with Omalu and Bailes "until your further studies are completed."

The NFL had brought in its own independent expert, but that expert had muddied the waters further. Davies had validated the magnitude of Omalu's findings. When he issued his final report, he differed only in that he thought some of the cases might have resulted from "either a toxicological or pharmacological cause, rather than traumatic events." That was scientific conjecture; there was no evidence that steroid abuse led to neurodegenerative disease (later, a Bailes study would show that it didn't). Davies also thought genetics might play a role. In light of the extensive history of mental illness in Webster's family, that certainly seemed plausible.

None of it was good news for the NFL. Davies was essentially telling the league it had two issues on its hands: head trauma *and* steroids.

At the time, in light of the way baseball had been consumed by the BALCO steroids scandal while football had stayed under the radar, the steroids scenario wasn't much better for the NFL. "Obviously this wasn't really what the head injury committee wanted to hear," Davies said. Interestingly, once the NFL realized that a steroids problem was in many ways preferable to the suggestion that the sport itself was to blame, committee members and league officials publicly latched on to the steroids theory as the possible cause of neurodegenerative disease.

Davies came away entertained by the experience. He wasn't certain football had caused brain damage in all of Omalu's cases, but it was clear that he had stumbled onto something huge. Casson hadn't gotten what he and his committee expected out of Davies.

"Rightly or wrongly, the perception of that original head injury committee was that they were downplaying the long-term consequences of concussion," Davies said. "Certainly, Ira Casson didn't believe that Omalu was right. And I don't think that anybody on that committee thought that Omalu would come out looking right. When he did, I think there was more of a panic mode, the realization that something was really going on here and it was very serious.

"I was kind of amused at the time. It was one of those things: Be careful what you wish for. You brought me in to find out if Omalu was right, and I said he was right in spades."

- - -

When Goodell took over from Tagliabue, he couldn't have foreseen how the concussion issue would overwhelm his tenure as commissioner and how damaging the discovery by an obscure forensic pathologist would be for his business. Omalu's conclusion that Webster had brain damage—and the implications that grew out of it—was quickly turning into the defining issue of Goodell's commissionership. After the precipitating event, the scandal continued to spin out in different directions, seemingly with a momentum of its own.

Omalu had become the fulcrum around which most of the action revolved. As the NFL continued to attack him, one of his closest friends, a Pittsburgh personal injury attorney named Jason Luckasevic, asked him one day: "What are you going to do about this?"

"I don't know. What do you mean?" Omalu said.

"Shouldn't you be doing something against the NFL, fighting back or whatever it takes?"

"I don't know. You're a good lawyer; you figure it out," Omalu said.

Jason Luckasevic was even greener than Omalu, a 30-year-old associate at the firm of Goldberg, Persky & White. He had a modest office near Duquesne University, where he had gone to law school. The two men had become friends through Luckasevic's older brother Todd, a pathologist in training at the Allegheny County coroner's office. The Luckasevics were from a sports-obsessed working-class family in the Monongahela Valley; their father was a machinist in a glass factory, and their mother worked at a credit union. Joe Montana had grown up down the street from their grandmother. The Luckasevics had Steelers season tickets and were devoted fans of the Pirates and the Pens. The family loved Omalu—his Nigerian perspective on life, his obvious smarts and religiosity. The Luckasevics invited him over for Christmas every year.

As Jason Luckasevic and Omalu spent more time together, Omalu began insisting that he would make a great expert witness and that Luckasevic should hire him. Luckasevic was dubious, for obvious reasons. Omalu was black, baby-faced, and foreign, not exactly the prototypical expert to persuade a jury to award millions. But Omalu was persistent and persuaded Luckasevic to use him on a major asbestos case. By the eve of the trial, Luckasevic was in a panic. What was he thinking? Omalu had never testified in an asbestos case. The trial was in a predominantly white rural county 90 miles east of Pittsburgh. He would get creamed.

Luckasevic tried to prep Omalu the night before, but Omalu just wanted to go out for a beer.

"Don't worry, don't worry," Omalu insisted

The next day, when Omalu took the stand, Luckasevic tried to lay the foundation to at least show the jury that his expert witness was qualified.

"Dr. Omalu, you are board-certified in anatomic pathology?" he asked.

"Yes," said Omalu, impeccably dressed, as usual.

"And you are board-certified in clinical pathology?"

"Yes."

"And you are board-certified in forensic pathology?"

"Yes."

"And you are board-certified in neuropathology?"

"Yes."

"And you have a master's in epidemiology?"

"Yes."

"And you're currently attending Carnegie Mellon University to earn your business degree?"

"Yes."

"And, do you have plans to be a lawyer."

"Yes," Omalu said, beginning to laugh, the jury joining in.

The judge finally asked Luckasevic to move on; he had made his point.

"They loved him!" Luckasevic said of the jury's reaction. "We won the case. I mean, it was a huge verdict for Indiana County. It was like almost $300,000. Ever since then I was a Bennet fan like beyond belief."

As Luckasevic watched his friend absorb repeated shots from the NFL, he grew protective. "Basically, I wanted to have his back as his friend," Luckasevic said. "They're saying that my expert and my friend is a quack, and he wasn't and he isn't. I wasn't gonna let his reputation go down the tubes for the NFL docs saying that there was nothing there."

"Maybe there's something that you can do from the legal side," Omalu suggested.

Luckasevic laughed. He was a lowly associate, spread ridiculously thin, with no time to tilt at windmills. Besides, whom was he going to find that would be willing to take on the NFL in court? And what was the case?

Omalu had a thought: What if you reached out to the families of all the players who had suffered, people like Terry Long's wife, Lynne, and the Waters family, and soon there would be others. Omalu noted that he knew some other potential expert witnesses who had been fighting the NFL for years, people such as Cantu, Bailes, Guskiewicz, and Nowinski. Omalu could make those introductions, laying a chronological history of the issue at Luckasevic's feet.

The young lawyer thought maybe it wasn't so far-fetched. He recognized he would have a long, long road before filing an actual claim, if it ever got to that, but it was *plausible*. In that way, Luckasevic was like Omalu—perhaps too confident and naive to know better.

It was yet another unlikely moment that soon would turn very bad for Big Football—two outraged young friends shooting the shit, thinking about how to sue the NFL.

Although such a lawsuit was still years away, its potential to wreak havoc unclear, the NFL found itself facing more immediate challenges that were also bad for business. To that point, the league's concussion policies had escaped regulatory scrutiny, but that too was about to change. The mounting press coverage—the steady stream of heartrending stories of former players who felt abandoned by the NFL—caught the attention of Congress, which began to examine the plight of retired players from different angles, putting more pressure on Goodell.

On September 18, 2007, the Senate Committee on Commerce, Science, and Transportation convened a hearing titled "Oversight of the NFL Retirement System." The hearing focused on the overall complaint that the retirement system was broken, that the league had abandoned the men who had built the modern NFL, but concussions and mental illness had become inextricably linked with that story.

One of the first witnesses was Garrett Webster. He had been invited to tell the story of his father's six-year battle with the NFL disability board, which had culminated with the appellate court's lacerating opinion and a $1.8 million judgment against the NFL rendered four full years after Webster's death. Garrett used the occasion to provide the Senate Commerce Committee with a sordid recounting of Webster's life after football. He asked if anyone in the room had any idea what it was like to shock one's father with a Taser to alleviate his pain; or if they had experienced receiving a desperate phone call from their dad, saying he was about to kill himself to escape the unending torture; or if they had watched a "once-proud, strong man" like Mike Webster beg for Kentucky Fried Chicken. But it was Garrett's story about how his father missed his tenth birthday without so much as a phone call—a man who once called him practically every night before bed—that left everyone in the room pondering the future of pro football.

"Later that month I found out why," Garrett told the rapt committee members, "when our family discovered Iron Mike Webster, bloated to over 300 pounds, shivering naked in a bed in a rat-infested motel, and at his side were not pictures of his kids, nor his Super Bowl rings, nor autographs or any glory that you associate with football, but a bucket of human waste, because he was too weak to make it to the bathroom."

Garrett was followed by a former player, Brent Boyd, who had played six seasons as an offensive guard with the Minnesota Vikings before retiring in 1986. Boyd had been looking forward to the opportunity to testify. It was a chance to tell the nation's policymakers, and by extension the public, his story.

"I do have brain damage," Boyd began. He asked the committee to please indulge his "invisible disability," which most affected him when he was under stress. Boyd explained that he had been diagnosed with football-induced brain damage in 1999. He said that he had been advised by a member of the disability board not to bother filing a claim because the NFL owners "would never open that can of worms by approving a claim for head injury."

The NFL's schizophrenic policy on concussions was beyond confusing at this point. The league had set up the 88 Plan for retired players with dementia, and the retirement board had distributed benefits to at least *some* players with brain damage. Yet its official concussion committee, cochaired by a neurologist universally known as Dr. No, continued to deny the connection between football and brain damage while

players like Brent Boyd testified under oath about what they perceived
as a conspiracy. Boyd likened the NFL to the "tobacco companies fighting against the link between smoking and cancer." He alleged that the
NFL had destroyed his medical files. His disability claim, he said, had
been denied by the board even though multiple doctors supported it.

One man took particular issue with Boyd's testimony. His name was
Dave Duerson, and he was also a witness that day. Duerson had spent
11 seasons as a defensive back in the NFL, mostly with the Chicago
Bears. He had earned a reputation as one of the game's fiercest hitters.
After retiring, he became a highly successful businessman, so popular
in Chicago that local power brokers recruited him to run for office.
During his playing days, Duerson was a player representative and took
the job seriously—an extension of a childhood that included standing
in picket lines with his father, who spent 38 years working for General
Motors and was active in the United Auto Workers. Duerson had been
one of the named plaintiffs in a federal lawsuit that led to free agency in
the NFL. After his final season, he stayed active with the union, eventually becoming so close to its director, Gene Upshaw, that some people
viewed him as an heir apparent. Upshaw made Duerson an alternate
trustee on the disability bsoard, and Duerson eventually became a voting member on disability claims such as Brent Boyd's, although it wasn't
clear how he voted in that case.

During the question-and-answer period, Boyd testified that NFL
players were never warned that concussions could destroy their lives.

Duerson came to the league's defense. There was no indication, he
said, that football caused brain damage. His own father, he pointed out
to the committee, "has Alzheimer's and brain damage, but never played
a professional sport. So, the challenge, you know, in terms of where the
damage comes from, is a fair question. . . ."

Duerson's defense of the NFL infuriated his fellow former players.
They found his argument—that his father had brain damage but hadn't
played in the NFL—bizarre and another indication that he was a sellout,
protecting the interests of the league. When Duerson walked out into
the hallway after his testimony, he got into a screaming match with Hall
of Fame linebacker Sam Huff and Bernie Parrish, a former Cleveland
Browns defensive back. Both players were critical of Upshaw, Duerson's

mentor. "Duerson was spewing profanities at Huff and Parrish," Boyd told the writer Irvin Muchnick, who ran the blog Concussion Inc. "He said, 'What the fuck do you know about the players union?' He was acting like he wanted to fight them physically." Parrish said he accidentally bumped Duerson during the melee, but Duerson "thought it was intentional."

Duerson had been charged with assaulting his wife in 2005 and, more recently, had run into financial problems. But to most people who knew him, screaming at a pair of respected former players in the halls of Congress wasn't like him. It seemed an extreme reaction, out of character.

No one had yet put it together that Dave Duerson—defender of the NFL, denier of football-related brain damage—was also losing his mind.

PART THREE

RECKONING

13

THE ART OF DISEASE

One weekend in June 2007, Chris Benoit, a 220-pound professional wrestler known as the Canadian Crippler, strangled his wife, smothered his seven-year-old son, and then hanged himself from the pulley of a weight machine at his home in suburban Atlanta. Details of the double murder-suicide spilled across the tabloids for weeks. Benoit, from Montreal (his name was pronounced Ben-WAH), left Bibles next to the bodies. Hours passed between the murders, during which Benoit sent cryptic text messages to coworkers with World Wrestling Entertainment, which alerted the police. Steroids were found inside Benoit's home, leading to speculation that he had committed the murders during an episode of "roid rage."

"I knew him well—nicest guy, plenty of concussions," wrote Nowinski, the wrestler formerly known as Chris Harvard, in an e-mail to his new colleagues at the Sports Legacy Institute. Nowinski had his own theory about what had caused Benoit to snap. The Canadian Crippler, he recalled, routinely allowed himself to be hit in the back of the head with a chair and often launched himself from the ropes, landing headfirst on his opponent or the mat. Within days of the murders, Nowinski was on the phone to the medical examiner and Benoit's father to secure his brain for SLI.

Shortly afterward, an ESPN crew showed up at Omalu's Pittsburgh condo for a story on Omalu and Nowinski—the odd couple suddenly giving the NFL fits. As they waited for Nowinski to arrive, the producer, Arty Berko, chatted up Omalu.

"I bet you would love to be involved in the Benoit case," Berko said.

Omalu smiled. "Can you keep a secret?" he said.

He led Berko to his hall closet. Tucked in the corner, beneath the winter coats and the umbrellas, was a large pail. It looked to Berko like a five-gallon paint bucket you'd pick up at the Home Depot. A towel was draped over the bucket. Omalu pulled it back to reveal a large piece of Chris Benoit's brain floating in a shallow bath of formalin. Omalu explained to Berko that he and Nowinski had driven to Atlanta days earlier to pick up the brain. Omalu planned to cut it up and study it once it hardened.

"It sounds like you guys had a busy weekend," Berko said to Nowinski after he arrived.

"What are you talking about?" Nowinski asked.

"I heard you're just back from Atlanta. Bennet showed me what's in the closet."

Nowinski was furious. "He wanted to kill Omalu," Berko recalled. The producer tried to persuade Nowinski and Omalu to let him report that they were studying Benoit's brain, but they refused. Nowinski didn't want to risk alienating Benoit's father with the disclosure, he said.

The Sports Legacy Institute had bigger plans for Chris Benoit's brain. After Omalu pulled it out of the closet, he found that it indeed was riddled with CTE. SLI used the diagnosis to further raise its national profile. Benoit wasn't a football player, but the case was consistent with the vision Nowinski had mapped out in his bullet points: to examine all athletes involved in contact sports. The organization hired a PR firm, Widmeyer Communications, which staged a press conference in New York to announce that Benoit had the same kind of brain damage that had been found in NFL players. That was followed by a round of national TV interviews, including a memorable appearance on *Larry King Live*. Benoit's father, choking back tears, told King the diagnosis was a revelation: "Larry, we were searching for answers. The world was black." But who would represent the Sports Legacy Institute? Larry could take only one brain researcher. The two neurosurgeons, Cantu and Bailes, bickered over who would get to do the Larry King interview.

Cantu prevailed on a coin flip, but like the flare-up at Omalu's condo, the tiff was another disharmonious sign for SLI.

To the outside world, the nascent research group, the first of its kind, looked like a natural alliance. The ESPN piece would portray Omalu and Nowinski as underdogs raging against the NFL machine. Omalu was shown cutting up brains. Nowinski pumped iron. The two men—one big and white, the other small and black—strode side by side, united. "The NFL has tried to discredit the work that Bennet and I have done, which has been pretty disappointing," Nowinski told ESPN reporter Steve Delsohn. "I wonder how many of these cases we're gonna have to put on their lap before they start taking it seriously." Nowinski tossed another grenade at the league: "I guess what we're dealing with is the issue that 32 billionaires are worried that they're gonna have the values of their franchises drop or that the game won't be as popular or else the players are going to start suing."

But when the cameras were off, SLI wasn't big enough to accommodate so many egos. The tension started with Nowinski and Omalu. Almost from the beginning, when Nowinski remarked offhandedly that Omalu looked younger and smaller than he expected, the relationship had foundered. Nowinski wanted a partner who was polished and reasonable enough to take on the NFL. He quickly determined that Omalu wasn't that person. He found him "unpredictable" and tactless, a feeling that was reinforced when Omalu revealed that he was keeping Chris Benoit's brain in a bucket in his closet or flashed pictures of Webster's corpse during meetings. "The seeds were planted early on that he wasn't going to be the right guy to carry the torch and be able to go toe to toe and stand up against the NFL or any other critic," said Nowinski.

For his part, Omalu came to see Nowinski as a condescending opportunist whose criticism about his ability to stand up to the NFL was laughable considering that Omalu already had withstood two years of attacks by the league. Moreover, Omalu was a licensed neuropathologist with three degrees and five board certifications. Nowinski, his concussion book notwithstanding, was a former pro wrestler and college lineman with a bachelor's degree in sociology. Omalu thought there was a whiff of racism about Nowinski's assessment of him. During their first meeting in Florida, he recalled, Nowinski told him: "You have a believability factor."

"He said that because I was not white and I was from Nigeria," Omalu said, "that Nigeria's not known for any breakthroughs, that I'm not an established scientist from an Ivy League school, that people are less likely to believe me."

Nowinski, though, said his issues with Omalu had nothing to do with race or culture. It was simply that Omalu was a "risk that needed to be managed."

From that crack in team unity, SLI began to split apart over a variety of issues, most of which revolved around money and control. Nowinski thought the Omalu Group lacked a cohesive plan. Fitzsimmons and Bailes were pushing hard to base the organization at West Virginia University, where Bailes still worked. Nowinski and Cantu thought Boston University was a much better fit, and they came to believe Bailes and Fitzsimmons were bullying them into going with West Virginia. "We were $150,000 in debt with no way of getting out of it, and I didn't understand what the game plan was," Nowinski said.

The members of the Omalu Group thought they understood Nowinski perfectly: He wanted to use their research—research he was unqualified to do on his own—to make himself rich and famous. The more they watched Nowinski try to seize control, the more resentment they felt. Bailes was one of the top neurosurgeons in the country. Omalu had discovered CTE in football players. Fitzsimmons was one of the most prominent lawyers in the Ohio Valley, the man who had beaten the NFL in court. Who was Chris Nowinski?

"There kind of was a feeling that the thing really was about Chris Nowinski, as opposed to the science and the research," said Fitzsimmons.

It all came to a head during a pair of conference calls with the founders. The group still hadn't resolved where to base the organization. Nowinski, meanwhile, was pressing to be compensated for his efforts. Fitzsimmons asked Nowinski how much he wanted. Recollections of the number Nowinski proposed varied between $110,000 and $160,000 a year. Nowinski told the group that he wanted to be paid retroactively to when SLI was formed.

Fitzsimmons laughed at him. "This is crazy," he told Nowinski.

The Sports Legacy Institute, which Fitzsimmons had helped fund with $10,000 of his own money, was broke, indebted from the public relations campaign and the creation of a website. Fitzsimmons had no interest in putting the fledging organization deeper in the hole. Bailes, too, began to object, but Nowinski "shut him down," according to Omalu. Nowinski suggested that Omalu was trying to shape the organization according to his own agenda. When Omalu started to protest, Bailes snapped: "Bennet, you don't have to explain yourself to Chris Nowinski."

Fitzsimmons had heard enough.

"I'm resigning," he said. "Good luck to you guys." The next sound they heard was a click. Bailes hung up, too. Omalu stayed on the line, chastising Nowinski for his impertinence to the two distinguished men.

Nowinski later said he and Cantu effectively ousted Bailes and Fitzsimmons from the new organization after deciding that "SLI would have a greater chance of success" without them. Nowinski said his salary demand was "a bluff" to test "their vision for who was going to lead this thing. It was, 'They're not looking out for me at all. If they're not worried about how I make a living, then there's nothing to [talk about].'"

It was an exit strategy, and it worked. Nowinski already had located another neuropathologist, someone who better met his criteria to "carry the torch" and be able to "go toe to toe" with the NFL. Not long after Bailes and Fitzsimmons resigned, Omalu said he received a call from Nowinski telling him he was no longer needed to analyze brains for SLI. Nowinski denied ever making such a call.

"Who are *you*?" Omalu said, incredulous. He said he found it hard to believe the source of the message, a layman who not long ago had called to ask for his help—or, as Omalu would put it, "this motherfucker who was begging me to talk to him."

Within a year, Nowinski had merged SLI with the Boston University School of Medicine to form the Center for the Study of Traumatic Encephalopathy. When that organization's website was created, it featured a history titled "Our Story." SLI was described as a "non-profit organization that was founded on June 14, 2007, by Christopher Nowinski and Dr. Robert Cantu in reaction to new medical research indicating that brain trauma in sports had become a public health crisis."

Omalu, Bailes, and Fitzsimmons found themselves erased from

history, as if they'd fallen victim to a coup. There was no mention of Bailes's labors or Omalu's research or even Fitzsimmons's $10,000 that had helped launch the organization that was now based in Boston.

To the world at large, the power struggle would have been unremarkable except for the consequences: It would determine who owned the issue of football and brain damage, a subject that continued to pick up steam.

The NFL was playing defense. Goodell's Concussion Summit in Chicago had been a disaster. Behind closed doors, the conference had only widened the chasm between the league and the Dissenters; publicly, it offered choreographed platitudes and nothing more. Coaches and parents were beginning to express concerns about the implications for youth sports. The specter of a lawsuit had suddenly become very real. When Nowinski and Omalu banded together to form the Sports Legacy Institute, they created an organization that would serve as a national voice for an issue that touched millions of Americans. Now divided, the two men and their associates were left to compete over attention, money, and brains.

In this respect, Omalu, Fitzsimmons, and Bailes had badly underestimated Nowinski. The savvy young activist had them outgunned. Through his relationship with Alan Schwarz, Nowinski had a direct pipeline to the *New York Times,* the most influential newspaper in the country. In Cantu, he had the support of the nation's preeminent concussion expert, a doctor with vast reserves of historical knowledge and an intimate understanding of the NFL's flawed research. Nowinski's alliance with Boston University was a masterstroke. It gave him instant credibility and access to the university's resources, including money and personnel.

Nowinski had made the connection through Bob Stern, a professor of neurology and neurosurgery at BU who also served as codirector of the school's Alzheimer's Disease Clinical and Research Program. Nowinski asked Stern if he could come by his office one afternoon to explain his new endeavor: an organization focused on athletes, especially football players, who appeared to have a form of dementia. Listening to Nowinski talk, "I had this gigantic reaction: I said, '*Oh, my*

God,' " Stern recalled. Stern found it "unbelievably fascinating from a public health standpoint, because if that's the case, football as we know it is going to be in trouble. And number two—and I think what turned me on most—was this is a disease that hasn't really been looked at. It immediately dawned on me that here's something that was a lifetime of research."

As the project began to gel, one key ingredient was missing: Nowinski needed someone to examine brains. In other words, he needed another Omalu. Stern could help there, too.

"Have I got a neuropathologist for you," he told Nowinski.

Her name was Ann McKee. Stern knew her from the Framingham Heart Study, a legendary project launched by BU and the National Heart Institute in 1948 to study heart disease in Framingham, Massachusetts. The study had continued through generations, branching out in different directions. McKee had studied the brains of Framingham patients after they died in an effort to map the origins of Alzheimer's disease. She had spent the previous two decades studying the intricacies of the tau protein, trying to figure out how the tangles first begin to form in Alzheimer's patients.

If Hollywood talent scouts set out to create a reality series on the search for football-related brain damage, they would start with Ann McKee. She was in her fifties, with blond hair and blue eyes, a Green Bay Packers nut from Appleton, Wisconsin, with a girlish giggle and a knack for making the brain accessible and fun. Describing how she removed the brain for study, McKee would say: "The brain is very delicate. You can't just pull it out or yank it out like sometimes you do with those other organs. You have to really deliver it. I mean, we deliver it like we deliver a baby." Seeing a fresh brain for the first time is "always a little bit like Christmas or your birthday," she said. "It's like, 'What do we have *here?*' " Watching the telegenic McKee slice into a formalin-fixed brain was a little like watching Rachael Ray carve up a cured ham.

McKee hailed from the sporting heartland of America. In 1986, *Sports Illustrated* dedicated 33 pages to Appleton in a search for the "essence of sport in mid-sized American towns." Appleton was "a town without a major league team or a major league garbage strike, a town that breathes clean air, sips fresh lemonade, does its shopping downtown and, with considerable relentlessness, pursues recreation when the work-day is done." McKee was not an athlete, but she was surrounded by them. Her father had played football at Grinnell College. Her older brother Chuck, whom she idolized, had been a three-sport athlete who turned down a scholarship at Wisconsin because he didn't want Division I football to distract him from becoming a doctor. He played quarterback at nearby Lawrence University, leading the Division III school to consecutive conference titles and earning All-America honors. McKee had been a cheerleader at Appleton East High. A tomboy, she played backyard football with her siblings and served as their regular punching bag. "Oh, Annie has her tough clothes on," the boys would announce, and then pounce on their baby sister.

McKee attended Wisconsin at a time when the university was the Berkeley of the Midwest, the heart of the region's counterculture movement. "I embraced it!" said McKee, laughing. A painter, she majored in art and married a musician. Neither her major nor her marriage lasted very long. She decided to follow her brother and become a doctor, enrolling in medical school at Case Western Reserve University in Cleveland. It was there that McKee developed her love of the brain. She found it endlessly fascinating, the source of all humanity. Everything else in the human body was "other stuff"; skin was facade. During autopsies, McKee liked to point out, "the face is actually inverted. That's a shock because everyone thinks their face is really, really important. But our face is just a layer of skin that you can actually roll down. And then you see the bony skull exposed, and you cut the skull and you lift off the skullcap, like a bowl. And then there's the brain: pink and gooey and gelatinous. It's kind of soft. If you poke it, you know, it's not rigid. And it's hard to believe that thing is what's controlling all this other stuff, that gooey, kind of pink thing. That's a real shock, I think."

McKee gravitated to neuropathology. She saw a connection between her interest in art and the patterns of brain disease. When she looked at the spread of tau, the tangles that strangled brain cells in the protein's destructive march, she couldn't help but admire it. She used words like *pretty* and *lovely* to describe the infinite patterns that tau formed, its "beautiful involvement" with neurons, even while recognizing the stark contrast between the disease's visual appeal and the havoc it wreaked on a person's life. "I was a fanatic about tau," McKee said.

That made her perfect for Nowinski. McKee would have a unique understanding of CTE, a tau-based disease, but she was the anti-Omalu. Omalu couldn't tell the Super Bowl from a cereal bowl, but McKee's entire life was steeped in football. Appleton is about 30 miles southwest of Green Bay, and McKee, almost by osmosis, had become a lifelong Packers fan, parking herself in front of the set every Sunday wearing an Aaron Rodgers jersey and a cheesehead. McKee also worked for the Department of Veterans Affairs. Her cluttered office at the redbrick VA complex in Bedford, Massachusetts, outside Boston, was filled with Packers memorabilia; she kept a Brett Favre bobblehead doll on her desk.

During her Alzheimer's studies, McKee had stumbled across a case involving a former boxer with dementia pugilistica. "I've been looking at oranges for years, and all of a sudden it was like, this is a banana," she said. "It was just thrilling." Later, she came across a fascinating presentation by Steve DeKosky, a fellow Alzheimer's researcher. It was the Webster case: "Chronic Traumatic Encephalopathy in a National Football League Player." McKee was jealous. She didn't recognize the principal author, Omalu, but the case fit the same pattern she had seen in the boxer. "I was really wishing I had that case," she said. She thought she could do better.

"Sorry!" she said, smiling sheepishly. "That's just my own . . . I thought I could do a much better job of lining up the pathology and really understanding it."

She looked for other cases, but they were hard to come by. Until now. Out of the blue, here was Chris Nowinski, telling McKee she could probably have as many Christmases as she wanted. Nowinski said he would go out and get the brains for her. McKee found him "handsome" and "impressive," a man of action around the same age as her kids. She couldn't believe her good fortune. She was fascinated by this area of research, and it involved football, a sport she loved. The players were her heroes. She might be able to help them, she thought.

"Yes! I would *love* to do that,' " McKee told Nowinski. She thought it was "like the greatest collision on earth."

- - -

Nowinski got McKee her first brain in February 2008. It belonged to an ex-linebacker named John Grimsley who had played in the NFL from 1984 to 1993, mostly with the Houston Oilers. Grimsley had a reputation as a hard hitter with a mean streak, the prototypical linebacker. When he retired, he launched World Class Expeditions, a company that organized hunting and fishing trips to places such as Texas, Mexico, and Argentina. For a time, Grimsley's business thrived, as did his relationship with his wife and his two sons. Then he began to lose his mind.

About a decade after Grimsley left the game, his wife, Virginia, who had been with him nearly 25 years, started noticing changes in her husband. First came short-term memory problems—forgetting why he went to the store, renting the same movie over and over. Then came the mood swings—anger and irritability. Grimsley always had been easygoing, relaxed with his family; now he would lose his temper without any warning or provocation.

The light bulb went off for Virginia Grimsley in May 2007. She and her sons happened to watch the HBO segment on football and brain damage that became famous for Ira Casson's denials, turning him into the NFL's Dr. No. But Virginia was less interested in what the NFL thought than in the description of the addled former players and their symptoms. "Mom, Dad is doing that already," her sons told her, and they were right.

Nine months later, Grimsley was dead at 45. He had shot himself in the chest. Police ruled it an accident. It appeared that Grimsley had been cleaning his pistol. Virginia told the *Houston Chronicle* that her husband, although he ran hunting trips for a living, had bought a new handgun with which he wasn't familiar. "Anyone could tell you that John would not take his own life," she said. "He was a happy guy. We had no financial problems, no marital problems, and the kids were doing well."

Two days later, Nowinski called.

When McKee got hold of Grimsley's brain, she was excited. Here finally was her chance to see for herself what was going on with these football players. Despite the previous studies on CTE, she needed to be convinced. "I trust my own work more than any other person's," she said. As she processed the brain, staining it for tau, she had no idea what it would look like. She thought the results might be inconclusive, reveal some other disease, or prove to be nothing at all.

Still, McKee was unprepared for what she saw when she peered into the microscope. She was stunned. This was the brain of a 45-year-old man, far less mature than the brains she typically saw in the Framingham Study. There was tau everywhere, "like disease on steroids," but unlike Alzheimer's, there was no trace of beta-amyloid, one of the main components of that disease. McKee would never forget that moment. In that respect, she was like Omalu, Hamilton, DeKosky, and Davies when they got their first glimpse of CTE. All had the same reaction. "It was like a scientific discovery," she said. "You feel like, 'Oh, my God!'"

Her first call was to her brother Chuck, the doctor. He had a family practice in Wisconsin and also was working as team physician at Lawrence University, his alma mater.

"You won't believe this," she told him.

She explained the disease she had found in John Grimsley's brain—the brain of a nine-year NFL veteran. It looked just like dementia pugilistica, she told her brother. The brain was riddled with disease, and he was just 45! Chuck's response would stick with McKee for years: "This is going to change football," he told her.

For his part, Chuck remembered not his own response but that of his sister, who seemed to grasp immediately how the news would be received. McKee didn't know Omalu and hadn't seen the NFL's attack on him, yet she sensed that many people would not be happy with her. "I think she had this feeling of, 'Oh, there are going to be a lot of people who really don't want to hear this and are going to be upset,'" said Chuck.

The case marked the coming out of Nowinski's reconstituted Sports Legacy Institute. Schwarz broke the story in the *Times,* revealing not only that SLI would announce the Grimsley findings at a press conference the next day but that the organization had established its own brain bank with Boston University. A dozen athletes, including six former NFL players, had pledged to donate their brains to SLI/BU upon their deaths. Among them was Ted Johnson, the ex-Patriots linebacker who had alleged that Bill Belichick had "played God" with his health.

Johnson told Schwarz: "I'm not trying to reach up from the grave and get the NFL. But any doctor who doesn't connect concussions with long-term effects should be ashamed of themselves."

The NFL, meanwhile, announced that its own study of the long-term effects of pro football probably would come out in 2010—16 years after the Mild Traumatic Brain Injury Committee was formed.

As Nowinski and his eager new neuropathologist were making news on the disease that Omalu had discovered in football players, Omalu was in Lodi, California, examining brains in his garage.

Omalu had beat a hasty retreat from Pittsburgh, a city he loved, after a Shakespearean drama that found him testifying in court against his mentor and father figure, Cyril Wecht. The celebrity pathologist had been indicted on 84 counts of abusing his position as Allegheny County coroner. Omalu became a star witness for the prosecution because Wecht, among other things, was charged with using his office to conduct private medical consultations and autopsies for personal gain—the same autopsies Omalu had performed for $300 a case, while Wecht, Omalu alleged, earned $5,000–$10,000.

Omalu was thrust into an impossible situation: He could testify for the government—and against the man he idolized—or he could refuse and face the possibility of being deported or even indicted.

"I was scared shitless," Omalu said.

Wecht understood Omalu's predicament—to a point. "His ass was going to be sent back to Africa; you know the way the feds work," he said. Omalu understood that Wecht didn't want him to testify. "He believed I should have sacrificed myself for him," said Omalu. Feeling like the world was closing in, Omalu quit his job and went into hiding. When the case went to trial, he testified for three excruciating days. Wecht never spoke to Omalu again, even after the trial resulted in a hung jury and the charges were later dismissed.

Omalu eventually landed a job as chief medical examiner in San Joaquin County, California, an agricultural hub about 80 miles east of San Francisco. While Nowinski gained power and recognition through his alliances with Boston University and the *New York Times,* Omalu and his colleagues were scattered around the country. The remnants of the Omalu Group re-formed as the Brain Injury Research Institute, a generic-sounding name they all vaguely disliked. The group was based in Morgantown, West Virginia, where Bailes continued to work as chairman of the neurosurgery department at West Virginia University. Fitzsimmons was still putting in 16-hour days in his Wheeling firehouse-office. The Brain Injury Research Institute's designated brain chaser became Garrett Webster, operating out of the two-bedroom apartment he once had shared with his dad in Pittsburgh's Moon Township.

There had always been a vampirish quality to the business of CTE. To survive and prosper, the researchers were on a constant search for fresh brains. But with concern about the disease growing, along with opportunities for money and prestige, the competition, now involving two research groups, grew more intense and macabre by the day. On May 25, 2008, another former NFL player died young: Tom McHale, 45, a 6-4, 290-pound offensive guard who had spent nine years in the league before retiring after the 1995 season. He died of a drug overdose. The story was too familiar: A successful restaurateur after his retirement, a Cornell graduate, at the time of his death the once thoughtful and friendly McHale "was very, very different from the guy I married," his wife, Lisa, said. "It was like he was a shell of his former self."

The brilliant smile, the charisma, and the polished presentation all disappeared, replaced by the often vacant and disheveled look of a man who no longer cared. Even more than becoming a football player, McHale had aspired to run his own restaurant. It was his passion, and he loved everything about it, from the cooking to the customers. Then one night, lying in bed, McHale told Lisa, "I'm not enjoying the restaurant business anymore. I think I want to get out." She couldn't believe it. The restaurant was "his baby, his brainchild." Gradually, McHale lost interest in everything. He stopped cooking and no longer went skeet shooting or bike riding. He began to distance himself from the people he loved.

The Omalu Group got to McHale's family first and made its pitch. Then BU stepped in and "convinced the wife to split the brain in two," Bailes informed the group in an e-mail. About a week later, Nowinski called Omalu to suggest that the two groups work together on this case. McKee and Omalu would analyze the tissue and then jointly contact Lisa McHale with the findings before making the announcement together. In fact, that was the scenario many researchers thought most appropriate. Sharing tissue and conducting independent analyses would help ensure the accuracy of the findings and provide a deeper understanding, especially for a scientific phenomenon that was not well understood.

However, by that point, there was too much bad blood between the groups. No one with the Brain Injury Research Institute trusted Nowinski. When Omalu e-mailed Fitzsimmons and Bailes to ask what they thought about Nowinski's proposal, Fitzsimmons wrote: "I suggest we do our thing & just disregard Chris." Bailes quickly agreed. The group moved ahead alone, without informing Nowinski. Omalu, who had set up a small lab in his Lodi garage, worked feverishly to make a diagnosis before his rivals. "I hope we can know the results before the Boston group. ☺," Omalu wrote in an e-mail to his colleagues. In another e-mail, he suggested that the Brain Injury Research Institute "may have to plan on how to optimize the utility of the case and possibly announce it before the Boston group. ☺"

On July 1, six weeks after McHale's death, Omalu sent an e-mail to his colleagues with the subject line "Thomas McHale, NEWS ALERT!!!!!!!!!!!!!!!!!!"

"THOMAS MCHALE IS POSITIVE FOR CTE," he wrote. "Please let us have a phone conference ASAP!! We have to announce this before the Boston group. We also need to inform the family. . . . Congratulations!!"

Bailes contacted Lisa McHale's father, David D'Alessandro, a surgeon who had become the point person for the family. He explained the significance of the results. Omalu followed up with his own call to D'Alessandro. But McHale's family was reticent about going public. "Lisa is still struggling with the diagnosis and it is my understanding that Lisa may be afraid of losing her benefits and rapport with the NFL and probably does not want to upset the NFL," Omalu wrote to his colleagues. (Lisa McHale said she never spoke to Omalu, and she didn't recall expressing to her father any fears about losing benefits or upsetting the league.) Omalu mailed her a copy of his report. Lisa was devastated. She hadn't expected brain damage. Her husband had had no history of concussions. She had thought his brain would be valuable as a "control," a healthy specimen to measure against diseased brains. In fact, McHale was sick, his brain riddled with CTE.

Bailes suggested giving the family time to digest the diagnosis. Meanwhile, Nowinski, believing he had an agreement to make a joint announcement, was trying to contact Omalu. McKee had completed her own analysis and had also found CTE. But Omalu wouldn't return calls or e-mails from Cantu or Nowinski. Finally, Nowinski contacted Lisa McHale, apologizing for the delay.

"Sorry, but we're having trouble getting in touch with the other guys," he said.

"Oh, they called me two or three months ago," Lisa said.

"Really?" said a surprised Nowinski. "Did they tell you the results?"

"Yes, they said he was positive for CTE," she said.

"At that point, I said, 'All right, fine, all bets are off,'" said Nowinski. "They broke the agreement." Among other things, Nowinski thought the Omalu Group had created a potential disaster if McKee had come up with a different conclusion than Omalu had. "If we didn't find it, it would be very confusing," he said. "And they wouldn't return our frickin' calls. I mean, what can we do?"

Nowinski told Lisa McHale that he believed it was important to go public with the results. Lisa, whatever reticence she may have expressed previously, agreed.

The plan Nowinski developed would put on full display his gifts as an activist. He proceeded to choreograph a piece of guerrilla theater on the NFL's biggest stage. He persuaded the McHale family not only to come forward but to make the announcement during a press conference the week before Super Bowl XLIII in Tampa, where McHale had spent most of his playing career.

In addition to Lisa McHale, Nowinski brought in the entire team for the announcement: McKee, Cantu, even Ted Johnson, the former Patriots linebacker. And, of course, Nowinski himself. The press conference was held at a Tampa Marriott. The turnout said a lot about the level of public interest at the time. Earlier that day, more than 4,000 people had attended the Super Bowl's annual Media Day. Less than two dozen showed up to hear that another dead football player had brain damage. But Schwarz was there for the *Times,* as was a reporter for the Associated Press, ensuring that the news hit the wires. A press release announced: "Leading medical experts at the Center for the Study of Traumatic Encephalopathy (CSTE) at Boston University School of Medicine (BUSM) reported today that nine-year NFL veteran, former Tampa Bay Buccaneer Tom McHale was suffering from chronic traumatic encephalopathy (CTE), a degenerative brain disease caused by head trauma, when he died in 2008 at the age of 45."

McHale was the sixth former NFL player to be diagnosed with CTE.

There was no mention that Omalu also had studied McHale's brain and reached the same conclusion. Omalu said he learned of BU's announcement on TV. Nowinski and the Boston Group had taken control of the issue and soon would be recognized as the leading authority on football-related brain damage. Omalu and his colleagues were destined to become an afterthought.

The SLI press release also noted that the group had discovered "early evidence of CTE in the youngest case to date, a recently deceased 18-year-old boy who suffered multiple concussions in high school football."

"This should be a wake-up call, especially to parents, coaches, and league administrators," said Nowinski. "We're exposing more than 1 million kids to early-onset brain damage, and we don't know yet how to prevent it."

Asked why the NFL had been so lax, Nowinski turned lawyerly: "I think it's because this is considered an on-the-job injury and it's a huge liability." He said he was in Tampa to recruit more players to donate their brains.

"I find these results to be not only incredibly significant but profoundly disturbing," said Lisa McHale, who would go on to sit on the Sports Legacy Institute's Family Advisory Board and serve as SLI's director of family relations. "We don't want to destroy the game. We want to make it safer." Even so, she said she was questioning whether she would let her sons, then 9 and 11, continue to play football.

But of all the people who spoke that day, none was more powerful than Ann McKee. In many ways, it was her coming-out party as a spokeswoman for the disease. She was a natural: thoughtful, reasoned, believable. She made it seem perfectly natural that on the eve of the Super Bowl, a neuropathologist was standing in a conference room showing slides of a diseased brain to a bunch of sportswriters. McKee pointed out the clumps of tau, the brown splotches that had eaten away at McHale's identity. This was not the normal brain of a 45-year-old man, McKee explained. It looked like the brain of a 72-year-old former boxer. McKee said she had been looking at brains for more than two decades and that what had happened to Tom McHale was not at all normal.

"I have never seen this disease in the general population, only in these athletes," McKee said. "It's a crisis, and anyone who doesn't recognize the severity of the problem is in tremendous denial."

Not long afterward, McKee's phone rang. It was the NFL calling.

14

BIG FOOTBALL

McKee would remember exactly where she was and what she was doing when she listened to Ira Casson's voice mail. It was that kind of call. She was taking part in a conference at the VA, and when she came out of a session, Casson had left her a message. "I was like, 'Oh, my God, what does Ira Casson want?'" McKee had never met Dr. No. She hadn't seen his virtuoso performance on HBO. She hadn't heard how he had mocked Bailes at the NFL Concussion Summit. And she had no idea that Casson, along with Pellman and Viano, had tried to get Omalu's work killed. But she had heard enough to be wary. "I knew he wasn't a friend," she said.

McKee returned the call nervously. Casson was pleasant and said the members of the NFL's Mild Traumatic Brain Injury Committee wanted to invite her to New York to present her work. They wanted to view the cases personally. McKee, though intimidated, welcomed the idea; she believed in the work, she knew it mattered, and she loved football. She hoped to convince the NFL that CTE was something it should pay attention to.

As they set a date for the meeting, McKee decided she "needed a little friendly accompaniment." She asked if Nowinski could attend, but the NFL refused. "Fine, I'm not coming," she said. The league relented, though it was suggested that Nowinski not speak during the meeting. McKee also decided to invite another expert in neurodegenerative disease, Daniel Perl, the director of neuropathology at the Mount Sinai School of Medicine and a consultant to BU's Alzheimer's Center. Perl was a heavyweight; among other things, he was the leading expert on a mysterious brain disorder found only on Guam. He had been fascinated by McKee's CTE cases. The disease clearly wasn't Alzheimer's, and the sheer amount of tau was stunning. Perl found he didn't need a microscope to see it: He could hold up some of the slides to the light and tell the brains were severely damaged.

On May 19, 2009, McKee, Perl, and Nowinski got together for breakfast in Manhattan before the meeting, not far from the NFL's Park Avenue offices. McKee was nervous but excited. She wasn't thinking about the future of football or even how the sport might need to change. She had important scientific information to pass along, and she hoped the NFL would take her seriously. Perl was expecting a straightforward academic presentation, like the hundreds he had participated in over the years, the audience respectful and curious.

"I didn't appreciate the political implications, okay?" he later said dryly. "That's the best way to describe it."

As they entered the lobby of NFL headquarters, McKee found herself in awe. It was cheesehead heaven. After being cleared through security, McKee, Perl, and Nowinski rode the elevator up to NFL Central, the inner sanctum, where America's richest and most popular sport was run. McKee saw the gleaming Lombardi Trophy, given to the winner of the Super Bowl; a trove of Green Bay Packers memorabilia; the legendary Jim Brown's old jersey. There was a waiting room with lined green turf that looked like it had been ripped from a stadium floor. There was no mistaking where they were. Even Perl, a casual fan, was impressed.

The trio was ushered into a huge board room with a lacquered table surrounded by plush chairs. Perl thought it was the fanciest conference room he had ever seen. There was high-tech equipment suitable for any type of presentation. As some two dozen participants took their seats, McKee noticed that she was one of just two women in the room; the other turned out to be an NFL lawyer. Along with the MTBI committee, there were a few other invited guests, including Peter Davies, the tau expert who to the league's chagrin had validated Omalu's work; John Mann, a Columbia University neuroscientist and psychiatrist who specialized in suicide research; and Colonel Michael Jaffee, the national director of the Defense and Veterans Brain Injury Center, which was seeking to collaborate with the NFL. One of the lawyers present specialized in class-action litigation, the visitors later learned. Nowinski believed the lawyers were present "to figure out what the researchers had and what to be prepared for down the road" in the event of a lawsuit. "They were clearly thinking about it already," he said.

McKee had prepared a PowerPoint presentation, but she also brought along a box of lantern slides with 4-inch by 5-inch slivers of brain the doctors could hold up to the light. She started with those, passing around the brains, and it immediately became clear that this was not going to be the academic discussion she and Perl had anticipated. Members of the MTBI committee seized on the absence of visible bruising to question how football-related head trauma could have caused the disease. If there was no contusion, there was no trauma. Of course, that was the point: Almost all the brains, from Webster's on, had looked normal from the outside. This wasn't a disease caused by a single blow or even a few. The brain was deteriorating from the inside as a result of repetitive, consistent pounding.

McKee turned to the slides. She pointed out the brown splotches representing neurofibrillary tangles of tau protein that had suffocated the cells. This always had been the most powerful evidence. The tangles were indisputable signs of disease, and there was little or no beta-amyloid, which meant it wasn't Alzheimer's. And these were relatively young men with one common trait: All had played football for years. To McKee and Perl, the experts, this suggested dementia pugilistica, the boxer's disease, now found in football players. Members of the committee again challenged her. Some wanted to know why the tangles weren't closer to the surface of the brain, where the trauma had occurred. It was a reasonable enough question, but it had an edge. To many in the room, Casson seemed especially combative. His questions were along the lines of "How can you possibly think that? How is that possible?"

"Casson interrupted the most," said Colonel Jaffee. "He was the most challenging and at times mocking. These were pretty compelling neuropathological findings, and so I guess to outright deny there could be a relationship, I didn't think that was really making an honest assessment of the evidence."

It was turning into Chicago all over again. Only now it was two years later, two years in which the NFL supposedly had made major changes in the way it addressed concussions. Hank Feuer, the Colts' physician and a charter member of the MTBI committee, said he was sitting directly across from McKee. He later said, "I honestly don't think we were any different with her than we were with anybody else. If we, for some reason, came across as being disrespectful, then I would say that everybody else we interviewed over the 15 years must have felt the same way." But as the meeting continued, the invited guests found themselves increasingly uncomfortable with the line of questioning. All had participated in sharp scientific debate. This was qualitatively different, they felt. McKee felt like it was more of an inquisition than a legitimate inquiry.

Mann, the Columbia suicide expert, had never met McKee, but he found her research compelling. It was obvious to him that she had found a serious brain disease in these players. After she was finished, Mann presented his own research, at one point describing data that showed how people who had had mild head injuries as children or adolescents were at an increased risk for suicidal behavior. Mann sought to connect his results to the cases McKee had presented.

Casson tossed up his hand and interrupted. "It would be impossible to link a disease like CTE to suicide," he asserted.

That wasn't true, said Mann: "It's not just possible, it's entirely plausible based on what I've seen from Ann McKee."

At one point, it was suggested to McKee that really, wasn't CTE just a "misdiagnosed case of frontotemporal dementia," a disease of the brain's frontal lobe? To which she replied: "Well, I was on the NIH committee that defined frontotemporal dementia's diagnostic criteria, so, no."

Perl studied the room. He, McKee, and Davies were the only experts in tau and neurodegenerative disease. He came to believe that no one else at the table truly understood the science. Or wanted to understand it. Casson and his colleagues—Viano and Pellman in particular—were most focused on proving that the cause of whatever they were seeing was *not* football. Perl described it as a "kind of unsophisticated denial. Now, admittedly it's not their field, okay? But we're the experts. Between Ann and myself, you had at that point maybe 50 years cumulative of look-ing at brains day in and day out." Perl did notice that McKee's message seemed to be sinking in with some of the other team doctors, particu-larly those who didn't have a background in the brain, such as the ortho-pedists and emergency room physicians.

They weren't saying anything, but what Perl saw on their faces said, "Holy shit!"

McKee had experienced heated debate before. Scientists in the Alzheimer's community weren't shy about attacking their colleagues. But this was different, she thought. It was almost personal.

"I felt that they were in a very serious state of denial," she said. "I felt like they weren't really listening. That's honestly what I thought. That's how it felt, like they had their heads in the sand. They didn't want to see it, so they didn't see it."

McKee also couldn't help noticing the preponderance of testoster-one in the room. She was surrounded by men. She already worked in a field dominated by men, and she was familiar with the look they were throwing her way. It said to her: "Is that girl saying something? Could we get a doctor in here, please? Could we get someone in here who actu-ally knows what they're talking about?"

Casson, Viano, and Pellman—the triumvirate that had run the NFL's concussion committee for years—bombarded McKee and Perl with alternative theories: steroids, nutritional supplements, high blood pressure, diabetes. On and on they went until finally McKee threw up her hands.

"You are delusional," she told the NFL's men.

Jaffee, the military doctor, had a sense of déjà vu. He had faced similar denials from Pentagon doctors who still couldn't accept the idea that concussive blasts in the field might contribute to mental health problems such as post-traumatic stress.

"There were certainly questions unanswered: Why everyone who played doesn't have this? What factors lead to it?" he said. "Those would be questions I have, as opposed to questioning if there is any relationship."

The two-hour meeting ended cordially, with McKee and the oth-ers receiving thanks from the MTBI committee but no promises for follow-up. As Mann prepared to leave, Casson told him how surprised he was that Mann had asserted that there was a relationship between head trauma and suicide. Mann couldn't tell whether Casson was genuinely curious or dismissive. "My reaction was, if he believes it, they'll be in touch pretty fast," he said.

Mann never heard from Casson or anyone from the MTBI committee again.

Out on Park Avenue, McKee, Nowinski, and Perl reflected for a few minutes, shocked by what they had just experienced. McKee was relieved it was over. It was clear to her that "we hadn't made a dent in anybody's opinion."

She couldn't wait to call her brother Chuck back in Wisconsin. He had to hear this not just because he was a doctor but because he was a sideline physician and a former football star. As McKee recounted the meeting, Chuck grew more and more angry that his sister had been attacked by those know-nothing doctors. Soon he and McKee were feeding off each other, blasting the league: *You wouldn't fucking believe these guys. These guys are such assholes.*

"Mental corruption, I think, is what we were talking about," Chuck McKee recalled. "That word never came up, that phrase never came up, but just that these people, what's the quote, 'A man will not believe something that his livelihood depends on his not believing.' You know, that's kind of what it's about. These people could not believe that because it meant that they were marginalized. And that was so clear, that this was about their protecting their own stake in the NFL and their positions as medical advisers. And they didn't give a damn about the data, and they didn't give a damn about the players."

The committee, of course, had already taken a public position on the matter in published papers and commentary. To acknowledge otherwise was to admit that the NFL's men were wrong, incompetent, or both.

As their conversation ended, Chuck McKee had one last message for his baby sister: "Just hang in there, kid. You're right and they're wrong."

By now, it was hard for the NFL to say it hadn't been warned. McKee, of course, was just the latest authority to go directly to the league with her concerns. Over the previous decade, the roster of neuroscientists making the case that football led to higher rates of depression, memory loss, dementia, and brain damage read like an all-star team of researchers: Barry Jordan, Kevin Guskiewicz, Julian Bailes, Bob Cantu, Bob Stern, Ron Hamilton, Steve DeKosky, Danny Perl, Bennet Omalu, Ann McKee. The warnings had come in the form of player surveys, research papers, autopsy studies, and innumerable public statements by experts and former players. Bailes and Guskiewicz had delivered the message personally to Goodell at the 2007 summit in Chicago. And now, two years later, McKee and Perl had brought the message to the NFL's doorstep. Meanwhile, the number of dead football players with CTE continued to mount.

Jason Luckasevic didn't know the half of it, but he still thought he had enough ammunition to sue the NFL. The young Pittsburgh lawyer originally had been motivated by his desire to protect his friend Omalu back when Omalu was under attack by the league's doctors. At the time, Luckasevic hadn't had the slightest clue to what kind of case he might bring. But as he looked at the situation more closely, Luckasevic thought that what had happened to Omalu was part of a pattern that went back at least to the publication of the first NFL papers and possibly as far back as the formation of the MTBI committee in 1994. One of the more curious aspects of the concussion crisis was that almost everyone who ended up taking on the NFL *loved* the NFL. Luckasevic was no exception. He bled Steelers black and gold. Yet he came to see himself as an advocate for the players, many of whom simply wanted the league to acknowledge their suffering.

From a legal standpoint, what Luckasevic was considering was by any measure preposterous, the ultimate David and Goliath story. He was a small-time personal injury lawyer, an associate at the Pittsburgh firm of Goldberg, Persky & White. The NFL was, well, the NFL: a multi-billion-dollar industry with a legal winning percentage that rivaled that of Lombardi's Packers. A cursory glance at the NFL's case history told Luckasevic that one major hurdle—among many major hurdles—was that the league could fall back on the collective bargaining agreement with the players to argue that the claims didn't belong in court. The contract specifically set up the Bert Bell/Pete Rozelle NFL Player Retirement Plan to deal with long-term health problems related to NFL combat. To the extent that the league might be liable, it was the individual teams, not the league, that managed injuries. The league would argue that the players' recourse was to appeal through the retirement plan or to bring workers' compensation claims against their teams.

Luckasevic thought that couldn't possibly be right. If the NFL had willfully denied or even concealed repeated warnings that football causes brain damage—and at that point there was no doubt in his mind that it had—that was a qualitatively different proposition. Luckasevic thought the collective bargaining agreement (CBA) couldn't protect the league from claims of negligence and fraud. "For me, it became an issue that, look, this isn't about a collective bargaining agreement," he said. "This is about something that they owe the players—as basic as the ball is to the game. I mean, you can't just hide from somebody that there's something inherently dangerous in my sport that's going to hurt you. You can't just lie to people about your sport." That became the core of Luckasevic's case: The NFL had had ample warning that football causes brain damage, but the league's response had been to deny that information and cover it up.

Even that, Luckasevic knew, would be a very tough sell. Who could possibly argue that the players didn't know what they were getting into when they strapped it on? But he would deal with that later. A similar claim had been made about smokers, after all.

Luckasevic began to look for cases that picked apart the argument that the CBA protected the league—a shield for the Shield. One such case, he felt, was *Brown, et al. v. N.F.L.*, a bizarre 2001 suit brought by Orlando Brown, a 6-foot-7, 360-pound offensive tackle who went by the nickname Zeus. While playing for Cleveland, Brown had been hit in the right eye by a penalty flag during a game against the Jaguars, temporarily blinding him. At the time, Brown was one of the highest-paid offensive linemen in the game, his contract worth nearly $35 million. The injury knocked him out of the sport for several years, though he did return in 2003 (Brown died at 40 in 2011 of an ailment related to diabetes). Brown sued the NFL for $200 million, arguing that the referee who hurled the penalty flag was a league employee whose negligence superseded the protection of the CBA. The NFL settled the case for an estimated $15 to $25 million in 2002.

Luckasevic began to line up consultants and expert witnesses. One of the first was none other than Nowinski. On September 19, 2007, the activist and author of *Head Games* quietly signed a $5,000 retainer to "perform litigation services relating to potential and/or actual claims that may be asserted by one or more of our clients against the National Football League and others." Those services included "performing primary and secondary research regarding, among others, concussions in the NFL and related medical care and policies, epidemiology, helmets, player contracts, collective bargaining agreements and the '88 Plan.'" Luckasevic later ended the contract, feeling that Nowinski had promised much and delivered little, but questions lingered about whether Nowinski continued his involvement in the suit. When Nowinski was asked in spring 2013 if he was still consulting for lawyers suing the NFL, he replied: "Where did you hear that?" After a long pause, he said: "I have no comment." A few hours later, he wrote in an e-mail that "all of my consulting agreements" are vetted by the Sports Legacy Institute's board. A few months later, when interviewed again—this time with a lawyer and a PR person on the line with him—Nowinski reiterated his no-comment. Asked specifically about the 2007 agreement, he said, "That doesn't exist; you don't have a contract." After he was read the specific language from the contract, which had been obtained by the authors, he said, "I don't have any recollection of signing that contract."

Other researchers who had challenged the NFL would stay as far away from the lawsuit as possible, fearing it could compromise their independence. Guskiewicz, for one, said he could have built "a beach house on both coasts" with the money lawyers offered him, but he turned them all down.

As he pressed forward, Luckasevic thought more and more that he had a viable case. He decided he was ready to take it to his bosses. He needed to convince them that it was worth his time and their money. He made his pitch during a meeting with the partners. Explaining the case, he told them he wanted to take on the National Football League.

They laughed at him. The players were simply crazy, they told him. Moreover, the players had known that football was dangerous; *everybody* knew that. How would he prove to a jury that their problems were related to some brain disease, much less a sport? "I'd love to cross-examine these experts," one partner told Luckasevic. "I'd have a field day if I was the NFL's lawyer."

"They practically laughed me out of the room, to put it nicely," Luckasevic recalled.

It wasn't that Goldberg, Persky & White was afraid of the NFL. The firm had helped pioneer asbestos litigation in the rust belt. But beyond the partners' howling skepticism about the potential for a lawsuit, the case probably would require a huge number of man-hours. It wasn't a case that one lawyer or even necessarily one firm could take on.

Finally, Luckasevic pleaded: "If I can pull this together, are you okay with it?"

The partners agreed to give him time to fish around as long as his other work didn't suffer. Here was a glimmer of hope. Luckasevic started cold-calling firms with a history of bringing class-action suits, but the reaction was much the same. "It was like being a musician and wanting to get your album bought or somebody to produce it," he said. The standard response was "We'll get back to you." At one point, Luckasevic thought he had a partner in a Houston-based firm, Lanier, which had won a $253 million judgment in the first lawsuit related to Vioxx, the notorious pain medication manufactured by Merck. But Lanier's lawyers ultimately pulled out after the NFL updated its concussion guidelines in 2007, telling Luckasevic they thought the move created timing and statutory problems.

By 2010, Luckasevic had neither clients nor a partner and was close to giving up. He was working closely with Jack Tierney, an older attorney in semi-retirement at Goldberg, Persky. Tierney had become Luckasevic's primary source of encouragement, "the only guy to support me, believe in me, believe in the case." When Luckasevic told Tierney he was ready to throw in the towel, Tierney said there was a lawyer in Miami that perhaps they should try. Herman Russomanno was just coming off a big win. He and another personal injury attorney, Stuart Ratzan, had won $11.5 million for O. J. McDuffie, a former Miami Dolphins receiver who had sued the team and its doctor for malpractice. McDuffie had led the AFC in receptions in 1998 and then sustained an injury to his left big toe that forced him to retire.

"Jack, I've already been told no about two dozen times," Luckasevic said, wallowing in pessimism and self-pity. "Is this a joke? Do you want me to be told no again? I mean, seriously, give me a break."

"Fine, I'll call them," Tierney said.

Tierney was right. Russomanno was prepared to join the fight. Not only that, he told Tierney and Luckasevic he had a big gun in Los Angeles who might be interested, too. His name was Tom Girardi, and he had extensive experience suing utility giants and pharmaceutical companies. Girardi had been part of the famous "Erin Brockovich" lawsuit that won a $333 million settlement from Pacific Gas & Electric for leaking a toxic chemical into the groundwater of tiny Hinkley, California. Girardi thought the cases were similar: PG&E, like the NFL, had ignored warnings for years. "You have these players that have been knocked around," he said. "You have studies that are done with respect to the constant hitting of somebody's head; they are well known in the medical community. And that was information we can prove was given to the NFL."

There was an obvious disconnect. The dire warnings from the experts, the stirrings of a class-action lawsuit, and the steady parade of diseased ex-players all pointed to a gathering storm. Yet the NFL mostly carried on business as usual. There were changes—the 88 Plan, mandatory neuropsychological testing, a blizzard of concussion literature distributed by the league—but the response was hardly commensurate with the industry-rattling developments in the air. It was like reeling in the laundry in the path of a giant tornado. The MTBI committee stood largely intact. Pellman, the former chairman, had been reassigned but continued to work as NFL medical director and remained part of the committee. The MTBI committee kept on publishing: NFL Paper Number 16 ran in the June 2009 issue of *Neurosurgery*. That study involved bashing rats in the head to simulate "impacts . . . experienced by professional football players." The results: "no or minimal brain injury" for the players, although the rats admittedly took a beating.

What would it take for the NFL finally to respond? That September, Schwarz, the intrepid *Times* reporter, came out with another confounding story. The NFL had commissioned a study that reported that former players between 30 and 49 years old were 19 times more likely to have Alzheimer's disease and other mental disorders than the normal rate among men that age. Bailes, whose own studies a decade earlier had shown the exact same thing, called the findings "a game-changer. . . . The ball's now in the NFL's court. They always say, 'We're going to do our own studies.' And now they have."

Aiello, the league spokesman, had the unenviable assignment of attacking the NFL's own work. The league-funded study by the University of Michigan's Institute for Social Research didn't formally diagnose the players with dementia, he said, and was limited because the information was derived from unreliable phone surveys. It was essentially the same argument Feuer had used to dismiss the work of Bailes and Guskiewicz as "virtually worthless" except that Aiello was using the argument against the NFL.

A few days later, in response to the latest disclosures, the House Judiciary Committee announced that it would hold hearings on football and brain damage.

Democratic committee staffers had been looking for an opportunity to bring the NFL back to Washington ever since the dramatic but obscure 2007 hearings on retired players in which Garrett Webster had described finding his addled father at a roach motel next to "a bucket of human waste." The NFL had managed to prevent the commissioner from testifying at those hearings, but this time the committee would insist on Goodell's attendance. The hearings held out the promise of drama and confrontation, a chance in many ways to put the NFL on trial for its handling of the concussion issue.

Weeks of not unexpected maneuvering preceded the hearings as committee staffers put together a roster of potential witnesses. Many were drawn from the neuroscience all-star team: Cantu, Bailes, Maroon, McKee. The fact that Omalu wasn't invited—and Nowinski was—was an indication of how far he had fallen and Nowinski had risen. After some resistance, the NFL agreed to send Goodell. But other potential witnesses—notably Casson, Viano, and Pellman—never got near the hearings. Committee staffers, working through the NFL's lobbyist, Jeff Miller, had asked for recommendations of NFL doctors who could testify. The league came back with three, none of whom were the current or former chairs of the MTBI committee. Eric Tamarkin, the counsel for the Democratic majority, said he personally reached out to Casson, who ultimately did not testify.

Right up to the hearing, the NFL worked to massage the imagery and the message. One of the witnesses scheduled to appear with Goodell was Dick Benson, an Austin, Texas, man whose 17-year-old son, Will, a high school quarterback, had died in 2002 several weeks after sustaining a concussion. Benson had spent four years pushing for passage of "Will's Bill," which mandated training for high school coaches and trainers. Benson's testimony would be a powerful reminder of how the issue trickled down to the 3 million kids who played tackle football. Tamarkin informed Miller, the NFL's lobbyist, that he intended to put Benson on the same panel with Goodell.

"He went apoplectic," Tamarkin said. "Having a picture of a kid who passed away from playing football, he didn't want that message to be on the same panel." Tamarkin agreed to change the order. "We didn't want to sandbag anybody," he said. Instead, Gay Culverhouse, former president of the Tampa Bay Buccaneers, was placed on the panel that included Goodell. Culverhouse, whose father, Hugh, had owned the Bucs, had become an outspoken critic of the league, referred to by some retired players as a "rebel with a cause."

On October 28, 2009, the packed hearing was called to order at 10:03 A.M. in the Rayburn Building. The chairman, Michigan Democrat John Conyers, began: "Everyone that plays football at any level knows it is a dangerous sport. In fact, everyone that watches it knows it is a dangerous sport. There should be no surprise when a football player separates his shoulder, twists an ankle, busts a knee. But over the past several years, an increasing number of retired players have developed long-term memory and cognitive diseases such as dementia, Alzheimer's, depression, and chronic traumatic encephalopathy."

Conyers added, "There appears to be growing evidence that playing football may be linked to long-term brain damage."

Tamarkin and others had hoped to get Goodell finally to concede the link. In his opening statement, the commissioner, wearing a light blue tie with thin white stripes, and a yellow ribbon in support of the military, gave a bland review of the league's accomplishments on player safety and head injuries during his first three years. Goodell told the committee that he expected the NFL soon would announce its support for research into CTE. Goodell mentioned nothing about the link between football and brain damage, though in his written statement he allowed: "It is fair to say head trauma may play a role."

"Commissioner Goodell, is there a link between playing professional football and the likelihood of contracting a brain-related injury such as dementia, Alzheimer's, depression, or CTE?" Conyers asked, getting straight to the point during the question-and-answer period.

Goodell said the league was not waiting "for that debate to continue" among medical experts but instead was doing everything "we possibly can for our players now." He continued for nearly a minute before Conyers interrupted.

"Well, you have testified to that. But I just asked you a simple question. What's the answer?"

"The answer is, the medical experts would know better than I would with respect to that. But we are not treating that in any way in delaying anything that we do. We are reinforcing our commitment to make sure we make the safest possible deal for our—"

Conyers again cut him off dismissively: "All right. Okay. I have heard it."

Goodell wasn't Casson, but in his own equivocating way, the commissioner was just as resistant. Then, toward the end of the session, Linda Sanchez, a perky Los Angeles Democrat, ruined the NFL's day. Sanchez had been a driving force behind the 2007 hearings. A former labor lawyer, she had been elected in 2002, joining Loretta Sanchez as the first sisters to serve together in Congress. Their father, a Mexican immigrant and former machinist, had Alzheimer's disease. Sanchez said she regretted that Ira Casson hadn't made it to the hearing "because there are a number of really great questions I would have loved to have asked him." She still managed to make his presence felt by showing a clip of Dr. No's rapid-fire denials to HBO.

Sanchez asked Goodell to read aloud from the NFL pamphlet telling players that "current research" had not shown that repeated concussions lead to permanent problems, a statement that seemed to contradict a lot of current research.

"Okay. Thank you," Sanchez said politely when the commissioner was finished. Then she cheerfully tore into him:

"I am a little concerned—and I hear the concern expressed by some of the witnesses on the panel today—that the NFL sort of has this kind of blanket denial or minimizing of the fact that there may be this link. And it sort of reminds me of the tobacco companies pre-1990s when they kept saying, 'No, there is no link between smoking and damage to your health or ill effects.' And they were forced to admit that that was incorrect through a spate of litigation in the 1990s. Don't you think the league would be better off legally, and that our youth might be a little bit better off in terms of knowledge, if you guys just embraced that there is research that suggests this and admitted to it?"

It was a nightmare scenario for the NFL: the comparison to Big Tobacco. Others had made it before. Nowinski drew the analogy in *Head Games*; on a shelf in his office at BU, he displayed a book, *The Biologic Effects of Tobacco*. Brent Boyd, the former Vikings offensive lineman, repeatedly made the case that the NFL was like the powerful tobacco companies "fighting against the link between smoking and cancer." But now Linda Sanchez had introduced the analogy to the House Judiciary Committee.

"Well, Congresswoman, I do believe that we have embraced the research, the medical study of this issue," said Goodell.

"You are talking about one study, and that is the NFL's study," said Sanchez. "You are not talking about the independent studies that have been conducted by other researchers."

It was the hearings' most powerful moment, the one that would haunt the NFL for years. Part of what made Sanchez's argument so powerful was that it rang true. There were, in fact, many similarities between Big Tobacco and Big Football. The NFL didn't have 400 law firms on its payroll or a database of 180,000 research papers that had cost hundreds of millions of dollars to assemble. But much like the tobacco companies, the NFL had used its power and vast resources to try to discredit scientists it disagreed with and bury their work, cherry-picked data to make selective arguments about concussions, and elevated its own flawed research. Playing on "the margins of science" was how Anthony Colucci, a former top researcher at R.J. Reynolds, had described Big Tobacco's strategy to the *Wall Street Journal* in 1993.

The tobacco fight's version of Omalu was Dr. Ernst Wynder, a public health researcher who was fresh out of medical school at Washington University in St. Louis when he published a landmark study in 1950 that identified smoking as a significant risk factor for lung cancer. As with Omalu's inquiry, Wynder's had started in the morgue: During an internship at New York University, he had watched the autopsy of a two-pack-a-day smoker who had died from lung cancer. Wynder followed up his first study by setting out to establish a direct link between smoking and cancer. He painted pure tobacco tar sucked out of Lucky Strike cigarettes onto the shaved backs of mice. Among the 62 mice still alive at the end of a year, 58 percent developed cancer.

That study, published in five parts beginning in 1953, prompted tobacco executives to form an "objective" and "disinterested" research group staffed by the public relations firm Hill & Knowlton. The Council for Tobacco Research—known originally as the Tobacco Industry Research Committee—soon began to churn out reports denying the connection between smoking and lung cancer. The council encouraged researchers to examine other factors such as "viruses and diet and car exhaust, to take contrarian positions, to savage the other side in the letters column of scientific journals," wrote Dan Zegart in *Civil Warriors: The Legal Siege on the Tobacco Industry.*

"The entire tobacco research council was a front put up by Hill & Knowlton," said Victor DeNoble, a former Philip Morris whistle-blower whose research proved nicotine is addictive, in an interview for this book. "They recruited scientists and paid them to make statements that just clearly were not true, couldn't be based in fact. They were opinions. And that went on for years."

The tobacco industry's researchers, foreshadowing the debate around football and brain damage, engaged in what Zegart called a "metaphysical quarrel over the definition of cause." There had long been an expectation that smoking heightened the risk for a variety of diseases, just as some scientists thought that the kind of brain damage seen in boxers might show up in other sports. But tobacco researchers continued to toss out a host of other possible factors that might be to blame, making it difficult to establish a clear causal link.

Of course, there were a lot of differences, too, between the retired debate over the hazards of smoking and the one that was heating up over football. Smoking, in the end, was a public scourge with no real utility to anyone who came in contact with it. Football promoted discipline, character, and mental and physical well-being and brought people together by the millions. It was an incredibly sophisticated, uniquely American sport, and entire books would be written about its appeal. Also, football, unlike cigarettes, wasn't addictive (although some Texans might disagree). The tobacco industry's manipulative fight against science went on for five decades and left zero doubt about the risks of smoking. The research into football, though ominous, was relatively new and far less conclusive about the ultimate risk and prevalence of neurodegenerative disease.

That was the point, Nowinski told the committee when he testified later in the day: "So much of this crisis has mirrored Big Tobacco and the link between smoking and lung cancer. And I ask you, if you were able to create all the smoking laws and awareness we have today back in the 1950s when the first conclusive pathological research was done linking smoking to lung cancer, would you save those millions of people who smoked without understanding the risks?"

To the question of whether football should be banned, McKee replied, "Football is an American sport. Everyone loves it. I certainly would never want to ban football. . . . We haven't banned cigarette smoking. People smoke. People make that choice. But they need to make an informed decision. They need to understand the risks and it needs to be out there if they want to pay attention to what those risks are.

"What I don't understand is why we are expecting that exposure to repetitive head trauma will cause disease in 100 percent of the individuals that suffer this trauma," she continued. "Do we expect 100 percent of cigarette smokers to develop lung cancer? Do we expect 100 percent of children who play with matches or even with chainsaws to get hurt? No. Even if the percentage of affected individuals is 20 percent, or 10 percent or 5 percent, there are still thousands of kids and adults out there right now playing football at all levels who will eventually come down with this devastating and debilitating disorder."

The comparison between the NFL and Big Tobacco had been planted in a public forum, and now the NFL was stained with it; it was as indelible as the tar that Ernst Wynder had smeared on his mice.

"Those hearings did one thing," said Bob Stern, one of the cofounders of the BU Group. "They said: 'NFL equals Tobacco.'"

Within three weeks of the hearing, Casson and Viano were out as cochairs of the MTBI committee. Goodell sent a memo to all teams stating that the two men had "graciously" resigned. The league announced several changes to its concussion policy, including a rule compelling teams to consult an independent neurologist after a player sustained any type of brain injury. Players with concussion symptoms were "no go" for practice or games and could not return to play the same day—a direct contradiction to the conclusion of one of the NFL's most controversial papers. A much-touted study to determine the long-term effects of playing football—originally scheduled to be released in 2010 and then pushed back to 2011 or 2012—was suspended indefinitely. Casson had been overseeing that study.

Then came the headline that the NFL never wanted to see: "Is Tackle Football Too Dangerous for Kids to Play?"

It ran atop a *New York Times* blog item written by Katherine Schulten, editor of The Learning Network. The piece referred to a guest column that had appeared in the *Times* a few days earlier in which a father, Adam Buckley Cohen, recounted his 10-year-old son Will's anxiety about playing football for his Pee Wee team. Cohen began the column with this quote from Will: "Dad, I'm scared. I only have one brain, and I don't want to hurt it playing football." Will had read about Troy Aikman's inability to remember his winning performance in the 1993 NFL Championship Game and was aware that Steve Young had retired because of concussions.

On the morning of December 20, Schwarz read a wire report that the NFL planned to donate $1 million to the Boston University Center for the Study of Traumatic Encephalopathy and would encourage current and former players to donate their brains to the institute. Schwarz was surprised, in part because Nowinski, his best source, typically notified him about all breaking stories related to BU. When he got Nowinski on the phone, Schwarz was told, "I don't know anything. I don't know what the fuck is going on."

Nowinski was aware that Goodell had reached out to Cantu about supporting BU's research by urging players to donate their brains after death. The commissioner had mentioned the discussion during the hearings. But the BU Group had heard nothing about money. Nowinski became concerned that the donation would be perceived as an attempt by the NFL to buy BU's support. The BU brain trust—Cantu, McKee, Nowinski, and Stern—spoke by phone. Cantu told Schwarz that BU wouldn't take any money from the league without assurances of its independence.

Nowinski didn't think the timing of the NFL's announcement was coincidental. BU and the Players Association were preparing to announce the next day that the union would be recommending that players pledge their brains to BU. Nowinski figured the league, still reeling from the hearings, had gotten wind of the plan and wanted to share in the attention for supporting CTE research.

Schwarz reached out to Aiello for comment on the NFL's overtures to BU. He asked the NFL spokesman the standard questions: What went into the decision? Who was involved? He then posed the more vexing question: Why would the NFL give $1 million to a group whose findings it had fought for years?

Aiello said matter-of-factly: "It's quite obvious from the medical research that's been done that concussions can lead to long-term problems."

Wait, what? Had the NFL's chief spokesman just acknowledged the link that Goodell had scrupulously avoided weeks earlier in front of Congress? The link that Casson, Pellman, and Viano had fought for years? How did Aiello's comment square with the pamphlet advising NFL players: "Research is currently underway to determine if there are any long-term effects of concussion in NFL athletes"?

"Greg, that's the first time you've ever said that or anyone with the league has ever said that," Schwarz said evenly, concerned that Aiello might back off.

"We all share the same interest," said Aiello, sounding miffed and slightly impatient. "That's as much as I'm going to say."

The next day, stripped across the top of the *New York Times* sports section, was the following headline:

N.F.L. ACKNOWLEDGES LONG-TERM CONCUSSION EFFECTS

Virginia Grimsley, the wife of John Grimsley, McKee's first CTE case, sent a bottle of champagne to BU. The group had brought about change.

"It was the turning point," said Nowinski. "I mean, the only way to say it is, you changed their mind. In a sense, it was a victory."

Aiello's statement, though, marked not only the first but also the *last* time anyone from the NFL has publicly acknowledged the connection between football and brain damage.

15

"PLEASE, SEE THAT MY BRAIN IS GIVEN TO THE NFL'S BRAIN BANK"

The magnitude of the wreckage soon became apparent. It wasn't just Casson and Viano. The entire Mild Traumatic Brain Injury Committee had been blown up by Goodell. It had been 16 years since Tagliabue had created the NFL's research arm in response to a concussion crisis the ex-commissioner had never quite believed in. Under the leadership of Pellman and, later, Casson and Viano, the committee had published 16 scientific papers and assorted other studies. It had conducted biomechanical reconstructions of concussions on crash-test dummies, completed a six-year epidemiological survey involving hundreds of players, performed thousands of neuropsychological tests, engineered a new helmet, and even re-created NFL-strength concussions in rats. All of that was now discarded as worthless. It was as if a factory had been shuttered. Mitch Berger, a prominent San Francisco neurosurgeon who was among the researchers the league brought in to begin anew, said he and his colleagues "essentially started from zero." Even the much-ridiculed name—the Mild Traumatic Brain Injury Committee—was scrapped. The research entity that replaced it was christened the NFL Head, Neck and Spine Committee.

The Dissenters had won. The world had been turned upside down. As the NFL began to spread money around, it recruited its biggest critics to help solve a problem it once had treated as fiction and now acknowledged as deadly real. One of those critics was BU. To assuage the group's concerns about maintaining its independence, the NFL drafted a two-page letter, signed by Jeff Pash, the league's general counsel, recognizing "the importance of preserving the Center as an independent and credible voice." The letter designated BU the NFL's "preferred" brain bank and pledged to encourage players to "donate their brains to the Center." Cantu, one of the original Dissenters, who had described the previous committee as stooges for the commissioner, was named a "senior advisor" to the new panel.

Not everyone was thrilled with the new arrangement. Bernie Parrish, the retired Browns defensive back, who had pledged his brain to BU, warned that the NFL was trying to buy off the researchers. He wanted no part of it. A year earlier, even before the NFL made its donation, Parrish had confronted Nowinski about this very possibility.

"Look, you can't do that," he told him. "Once you accept money from them, they *own* your ass."

"We would never take money from them," Nowinski responded, according to Parrish.

Now BU was doing exactly that. Parrish wasn't happy.

"I want my brain back!" he declared during a follow-up hearing before the House Judiciary Committee. Not long after, he rescinded his pledge to BU.

Guskiewicz, who had savaged the NFL in a commencement speech and later compared Tagliabue's slapdash creation of the MTBI committee to an airport security breach, was brought on as a full-fledged member of the new panel, overseeing rules and equipment. From his days taping ankles for the Steelers, Guskiewicz had come far. His groundbreaking work would garner a $500,000 "genius grant" from the MacArthur Foundation for "major advances in the diagnosis, treatment, and prevention of sports-related concussions." Guskiewicz had to think long and hard before accepting the NFL's invitation. The league had approached him once before, an overture he had perceived as "damage control" to show that the NFL was doing something "without canning Casson and Viano and admitting we were fools." Guskiewicz had said no that time, but now Casson and Viano were gone and everything was different, he believed. It was a total reversal. Guskiewicz signed on as an unpaid member of the committee, although he recognized that one of the first questions people would ask was "Did the NFL buy Kevin Guskiewicz?"

For years, the old committee boasted just one neurosurgeon, Hank Feuer of the Colts. It had been just another sign of the NFL's lack of seriousness about concussions—the virtual absence of the doctors most intimately familiar with the brain. Now the NFL was appointing brain surgeons to head the new committee. The cochairs were Richard Ellenbogen and Hunt Batjer, respected neurosurgeons with no previous ties to the NFL. Ellenbogen was chief of neurosurgery at Seattle's Harborview Medical Center, one of the country's busiest brain trauma facilities. His specialty was children. Ellenbogen had helped pass the Zackery Lystedt Law, which set strict return-to-play guidelines in Washington State, mandating the removal of any young athlete suspected of having a concussion. The law was named after a middle schooler in Maple Valley, Washington, who had returned to play after a concussion and developed a brain hemorrhage that almost cost him his life. Ellenbogen's team had performed several surgeries on the boy.

Goodell had recruited Ellenbogen personally. The brain surgeon was on his way to the emergency room one morning when his cell phone rang. The caller identified himself as the NFL commissioner. Ellenbogen thought it was one of his colleagues or an old friend having some fun with him, so he proffered Goodell an obscenity. Goodell assured him that he was in fact the NFL commissioner and was looking for a doctor to chair his new concussion committee. "I felt like such a dope," Ellenbogen recalled. He met with Goodell and agreed to take the job.

Batjer, a native Texan, was just completing a 17-year run as chairman of neurosurgery at Northwestern University's Feinberg School of Medicine in Chicago. When Batjer got the call from the NFL, it immediately touched a nerve. He reflected back on an experience he'd had two years earlier while watching an exhibition soccer match in Lake Forest, Illinois. During the game, a player was knocked unconscious.

After spending several minutes on his back, the player returned to action only to collapse face-first on the turf. Batjer rushed onto the field. He feared the young man was dead.

"I'm a neurosurgeon," Batjer said as he approached the player, who thankfully was beginning to stir. "This kid is out of here. He needs to get to the Lake Forest emergency room. I'll drive him. He needs a CT scan now."

"I'm sorry, Doc, thanks for introducing yourself," someone told him. "But it's the coach's call."

Batjer and Ellenbogen professed to know very little about the old NFL committee—or "the MB, whatever, TI committee," as Ellenbogen referred to it—and the contempt it had engendered before its ignominious dissolution. In an interview for this book, Ellenbogen said he had reviewed one of "Elliot Pellman's articles" for *Neurosurgery*—Paper Number 14, on biomechanics—but claimed, "I never knew there was a committee." That statement appeared to be at odds with Ellenbogen's review, in which he wrote that the authors and "the NFL MTBI committee are to be congratulated on the 14th contribution in a superb series of the analysis of concussions in NFL players."

The two neurosurgeons got an early crash course in what they were facing courtesy of the House Judiciary Committee. The football hearings the previous October had been so successful, the NFL so thoroughly demoralized, that the committee decided to take the show on the road in a series of forums across the country. One was held in New York. Linda Sanchez and her colleagues appeared slow to accept the legitimacy of the league's new doctors. After listening to Batjer and Ellenbogen talk about their goals, Sanchez said they sounded "like the same old NFL." The two men had been on the job two months and felt they were being criticized for not solving the problem. Referring to the recent Deepwater Horizon disaster, Ellenbogen turned to Batjer and whispered: "That's less time than oil has been spilling into the gulf."

It was an early indication of the scrutiny they would find themselves under. Ellenbogen and Batjer wanted to ignore the NFL's recent past, but because of it they wouldn't get the benefit of the doubt—not for a while, perhaps not ever.

"The NFL has had its four stages of grief: denial, more denial, some level of recognition, and now research," said New York Democrat Anthony Weiner.

The NFL's previous work was "infected," Weiner told Batjer and Ellenbogen. Their immediate task was "to mop up."

Ellenbogen decided the committee had to accomplish something, "one thing," quickly. Even that, though, would not prove easy. The decision was made to produce a poster warning players about the dangers of concussions—a poster that would replace the NFL's pamphlet insisting that "current research" hadn't shown that repeated concussions could lead to long-term brain damage. Ellenbogen said as many as 30 people took part in crafting the new poster, including representatives of the new NFL committee, the NFLPA, and the Centers for Disease Control, as well as several lawyers. The poster they finally settled on was titled "CONCUSSION—A Must Read for NFL Players . . . Let's Take Brain Injuries Out of Play." The poster listed a series of concussion facts and symptoms, and it warned, "Repetitive brain injury, when not treated promptly and properly, may cause permanent damage to your brain."

Ellenbogen said about the process of coming to agreement on the poster's language: "It was the most painful thing I think I've ever done."

There was no place for Bennet Omalu in this brave new world. While Nowinski and McKee were soaking up the spotlight, the man who had set the NFL's concussion crisis in motion was carrying out his duties as San Joaquin County medical examiner, cutting up bodies at the dank coroner's office in tiny French Camp, California, and moonlighting in the lab he had set up in his garage.

Omalu seemed like a man in exile. His moods vacillated between a self-pitying desire to stay as far away from the NFL as possible and a yearning to be recognized for his historic discovery. One day Omalu would say, "To be honest with you, I really wish I never touched Mike Webster's brain." The next day he would rage against all the attention now going to the BU Group, whose members frequently downplayed the significance of his work.

BU's researchers literally kept a file on what they alleged were Omalu's exaggerations, primarily his claims that he had discovered

CTE. (In fact, Omalu discovered brain damage in pro football players and applied the preexisting term *chronic traumatic encephalopathy* to the disease.) "Bennet has done a marvelous thing and deserves all the credit in the world," said Cantu. "My problem with him is that he is not scrupulously sticking to the facts, ma'am. He embellishes remarkably. And that will bring him down." Of course, some research scientists would soon level the same criticism at Cantu.

Nowinski was no more charitable. Speaking on the popular *Dennis & Callahan* radio show on Boston's WEEI one day, he was asked, "What woke up the NFL?"

"I honestly believe having been in the meetings with the NFL last year that it was Dr. McKee," he said, "because the first pathologist who looked at this work overinterpreted the findings and was not as credible."

When Jeanne Marie Laskas, a writer for *GQ,* contacted Nowinski in spring 2009 and asked where she could find Omalu, Nowinski replied, "Oh, he's not in it anymore," according to Laskas.

"It sounds like he discovered it," she said.

"Well, he had a lot to do with it then, but he's just not in it anymore. He moved," said Nowinski. (Nowinski later said he told Laskas that Omalu wasn't doing research with *him* anymore, not that he wasn't doing it at all.)

Laskas eventually tracked down Omalu in French Camp. She discovered the "happiest man alive that I was asking" about CTE.

"But Dr. Omalu, I heard you aren't in it anymore," Laskas said.

"No! No!" Omalu said, his voice rising. "Dr. Omalu is in it! Dr. Omalu is in it!"

Omalu's third paper on CTE in an NFL player—Andre Waters— was ultimately rejected by *Neurosurgery,* even though the diagnosis had made the front page of the *New York Times.* Omalu believed, without evidence, that this was because the three cases would have represented a series, and Apuzzo, doing the NFL's bidding, didn't want to acknowledge they were anything more than random. The Waters paper eventually appeared in *The Journal of Forensic Nursing,* a fact that was privately ridiculed by doctors affiliated with the league.

But Omalu brought many of his problems on himself. He couldn't seem to get out of his own way, never recognizing the need to filter.

In January 2010, he was invited to speak at the first meeting of a new concussion committee that had been formed by the Players Association. The meeting took place at a Palm Beach resort and drew dozens of current and former players, union officials, doctors, and widows. Hall of Fame defensive end Jack Youngblood stood by with a stopwatch, with instructions to sack any speaker who went over seven minutes.

Omalu droned on for 45 as Youngblood stood by, seemingly helpless to stop the cherubic African researcher. "What happened, Jack, your stopwatch break?" somebody asked Youngblood. Omalu left the crowd numb and murmuring. He again showed the grisly autopsy photos of Webster. "It was like crime photos, like Dillinger, you know?" said Lovell, who attended. "He had no idea how inappropriate that was or didn't care." Omalu then proposed that NFL players sit out at least 99 days after a concussion, at which point the players in attendance "started laughing in his face," said Lovell. Even people originally sympathetic to Omalu's cause were appalled. "He was just going on and on," said Guskiewicz. "He put up those pictures of Mike on the slab. That may be very appropriate in a pure medical meeting where you've got a bunch of pathologists or even physicians. But you've got players in there. You had former teammates in there. You had some coaches. You had some former wives."

Guskiewicz thought the event had the effect of further legitimizing BU and confirming some people's worst fears about Omalu. "I think it exposed him in front of an audience and confirmed what some people had heard about him," he said. "It's like, 'Ah, I've heard about this guy. And now I see. Now I understand.'"

But some people thought the backlash against Omalu went deeper than his indiscretions and outside-the-box proposals. Certainly, other researchers were unconventional and took provocative stances. Cantu would call for a complete ban on tackle football for children under 14, a recommendation far more controversial than Omalu's proposed three-month recovery period. And Omalu was vastly more qualified than many people now sitting at the NFL's table, notably Nowinski.

Even people who didn't sympathize with Omalu's views marveled at the swiftness with which he was dispatched. "He got steamrolled," said Micky Collins, never a huge Omalu fan. "Completely. He was really the first guy that did all this stuff, you know? He got rolled—rolled and put away wet."

Bailes thought the NFL identified Omalu early on as the league's biggest threat, a bomb thrower who knew nothing about football and was therefore beholden to no one. That was one reason, Bailes believed, the league had invited him to the Chicago summit to present Omalu's work but not Omalu himself. "I don't think they liked the whole scene from the beginning," said Bailes. "He was perhaps perceived as not mainstream, certainly not an American. It's like, 'How can a Nigerian doctor tell us what's wrong with our sport?'"

Harry Carson, the Giants Hall of Fame linebacker, thought Omalu's marginalization was easy to understand: He looked and sounded different from every person in the medical establishment, the NFL, and the concussion committees. "I think it's because he's a black man, I honestly believe that," Carson said. "And he's not an American black man; he's from Africa." Before arriving in the NFL, Carson had attended South Carolina State, an obscure black school. He saw parallels between his life and Omalu's. "It was up to me to prove people wrong, and I think with him it's the same way," he said. "People will think less of him because of his skin color. And it's not because I'm black and he's black. It is because he did the groundbreaking work."

"This is something that is too big for everybody to not be included," said Carson. "And when you have an authority like him on the outside looking in when he was the one who provided the information, there's something wrong with that picture."

On February 17, 2011, police were summoned to a luxury condo in Sunny Isles Beach, Florida, a spit of land north of Miami. The condo, Ocean One, towered over the turquoise water. At 2:51 P.M., the police entered Unit 603. The tenant hadn't responded to his fiancée's calls or the building manager pounding on the door. Once inside, officers found the apartment immaculate, the air tinged with the smell of a cigar. The police announced their presence, but no one responded. The officers made their way through the apartment room by room, arriving finally at the master bedroom, where a large man lay nude on top of the bed, a blanket drawn up to his neck, a chrome Taurus .38 Special by his side. The man had a single gunshot wound on the left side of his chest, just below the nipple.

Up to that moment, to the extent that Dave Duerson had played a role in the NFL's concussion crisis, it was as a lightning rod for many retired players, who saw him as a traitor and a fellow traveler with the worst of the league's deniers. The former Bears safety had been very much a part of the system. As a player rep on the Bert Bell retirement board, he had turned down numerous disability claims from broken men. Records show that Duerson cast a proxy vote when the board unanimously rejected Webster's appeal for full benefits in 2003. During the 2007 congressional hearings on the retirement system, Duerson invoked his 84-year-old father's Alzheimer's disease as proof that football didn't cause brain damage.

But that wasn't the message Duerson was sending now. Before pulling the trigger, he had staged his condo meticulously. On the living room table were assorted clues, "as if someone's trying to tell you a story in a room," said Duerson's son Tregg. There was a copy of *Sports Illustrated* from three months earlier with a headline on the cover: "CONCUSSIONS." The word was superimposed over Steelers linebacker James Harrison demolishing a helpless receiver. "THE HITS THAT ARE CHANGING THE GAME . . . AND THE HITS NO ONE IS NOTICING," the cover said. Next to the magazine were two identical binders filled with documents from the retirement board's Traumatic Brain Injury Evaluation Program. There was a DVD case for *Trapped: Haitian Nights,* a "psychological thriller that delves into the dark world of Voodoo, deception, and the fragility of the mind." Duerson had laid out all his disability files, as well as documents indicating that he was preparing to file a workers' compensation claim related to brain trauma. He was scheduled to fly to California the next month to be assessed by four doctors, including a neurologist.

"It was eerie because you almost kind of felt his presence in the place," said Duerson's ex-wife, Alicia, the mother of his four children.

Duerson's family and friends thought it was as if he were trying to explain himself, to make one final plea for understanding. His suicide note ran five typed pages and had the feel of an instruction manual, which some relatives thought fitting, since Duerson was always telling people what to do. The note contained no salutation and was titled "REFERENCE TOPICS FOR LATER." Those topics included notes on his finances and possessions. Only a small portion addressed Duerson's thoughts on how football had destroyed him. It was the only part of the note in all caps:

MY MIND SLIPS. THOUGHTS GET CROSSED. CANNOT FIND MY WORDS. MAJOR GROWTH ON THE BACK OF SKULL ON LOWER LEFT SIDE. FEEL REALLY ALONE. THINKING OF OTHER NFL PLAYERS WITH BRAIN INJURIES. SOMETIMES, SIMPLE SPELLING BECOMES A CHORE, AND MY EYESITE GOES BLURY. . . . I THINK SOMETHING IS SERIOUSLY DAMAGED IN MY BRAIN, TOO. I CANNOT TELL YOU HOW MANY TIMES I SAW STARS IN GAMES, BUT I KNOW THERE WERE MANY TIMES THAT I WOULD "WAKE UP" WELL AFTER A GAME, AND WE WERE ALL AT DINNER.

On the last page, almost as if he had just remembered something he had forgotten, Duerson provided a handwritten addendum:

PLEASE, SEE THAT MY BRAIN IS GIVEN TO THE NFL'S BRAIN BANK.

A week after Duerson killed himself, *Time* called him "Football's First Martyr." That was a stretch. Webster, after all, had died nine years earlier. Andre Waters also had turned a gun on himself, and Justin Strzelczyk had chosen to go up in flames. But the act was chilling. Duerson had shot himself in the chest to preserve his brain for study. The cool preparation and the contrition his death seemed to signal to all the players he had judged harshly spoke to the horror of the disease.

Duerson didn't seem like a man who had been destined for this, as if anyone were. He had grown up in Muncie, Indiana, a star scholar-athlete who was scouted by the Dodgers and chose to play football at Notre Dame. His father spent nearly four decades working on an assembly line for General Motors. Awed by the machinery, Duerson as a small child would tell his dad: "I want to do that." "No, son, you want to *own* that," his father would say. Duerson made the National Honor Society, displaying great drive and ambition and a meticulous attention to detail that would later seem in contrast to his savage approach to the game.

Alicia met Duerson during his freshman year at Notre Dame, and it was hard for her to reconcile the smart, reserved young man she had come to love with the beast he became on the field. On Fridays before game day, Duerson liked to read Jack Tatum's autobiography, *They Call Me Assassin,* in which the former Raiders safety bragged: "I like to believe that my best hits border on felonious assault." When Alicia went to meet Duerson after the game near the locker room, she was scared of him, wary of coming close. Duerson was irked and confused. "Get over here and give me a hug," he said. "I was just playing a game," he assured her. "I'm fine now. It's out of my system."

A third-round pick in the 1983 draft, Duerson became one of the hardest hitters on a Chicago Bears team built around one of the best defenses the game had ever seen. One of Duerson's closest friends on the Bears was linebacker Otis Wilson. When the two men joined forces on a big hit, they hovered over their victims, barking and howling. The defense became known as the Junkyard Dogs. Duerson, like Tatum, viewed the defensive backfield as a free fire zone. "That was Dave's thinking," Alicia said in an interview for this book. "Make them remember the hits and they won't be coming up the middle that much."

It didn't seem to matter if Duerson couldn't remember the hits as long as they had their desired effect. That was part of the job description: headaches, nausea, "dings," and, at times, huge gaps in his memory.

"He had a lot of concussions," said Alicia. "But back then, you know, there was nobody pulling you off to the side. It was just, 'Shake it off, go back in.' And I think because there was no real free agency—this is just my opinion—I just think everybody probably tried to kill themselves because you don't want to not play, then you don't get the money next year."

Duerson graduated with honors from Notre Dame and earned a degree in economics. He contemplated running for office someday. He and Alicia saw themselves as a power couple, driven to help others. Duerson ended up playing 11 seasons in the NFL, making the Pro Bowl four times. He served as a Bears player rep and played an important role in the fight for free agency, gaining the trust of Gene Upshaw, the head of the players union. Duerson thought someday he might succeed Upshaw and told people that Upshaw was grooming him for the position.

After Duerson retired in 1993, he started a career in the food industry. He first bought McDonald's franchises and then purchased a food distribution company called Fair Oaks Farms. He doubled the company's annual revenues to more than $60 million, according to a story in *Men's Journal* magazine that chronicled his rise and fall. Stogie in hand, Duerson looked the part of a successful businessman. He and Alicia were living the high life they had always envisioned for themselves. When they vacationed in Paris, they stayed at five-star hotels, rented a BMW, and flew on the Concorde. Duerson bought a 17-room, 8,000-square-foot house with a four-car garage and a swimming pool in the same neighborhood as Michael Jordan.

Duerson was named to the board of trustees at Notre Dame and also served on the board of the Boys & Girls Clubs of America. He earned an MBA through Harvard's executive training program. He had a beautiful wife and four kids.

"We always knew that the next level we were going higher," Alicia said of Duerson's life after football. "David never, ever thought the next level would be going lower."

When Duerson decided he wanted to be bought out of his ownership stake in Fair Oaks Farms, it was to start his own company, Duerson Foods. That made sense; Duerson always thought he could do things better than everyone else and had had great success with Fair Oaks. But Harold Rice, one of his closest friends, thought it was odd that he was complaining so much about his Fair Oaks partner, Shelly Lavin. Duerson sounded irrational. "He thinks I'm some nigger he can control," Duerson would say of Lavin. "I'm not his boy." But Rice chalked it up to Duerson's bluster and need to demonstrate that he was in charge.

The new business buried Duerson financially. He had leveraged all his assets to create what he hoped would be a meat-distribution empire. Rice said Duerson spent $24 million to launch the company, when he probably should have spent $5 million. "He had emptied all the accounts for Duerson Foods, put everything in that one deal," Alicia said.

The people closest to him began to see him as reckless and occasionally disconnected from reality. They noticed that Duerson seemed less able to control his emotions, more prone to fits of rage. He lost his temper with employees or exploded in anger at business meetings. During one meeting with Marriott to discuss servicing the hotel chain's restaurants, Duerson became confrontational. "You guys are looking at me like I don't know what I'm talking about," he said. Alicia, who was working with her husband, watched as the room fell silent. "You got to understand, Dave was 6-2, maybe 230, 240 at that time," she said. "In a room with little bitty white men, you know what I mean? Sometimes when he got mad, he would have that glare in his eyes. I can't explain it. It's like you're dealing with somebody that's not rational."

In February 2005, Duerson traveled to South Bend for a Notre Dame board of trustees meeting. Alicia went with him. They had a nice dinner together and then returned to the hotel, the Morris Inn, where they went to the bar for a drink. Alicia was tired, and so she headed upstairs while Dave stayed to hang out with friends. Shortly afterward, Dave shook her awake. Alicia was certain he wasn't drunk, but he wasn't himself. Duerson had grown paranoid that she was having an affair, and now he wanted to confront her.

"He wanted to discuss something that was in his head that wasn't real," she said. "I was trying to walk him through it to show him how it was not real, but his mind was just so screwed up. And he didn't believe me, and one thing led to another."

Duerson had that glare in his eyes. Alicia became scared and tried to get away. A witness described seeing the door fly open and then Alicia being pushed out, her body slamming into the wall. Then, just as quickly, Duerson was calm, aghast at what he had done. Alicia was taken to the hospital for cuts to the head and dizziness. Duerson was charged with misdemeanor battery. The incident cost him his spot as a Notre Dame trustee. Later, he described the incident as a "one-time event" in which he lost control for "three seconds" and his "biggest regret."

By 2006, Duerson's life was in free fall. He was forced to shutter Duerson Foods, the big house went into foreclosure, and he divorced Alicia. He moved down to Florida, into the ritzy condo he and Alicia had purchased as a winter getaway when their life was going so well.

Gradually, he began to withdraw from family, friends, and former team-mates, creating a new life in Florida built around a facade: He was fine, had plenty of money, and was on the verge of resurrecting his career.

Tregg, a private banking analyst, knew his dad was going through a rough time, and he would call him in Florida and ask, "How's it going, anything I can do?"

"No, things are going fine," Duerson would say. "I'm looking at this business. I might buy this business with this guy."

In reality, Duerson was deep in debt. Alicia claimed he owed her $70,000 in child support, one bank was after him for $9 million, and he was behind on his condo fees. Five months before his death, he filed for bankruptcy.

Duerson had maintained his connections with Upshaw, still hoping against all reason that he might someday lead the union. When Upshaw died suddenly in 2008, Duerson's dream was revealed to be just that—a dream. But he was allowed to keep his appointment as one of the union's three voting members on the disability board. The position put him in contact with the growing number of retired players who were seeking benefits for cognitive problems stemming from football. He also was familiar with the league's ongoing attempts to deal with the problem, mostly through rule changes and fines to limit blows to the head.

If there was a point when Duerson became conflicted by his own worsening condition and his disdain, public and private, for the claims that football caused brain damage, he didn't show it. Nor did he hide his contempt for what he saw as the softening of the game.

Duerson had a radio show, *Double Time with Double D,* that ran on VoiceAmerica. On October 21, 2010, Duerson told his listeners, "I'm pissed today."

He lamented the NFL's crackdown on dangerous head-to-head tackles. He read one of his own Facebook postings: "The Big Hit has been told to turn in his pads and jockstrap." He read several comments from readers ridiculing the league for trying to "sissify" the sport. At one point, Duerson recalled a 1984 playoff game in which his teammate Todd Bell blasted Redskins running back Joe Washington. "He helicop-tered this brother, *helicoptered* him," Duerson said. "It was a wonderful hit, it was clean, but based upon what the commissioner is talking about today, they would have suspended Todd on the spot." Later he added, "I have expressed several times, there is nothing like hearing the air rush out of a man's body."

At no point during the one-hour show did Duerson address the issue behind the rule changes: the possibility that football was causing neurodegenerative disease in his fellow retired players.

Four months later, Duerson was alone in his Florida condo, carefully plotting his suicide. He laid out a Bible, set aside books for various family members, and smoked one last cigar. At 2:52 A.M.—just before he shot himself, authorities concluded—he sent a text message to Alicia. The last line read: "I really do think there's something going on in my brain in the back left side. Get it to the NFL. Please."

Duerson sent a similar text to his fiancée and scribbled the same message at the end of his typed suicide note. Clearly, he wanted to leave nothing to chance.

The task fell to Tregg, but Duerson's son had no idea how to go about donating his father's brain to science. Like every other football fan, Tregg knew that concussions were a hot topic, but he hadn't heard about CTE or the initiative to create a brain bank for NFL players. Tregg had only questions, most of which he thought were bizarre: How does one donate a brain? What is the NFL's brain bank? Does the coroner need to do something special to keep my dad's brain? What does this do to our funeral plans?

In his search for answers, Tregg called the Players Association, figuring his dad had worked with the union and someone there would be able to help him. He reached one of his father's former teammates.

"My dad committed suicide and I'm trying to donate his brain to the NFL," Tregg said. "Can you help me?"

"Okay, I'll get on this and call you back," the man said.

At the same time, Alicia Duerson sought help from Connie Payton, the wife of Bears great Walter Payton, another former teammate of Duerson's. On the Duersons' behalf, an employee from the Paytons' foundation contacted the NFL's offices and explained the family's desire to donate the brain to science.

Despite Duerson's last words—"Please, See That My Brain Is Given to the NFL's Brain Bank"—no such place existed. But it was hard to imagine that any other research institution except Boston University— the league's "preferred" brain bank—fit that description. Both the union and the league had pledged to encourage players to donate their brains to BU after death. The NFL's $1 million gift was intended to under-write the BU Group's research. Shortly after the donation, the group presented Goodell with its "Impact Award" during a gala fund-raiser at the Boston Harbor Hotel. Guests were treated to a large cake adorned with a football-shaped "brain" that appeared to be made of fondant.

Tregg was directed to Nowinski, who explained the process and sent him the paperwork. Fighting through a haze of sadness and exhaustion, Tregg read the documents. He stopped at the language describing how even his father's eyes would be part of the donation.

"You want to take his eyes?" Tregg asked Nowinski.

"Yes, we need to take the eyes; they are actually really important to our study," Nowinski said. BU was exploring whether an examination of the optic nerve might help with the diagnosis of CTE.

"Okay," Tregg recalled saying, "and then I just signed it. And then we faxed it off. And that was it."

But the NFL wasn't nearly as unified behind BU as the league's let-ter of support and million-dollar gift suggested. Top members of the reconstituted concussion committee were already expressing doubts about BU and, unknown to the BU researchers, were working to keep Duerson's brain away from the group.

The new NFL doctors said they had four primary concerns about BU, which they voiced to fellow researchers, journalists, and the fami-lies of former players: (1) There wasn't enough research for BU to state conclusively that football-related head trauma was causing CTE. (2) BU had oversold its findings, feeding a growing hysteria about the risks of playing football. (3) BU refused to share brain tissue with other scien-tists, making it impossible to validate its conclusions. (4) The group's growing fame and funding were predicated on establishing the link between football and brain damage, creating an inherent bias.

By then, Ann McKee had emerged as BU's rock star, eclipsing even Nowinski. Her appeal as a spokeswoman seemed boundless. The sudden attention had yanked her out of her "rabbit hole" of self-imposed scientific isolation and cast her into the spotlight, where she was sought out by everyone from *60 Minutes* to HBO to explain the new football disease. Laypersons, journalists, neuroscientists, athletes—all seemed fascinated by her dazzling looks and her ability to make CTE understandable. Much was made about how McKee studied the brains of dead players during the week, then put on her cheesehead and her Packers jersey to watch Sunday's game. "She's a brilliant scientist who happens to be a little blond bombshell," said Eleanor Perfetto, the widow of a former player, Ralph Wenzel, whose brain was studied by McKee. Introducing McKee at a conference in Las Vegas, a fellow researcher gushed: "In addition to having golden features, she has a gold standard. If it doesn't meet her gold standard, it ain't CTE."

McKee and her colleagues had used their platform to become increasingly assertive about the dangers of football. One of their most ominous assertions was that full-blown concussions weren't what was triggering the disease. Rather, McKee and her group believed that CTE was essentially dementia pugilistica—boxer's dementia—now being found in other contact sports, especially football and hockey. As in boxing, it was the accumulation of hundreds or thousands of "subconcussive" blows that caused the damage, not one big knockout punch or open-field collision. "We don't think it's because of direct blows," McKee said. "This is a very internal part of the brain. I mean, it's really deep inside." Cantu called CTE "a dose-related phenomenon" involving "total brain trauma."

These assertions had obvious implications for the NFL. The league could change the rules to cut down on helmet-to-helmet hits. It could monitor the number of concussions in an effort to reduce them. It could put independent neurologists on the sidelines to look for concussions and try to end the culture of pain that pressured players to play through it. But if CTE was occurring at a deeper level, as the BU Group believed, that raised questions about the very essence of football.

One of BU's main critics was Mitch Berger, the chairman of the neurological surgery department at the University of California San Francisco Medical Center. Berger, a strapping former Harvard defensive end with wavy salt-and-pepper hair, had been brought onto the new NFL committee to conduct a longitudinal study on football-related head trauma—the long-term study that had been started and then abandoned by the original MTBI committee. Berger, who once had a tryout with the Bears, was so prominent and well regarded within the neurosurgery community, UCSF put his face on a billboard off Interstate 80 near the San Francisco side of the Bay Bridge.

Berger didn't doubt that McKee had seen CTE in some former players, but he was troubled by what he perceived as the BU Group's agenda. The group's survival, he felt, depended on proving that CTE was a major health problem. "I mean, their whole existence, their funding, relies on this [idea] that they're perpetuating that it's a fact if you play football you're going to have some form of cognitive impairment," he said. "So it's very, very difficult to accept it because it is so biased. I mean, anybody would say the same thing: You can't help but believe there's a bias. This is what they're there to do—to show that there is a link." He called BU's reluctance to share brain tissue with other scientists "suspect."

Berger likened the hysteria generated by BU to fears that cell phones caused brain tumors. For BU to suggest an absolute link between football and brain damage was "irresponsible," he said.

Berger's criticism was a common refrain: How could McKee be certain that head trauma was causing this disease? In fact, she couldn't be sure. It was all too new, and there weren't enough cases. The mechanism by which head banging turned into brain disease was unknown, though it was well established in the scientific literature that head trauma could lead to long-term cognitive problems.

Yet there wasn't a single recorded case of CTE in someone who had not sustained some form of brain trauma. To scientists such as Omalu, Bailes, McKee, Cantu, Hamilton, and DeKosky, along with numerous others, that alone was overwhelmingly persuasive. There was simply no other common factor. It was true, as critics like Berger noted, that there was a self-selecting quality to the cases: McKee was getting the brains of people who had been profoundly impaired, and their families wanted answers. The BU Group was drawing from a sample size that was "skewed beyond belief," Cantu acknowledged. But the sheer number and variety of cases was impossible to ignore, he felt.

"Mitch Berger, with all due respect, is full of shit," said Cantu, defending the BU Group when the criticism surfaced publicly.

"No, *not* with respect," Cantu added testily. He suggested that Berger and others were jealous about the publicity the BU Group and McKee had received. "This is a neuropathological diagnosis that's black-and-white, and one confirmed by anyone who has looked at the tissue," Cantu said. "It's not something with bias. It's not like if this brain doesn't have it, we'll duck it or stick it in a bucket."

Nowinski called Berger's comments "bizarre. I mean, the facts are the facts." He noted that the criticism had come from "somebody connected with the group that profits from the sport."

Berger and other members of the NFL committee wanted to steer Duerson's brain away from the BU publicity machine. The designation of BU as the NFL's preferred brain bank and the $1 million donation had predated the new committee by several months. The doctors thought it was irrelevant. Almost from the new committee's inception, Ellenbogen and Batjer had advised Goodell to start funneling the NFL's money to the National Institutes of Health. Their argument was that the NIH could play a neutral role—"like Switzerland"—and farm out the research to independent scientists who didn't have a vested interest in proving that CTE was connected to football.

The conflict put Duerson's family in the cross fire of a highly unusual situation. Duerson had asked to make sure that his brain was turned over to the NFL's brain bank. The NFL had designated BU as its "preferred" brain bank, and league officials had even directed Duerson's family to Nowinski. Yet the NFL's doctors wanted to divert Duerson's brain away from BU to the NIH.

"We had Dave Duerson's brain," Hunt Batjer, one of the committee cochairs, would later complain. "We talked to the family, the coroner, we had two outstanding neuropathologists waiting via NIH. But Nowinski flew into Chicago and told the family he represents the NFL, and they got it."

It hadn't gone exactly that way. But Batjer's tone reflected the new NFL committee's disdain for the BU Group. It was a fight that was far from over.

Two and a half months after Duerson's suicide, BU held a press conference to announce that he had CTE. Alicia, Tregg, and Duerson's other three children attended.

McKee said the case was indisputable evidence that the disease was connected to football. She added: "I think in Dave Duerson's case it drove him to suicide."

For McKee, Duerson's death was simply more proof that the NFL—and, by extension, the entire football-mad country—was facing a huge problem. Including Duerson, McKee had examined the brains of 25 deceased NFL players; 24 had CTE. McKee understood the lingering doubts. She herself had once had them. With each new case of CTE, she thought: "I just can't even believe this."

"There's definitely this feeling like, 'I must be making this up,'" McKee said. "You know, you're pushing credibility so far. You're thinking, 'This can't be true.' But then I kept saying: 'It is true. It is true. I've been doing this for too long. I've never seen this thing before, and it's really there.'"

McKee found herself thinking: "I'm really wondering where this stops. I'm really wondering if every single football player doesn't have this."

16

CONCUSSION, INC.

The NFL's concussion crisis continued to metastasize, spread by a growing army of former players, doctors, and lawyers. In Los Angeles, a prominent workers' compensation lawyer named Ron Feenberg began meeting former players with cognitive problems and saw another way to go after the league. California has some of the most lenient workers' compensation laws in the country. Any employee who works in the state for any length of time is eligible to file a claim regardless of where the company he or she works for is based. That meant any former NFL player who played even one game in California could file a claim against his team if he could show that he suffered debilitating injuries during his career.

Feenberg, a voluble man with a full head of gray hair, soon found himself drawn into the horrifying world of gridiron dementia. The lawyer recruited some two dozen clients who claimed to have traumatic brain injuries or some combination of orthopedic injuries and neurological disorders that stemmed from their careers. On one level, Feenberg thought these were garden-variety workers' compensation cases, not much different from "someone falling down a flight of stairs, getting your finger caught in a machine." But what struck him was how devastating the injuries were to the men and their families. It was like a siege on their identities. "I have players who have been shown pictures of themselves in uniform, and they don't even recognize the photograph and they can't tell you who that picture is even though it's themselves," he said.

Feenberg thus began to file claims with the California Workers' Compensation Appeals Board. The forms were straightforward, full of checked boxes and brief explanations. In the section where the former NFL player was asked to identify which body part had been injured, Feenberg would write in "brain." The players sought compensation from individual teams, not from the NFL. "McDonald's franchises answer to McDonald's corporate, but if you slip and fall at a fast food store on water or grease and break your leg, you bring your action against your direct employer," he explained. Within two years, hundreds of former players had lined up to file workers' compensation claims in California for brain injuries, opening up a new front against the league. In response, the NFL mounted a fierce lobbying campaign to close the loophole while teams and insurers fought the individual claims. The league had exerted the same pressures in an attempt to change the laws in other states. The battle became so heated that Patriots quarterback Tom Brady and Saints quarterback Drew Brees wrote a joint letter to the *San Francisco Chronicle* in opposition to the proposed change.

Jason Luckasevic, the young Pittsburgh lawyer, was out for bigger game than Feenberg. Relatively speaking, the workers' compensation cases were small legal matters, often involving thousands of dollars. His fight was against the entire NFL, with the stakes potentially in the billions. But the workers' compensation cases were not entirely unrelated to the whale Luckasevic was pursuing. To mount a case that the NFL had denied and concealed evidence that football causes brain damage, Luckasevic needed actual living players (or the families of deceased players) who were willing to come forward. This had proved one of his more difficult hurdles. During his three-year journey, Luckasevic had found numerous players who initially expressed interest, but when push came to shove, they were ambivalent about taking on the league or fearful of exposing their grotesque afflictions to a public that admired them for their mental and physical toughness. The workers' comp cases provided a potential feeder system to lawyers such as Luckasevic who were girding for the bigger fight ahead.

One of the first brain-related workers' compensation cases involved Fred McNeill, a quiet and thoughtful former Minnesota Vikings linebacker who played from 1974 to 1985. Ironically, McNeill himself had been a lawyer—even handling some workers' comp cases on behalf of former Vikings—until the deterioration of his brain abruptly ended his legal career. He had started attending law school just before his retirement, and by his late thirties he had made partner at Zimmerman Reed, a Minneapolis firm. Then, at 44, he was fired. McNeill managed to get other jobs and lost them, too. "It seems like it started that I was taking a longer time to do the work," said McNeill, his voice slow and gentle, edged with a kind of bewilderment at what had happened to him. "What I found is that in those firms, the attorneys that were managing me perceived that it was taking me longer to do the work than it should have been taking." Before long, McNeill was bankrupt, no longer practicing law, his loving family broken apart. He drifted through his days in intermittent states of lucidity and confusion. McNeill was still able to recall in great detail pieces of his distant past, such as his blocked punt on Oakland's Ray Guy in the first quarter of the 1977 Super Bowl. But his short-term memory was shot. He often couldn't remember people he just met or conversations he just had. He was living with his 23-year-old son, Gavin, who managed most of his father's needs out of their Los Angeles apartment. Gavin compared the experience to "seeing Superman lose his powers. But, in the brighter side of things, I'm gonna save him now."

Asked what he feared most about the future, Gavin said: "You know, I don't even want to talk about it. I don't even want to put it out there in the universe."

Luckasevic met Fred and his ex-wife, Tia, at a meeting of retired players in Las Vegas and recruited them to his cause. On July 19, 2011, the McNeills joined the 75 former players and their relatives suing the NFL for concealing the link between football and brain damage. The other players included Mark Duper, a longtime wide receiver for the Miami Dolphins; former New York Giants running back Rodney Hampton; and Steve Nelson, who played linebacker for 14 years with the New England Patriots.

Luckasevic finally had his lawsuit. It had grown out of an idle conversation with his friend Bennet Omalu one morning in Pittsburgh five years earlier. Along the way, Luckasevic had been laughed out of a conference room by the partners in his own firm and turned away by countless other lawyers. Now the 34-year-old associate was the coauthor of an

86-page complaint that would precipitate a tsunami of litigation against the NFL.

The complaint, written by Luckasevic and edited by his more experienced cocounsels Tom Girardi and Herman Russomanno, and Russomanno's partner, Bob Borrello, alleged that the NFL had created a fraudulent research arm to whitewash a problem that directly threatened its bottom line. At the center of the allegations was the league's MTBI committee. The complaint claimed that the NFL, "to further a scheme of fraud and deceit, had members of the NFL's Brain Injury Committee deny knowledge of a link between concussion and cognitive decline." Most of the major players in the drama of the previous decade figured prominently in the legal narrative: Omalu, McKee, Pellman, Casson, Guskiewicz, Lovell. Riddell, the NFL's official helmet maker, was named as a codefendant over allegations that its product was unsafe and the company had failed to provide sufficient warnings about the potential for long-term brain damage. In a cover sheet that outlined the nature of the filing, the lawyers checked the box for "Product Liability" in which bodily injury, death, or damage occurred.

When the complaint was filed, the lawyers had no idea where it might lead and whether other players would follow. "We thought maybe there was a body out there of two or three hundred players who've really been significantly harmed," said Girardi. Right up until they filed, their suit included only a few players, but as word spread that it was about to become a reality, more and more players signed on.

After the case was filed, players (and, with them, lawyers) continued to come out of the woodwork. It was as if an unspoken taboo had vanished. Luckasevic and Girardi had filed their case in California Superior Court, the logic being that the case might do better in state court. The next month, though, a Philadelphia personal injury lawyer, Larry Coben of the firm Anapol Schwartz PC, filed the first suit in federal court on behalf of seven more players. Coben previously had won cases against helmet makers Riddell and Schutt, and he had been exploring a lawsuit against the NFL for some time. Now, among his clients was former Chicago Bears quarterback Jim McMahon, who the previous year had acknowledged that he was having memory problems at age fifty-two. McMahon's admission was particularly jarring: Most fans still

remembered him for his rebellious leadership of the 1985 Bears, moon-
ing reporters, snubbing his nose at NFL Commissioner Pete Rozelle,
and leading with his head. When he appeared in public now, McMahon
still wore his trademark sunglasses, but it was generally to talk about
how he had trouble finding his way home.

"I won't remember a helluva lot about this interview in ten minutes,
probably," McMahon told ESPN's Steve Delsohn.

The lead plaintiff in the federal suit was a former Atlanta Falcons
safety named Ray Easterling. The suit did not provide much detail about
his plight, but the litany of Easterling's problems was by now painfully
familiar: mood swings, inattentiveness, business failures, erratic behavior. Easterling's hands shook. He had impulsive urges to run for miles
in the dark or to chop wood, which he stacked in his driveway in Rich-
mond, Virginia; once, while chopping, he accidentally took off part of
his thumb.

Eight months after the lawsuit was filed, Easterling shot himself to
death at the home he shared with his wife of 36 years. He was 62. His
brain, it was later discovered, was riddled with CTE. By the time the
results were released, one year after Jason Luckasevic and his colleagues
filed the first lawsuit, more than 3,000 retired players and their relatives
were suing the National Football League—nearly one quarter of all living former NFL players. And counting.

Every few days, Fred McNeill would travel to a clinic in Newport
Beach and stuff his 6-foot-2 frame into a small space-age room while
100 percent oxygen was pumped into his lungs. The hyperbaric oxygen
therapy had been recommended by a psychiatrist and author, Daniel
Amen, whose Amen Clinics around the country had attracted the attention of numerous retired NFL players who were concerned about their
brains. Many players swore by the treatments, which were said to promote healing and improve memory, but to date there was no conclusive
evidence that the process worked. A November 2012 study of 50 military service members with post-concussion syndrome found "no efficacy
in symptom relief" after 30 straight days of 90-minute treatments in the
hyperbaric chambers.

No longer a backwater of medical research, concussions had become a booming industry, attractive not only to the world's most prominent researchers but also to any number of entrepreneurs. No one could keep up with the array of products and gadgetry suddenly flooding the market. There were dietary supplements to treat brain swelling and others to prevent brain cells from dying. There were soft protective coverings that fit over helmets and hard skullcaps that sat beneath them like Kevlar yarmulkes. There were mouth guards and neck braces and helmet sensors that recorded the magnitude and frequency of each hit. After producing a few concussion stories for ESPN, the authors of this book found themselves bombarded with creative proposals. One read: "I would like to talk to you about the last 7 years of development of a Physics and Engineering foundation I have discovered. It is an Energy Absorption System that only allows 10 to 15 G's to the end user of all helmets. I have found the Holy Grail that will protect and preserve football, our troops and so much more."

It was a strange new world of experimentation and opportunism. The rapid pace of the research and the high-profile disclosures of prematurely demented football players were provoking a wave of anxiety among parents, coaches, athletes, and medical professionals. Everyone wanted answers to the proliferating questions: Since CTE could be diagnosed only postmortem, was there any way to detect the disease in living patients? Was there a way to predict—through genetic profiling or other means—who was more likely to get the disease (and get them out of harm's way)? How many concussions were too many? What products, if any, might reduce the effect of head trauma in football? The questions produced more questions, which in turn produced more opportunities.

No one was better positioned to cash in than the early pioneers, researchers such as Bailes and Maroon and Lovell. Each staked out new territory that presented opportunities for (1) scientific discovery and (2) financial gain. Bailes was researching a medieval-sounding device that he said could potentially prevent the brain from rattling around inside the skull. "You have to indulge me a little bit here," he said one afternoon in his office outside Chicago, displaying what appeared to be a form of neckwear with two large rubber beads in front. "So this is a new device. It's a first attempt ever to prevent brain injury by using a collar that compresses the jugular veins, which back up the blood in the brain some, and it decreases the room for slosh."

Some of Bailes's other initiatives sounded more promising. He and Omalu coauthored a pilot study that used brain scans to detect tau protein in five former NFL players—including Fred McNeill—the first time researchers were able to show signs of CTE in living patients. The scans, developed by Gary Small, a UCLA professor of psychiatry and behavioral sciences, had previously been used to detect Alzheimer's disease. "I've been saying that identifying CTE in a living person is the Holy Grail for this disease," Bailes said. "It's not definitive, and there's a lot we still need to discover to help these people, but it's very compelling. It's a new discovery." The announcement produced a cascade of new questions, in particular: If CTE could be diagnosed in living players, could the NFL force them to be tested? Would brain scans become mandatory at the NFL Combine? Was it a collective bargaining issue? Would children have to be tested before playing contact sports? Before every season or even every game? After a concussion? What was the threshold for banning a player? The mind reeled at the implications.

Concussions had become a full-time profession. ImPACT was so successful that Mark Lovell left his job at UPMC to run the company full-time. Fifteen years after Lovell and Maroon administered crude neuropsychological tests on Merril Hoge and 26 of his Steelers teammates, ImPACT had become a global phenomenon, the default standard for concussion testing. There were occasional skeptical studies and people such as Bill Barr and Chris Randolph, a Chicago neuropsychologist, who railed against the claims that ImPACT was better than any of the myriad other neuropsych tests that were out there. But it was like complaining about the domination of Kleenex over all the other facial tissues. ImPACT was what people turned to when a concussion occurred. The test was used by nearly every NFL team, all NHL teams, all Major League Baseball teams, all Major League Soccer teams, and the U.S. Olympic boxing, soccer, and hockey teams, not to mention rugby, soccer, and auto racing leagues around the world. ImPACT was used by Cirque du Soleil, the Pittsburgh Ballet, and the Lingerie Football League. It was used by 62 colleges and universities in California alone. Lovell and Collins insisted that ImPACT was just "a tool in the toolbox" for treating concussions, but it was marketed to schools as a tool no less indispensable than a screwdriver or a hammer. An army of ImPACT trainers stood by to ensure, for a small fee, that the test was administered correctly.

Lovell's reputation as a researcher had taken a big hit because of his association with the MTBI committee. The obvious conflicts of interest—pushing his own company to teams while running the NFL's neuropsych testing program—also had caught up with him, and the league finally cut him loose, like Casson, Viano, and most of the other original MTBI members. "Mark was canned," said Guskiewicz. Unlike the combative Collins, who took the attacks on ImPACT personally, Lovell seemed not to care much about the criticism anymore. In many ways, that was easy: ImPACT was a success beyond anyone's wildest dreams, and Lovell was in demand from Europe to South Africa. But he also had suffered two heart attacks—one at 43, another at 59—for reasons no one could explain, and the experience made him more laconic and philosophical than ever. "I'm not out to get anyone," he said over dinner one evening. "I've moved on, you know? I don't want to spend the rest of my life chasing down Bill Barr. I just don't care."

After leaving UPMC, Lovell, often wearing jeans and a fleece pullover, spent most of his days at ImPACT's new headquarters, a largely vacant suite in a business park down the road from the Steelers' practice facility. In the afternoons, a flock of geese often settled outside his window, which looked out on the Monongahela River. Lovell, still youthful-looking at 60, knew his legacy in the NFL saga was mixed at best. His research had helped bring attention to the problem. He had created the most widely used concussion test in the world. But he also had played a key role on a discredited committee whose major findings he now disavowed. Lovell continued to see himself as a marginal figure in the drama, the MTBI committee a product of its ignorant times and no more.

"You publish stuff," Lovell said, shrugging. "I always thought we were publishing a snapshot of things. And people tried to say we were publishing a movie. It's not the way it works. But it got interpreted that way."

Lovell and Maroon would live on in the gray areas of the concussion crisis—not Pellman or Dr. No but still part of the NFL's denial machine. Maroon had undergone an almost complete transformation. After famously dismissing Omalu's findings and then waking up to the implications ("Bennet, do you know what this really means?"), he now so embraced the idea of CTE that he was conducting his own research into the disease. That research often combined some of his favorite topics, including the health effects of products such as fish oil and red wine, which Maroon believed could help stave off neurodegenerative disease in the same way he believed they could stave off aging and death.

Maroon was perfectly suited to this next phase of the crisis, which favored entrepreneurship and not a little bit of self-promotion. The diminutive neurosurgeon was never more his father's son than in these moments. Maroon's dad had made his mark in the Ohio Valley providing diversions and respite to miners and travelers: a pack of cigarettes, a pull at a slot machine, a cheeseburger, and a fill-up along the interstate. Maroon, too, would prove himself an expert marketer. ImPACT, the product of his long-ago conversation with Chuck Noll, was, of course, a gold mine. Now, in response to the science he once had resisted, Maroon was endorsing concussion-resistant caps and repurposing his advocacy of wine and chocolate as the secrets to a long and healthy life.

It brought Maroon new adherents to his brand of alternative medicine, along with other attention he hadn't been seeking.

The soaring concern about concussions led to a wave of state regulations designed to protect children, regulations like the Zackery Lystedt Law that Ellenbogen and others had helped pass in Washington and that the NFL had pushed in other states.

One of the first states to adopt the legislation after Washington was New Mexico, and the issue caught the attention of Tom Udall, the state's Democratic senator. Udall, a nephew of 1976 presidential candidate Mo Udall, once had been New Mexico's attorney general. He had used that position to crack down on consumer fraud, going after telemarketers and other scourges. It was that aspect of the burgeoning concussion crisis that Udall thought most needed regulation, because so many of the new products making wild claims were aimed at children and their parents.

Udall was drawn immediately to Riddell's ongoing advertising campaign for the Revolution helmet and the company's claim that the youth line of helmets reduced concussions by 31 percent. The claim, of course, was the by-product of the controversial NFL research now at the heart of the lawsuits. It also stemmed from the notorious UPMC study that had been funded by Riddell and coauthored by the company's vice president of research and development, along with the ImPACT crew: Collins, Lovell, and Maroon. Udall focused on the potential conflicts of interest and the truthfulness of the claims, including the admission by UPMC that Riddell had distorted and misused the results.

Udall sat on the Senate Commerce Committee, which provided oversight of the Federal Trade Commission. He sent a letter to the FTC requesting an investigation, expressing concern "about potential unfair and deceptive practices related to the sale of football helmets, especially those advertised for children's use." The letter included page after page of Riddell advertising—on the company website, in print, on YouTube—boasting that the Revolution helmet line reduced concussions by 31 percent. Udall cited as particularly egregious Riddell's online description of the Revolution Youth helmet, in which the company touted an "extensive long-term study by the University of Pittsburgh Medical Center" as the basis for the claim. The study in fact had never tested the youth version of the NFL-inspired helmet.

"These prominently displayed claims citing a prestigious medical institution and scientific journal give the overall impression that these helmets provide a significant safety improvement over other helmets and that this is strongly supported by research," Udall wrote. "Yet there is actually very little scientific evidence to support the claim that Riddell Revolution helmets reduce the risk of concussion by 31 percent."

The FTC immediately opened an investigation into Riddell and other helmet companies that made similar claims. Udall and his aides thought the Riddell campaign had launched a wave of fanciful claims by companies seeking to capitalize on fears about concussions. "I really look at the UPMC study as what launched this whole era of concussion marketing claims in the area of sports equipment," said one Udall aide. The senator and his staff ultimately would flag dozens of suspicious products. The makers of one mouth guard that Udall targeted,

Brain-Pad, claimed that it could eliminate concussions entirely by creating what it called a "brain safety space."

Udall regarded Maroon as one of the industry's worst offenders. In addition to his participation in the flawed Riddell study, Maroon had endorsed a dietary supplement called Sports Brain Guard that purported to "maximize the brain's ability to heal and reduce inflammation."

An endorsement from Maroon—described as "part of the NFL's Traumatic Brain Injury Committee"—ran on the product's website: "Over the past 30 years, as a practicing neurosurgeon, I have treated thousands of athletes with sports related concussions—players from the NFL, NHL, NBA, NCAA and all the way down to kids playing youth sports. . . . A major consequence of a concussion is inflammation of the brain and the subsequent cascade of biochemical events that results in brain damage. . . . I have personally recommended [this] product, SPORTS BRAIN GUARD, to athletes at all levels following concussions."

On October 19, 2011, the Senate Commerce Committee gathered for a hearing on "Concussions and the Marketing of Sports Equipment." At one point, Udall asked Jeffrey Kutcher, an associate professor of neurology at the University of Michigan and chair of the American Academy of Neurology's sports neurology section, about the truthfulness of the Riddell/UPMC study. Kutcher replied that "there is no significant data" to make the claim that the helmet reduced concussions 31 percent.

"And you can see why a parent who would be concerned about concussions with all the increasing awareness that is out there would see something like this and think, 'I am going to get a really protective helmet for my child,'" said Udall. "And really, what we are talking about is something that is very, very misleading."

"Well, I can see that, and I do see that every week in my clinic," said Kutcher. "I see patients coming in with their parents saying they want to buy the new helmet: 'This is the concussion helmet. What do you think about it?' That is a very real conversation I have all the time."

"And they are asking you that question over and over again?" said Udall.

"Correct."

As for the Maroon-endorsed Sports Brain Guard, Kutcher said:

"There is no data that this type of thing will help prevent concussion at all, really."

Maroon wasn't asked to testify. Not surprisingly, he saw it differently when interviewed for this book. Like Lovell, Maroon claimed to have played little role in the Riddell study even though his name was on the paper and he was a cofounder of ImPACT. He remained unapologetic about the products he endorsed, including Sports Brain Guard, which soon was taken off the market amid the controversy. After decades in medicine, Maroon said he truly believed in the healing properties of the products he was touting. In the middle of helping the NFL figure out the implications of CTE, he sent a copy of his book *The Longevity Factor,* along with a supply of dietary supplements, to Peter Davies, the neuropathologist brought in by the league to evaluate Omalu. "Now just don't forget to take your fish oil!!" Maroon wrote in an e-mail. Maroon ingested the products he endorsed. He prescribed them for his patients and wrote about them in his books. Besides, he reasoned, what was the alternative? "Tell me what medicine is going to prevent concussion or treat concussion, what medicine is out there?" he said.

"I'm 72 years old; I'm 72 years old," said Maroon, looking trim and dapper one afternoon in his office at Pittsburgh's UPMC Presbyterian Hospital. "I'm doing what I believe. And I really mean it that way. I believe this. This is what I would do for me. This is what I'd do for my kid and what I do for my patients. So it can be said to be crackpot. But tell me what you're doing better?"

In November 2012, the FTC ordered the makers of Brain-Pad, the mouth guard, to stop making claims that their product reduced concussions. The agency also sent warning letters to 18 other marketers of "anti-concussion" products. Six months later, the FTC closed its investigation into Riddell and other helmet companies. In a letter to Riddell, Mary K. Engle, the FTC's associate director for advertising practices, wrote that the agency had concluded the UPMC study "did not prove that Revolution varsity football helmets reduce concussions or the risk of concussions by 31%." The UPMC study also didn't prove, as Riddell had claimed, that the Revolution Youth helmet had that effect, because the study never looked at those helmets.

But the FTC had decided not to sanction Riddell. That was partly

because the company, after years of making the UPMC study the centerpiece of its national marketing campaign, had "discontinued use of
the 31% claim," Engle wrote.

T he NFL had long prided itself on its PR machine. Now the machine
was facing its greatest challenge. Since its inception, the NFL had
played on the country's primal urges, promoting itself as a refuge for
legally sanctioned violence. That would obviously have to change. With
former NFL stars shooting themselves in the chest to spare their brains
and thousands of players suing the league, the task of remaking football's image would not be an easy one.

In 1970, when the NFL and the AFL officially merged, the league
produced a coffee table book that offered an unusually frank assessment
of life in the NFL. Half-naked players were seen lounging in a trainer's
room next to miles of athletic tape and drawers filled with painkillers;
armored gladiators walked single file toward an unseen battlefield; piles
of humanity fought in the muck, a boiling mass of indistinguishable
arms and legs.

The NFL let the players tell the story in their own words, interspers-
ing their quotes with meditations on war and aggression from philoso-
phers and psychiatrists:

"Football is a violent game. You are physically attacking another person. To do this, you almost have to change your personality, to break down some of the things taught you, because
this is not accepted in our society."
—Howard Mudd, guard, San Francisco 49ers

"Violence, in its many forms, [is] an involuntary quest for
identity. When our identity is in danger, we feel certain that we
have a mandate for war."
—Marshall McLuhan, *War and Peace in the Global Village*

"It's a feeling of exhilaration. Boy, you really knocked the hell
out of that guy. You just feel great because you hit somebody."
—Ernie Stautner, tackle, Pittsburgh Steelers

"There is, in the modern community, no legitimate outlet for aggressive behavior. To keep the peace is the first of civic duties, and the hostile neighboring tribe, once the target at which to discharge phylogenetically programmed aggression, has now withdrawn to an ideal distance, hidden behind a curtain, if possible of iron. . . . The main function of sport today lies in the cathartic discharge of aggressive urge."

—Konrad Lorenz, *On Aggression*

The NFL took the violence at the core of the sport and turned it into art. The book, *The First Fifty Years,* was produced by "the creative staff of National Football League Properties, Inc.," the league's licensing arm. It had the same raw and hagiographic feel as the work produced by NFL Films, another project Commissioner Pete Rozelle had funded. *Sports Illustrated* would famously call NFL Films "perhaps the most effective propaganda organ in the history of corporate America." The company's origin story has been told and retold, mirroring in many ways the birth of the modern NFL. The founder, Ed Sabol, was a former overcoat salesman who received a 16-millimeter Bell & Howell movie camera as a wedding present and later used it to film his son's high school football games. Sabol ultimately left his job and created a production company. He somehow persuaded Rozelle to let him shoot the 1962 NFL Championship Game between Green Bay and New York; the 28-minute production was a wild success, and thus was born NFL Films.

Sabol soon joined forces with his son Steve, an art major and film lover who infused the enterprise with a style that combined pieces of his favorite artists and movies: the tight close-ups of clawing hands and rock in the 1946 film *Duel in the Sun*; the use of light and shadow by the Renaissance masters; Leni Riefenstahl's epic presentation of the 1936 Olympics; the sweeping musical scores of movies like *Gone with the Wind*. The highlight reels produced by NFL Films were tales of heroism and sacrifice. Amid the martial music that stuck in every fan's head came the "Voice of God," John Facenda, who made a recap of a midseason game between the Chiefs and Vikings seem like the Battle of the Bulge. NFL Films would win more than 100 Emmys. *They Call It Pro Football,* the Sabols' magnum opus, released in 1967, was recognized by the National Film Registry of the Library of Congress, which called it the "Citizen Kane of sports movies." The film opens with Facenda intoning: "It starts with a whistle and ends with a gun."

Violence, stylized and exquisitely rendered, was always an inextricable part of the show, no less than was the case in the Martin Scorsese and Francis Ford Coppola films of that era. NFL Films pumped out titles such as *Crunch Course, Strike Force, Moment of Impact,* and *The Best of Thunder and Destruction: NFL's Hardest Hits.* "In the NFL's war zones, the most explosive weapon that can be deployed is a man's body," Facenda declares in *Crunch Course.*

There was always one major difference between the NFL's brand of art and everything else: "Unlike other forms of popular entertainment, NFL football is *real*—the players actually do what they appear to be doing—yet at the same time it is a creation of the media, and it generates some of the most powerful fantasies in our culture," wrote Michael Oriard, a former Notre Dame and Kansas City Chiefs offensive lineman who went on to become Distinguished Professor of American Literature at Oregon State University. "The actuality of football is the source of its cultural power, but media-made images of that reality are all that most fans know."

The images are seductive yet deceptive. Like war movies, the images soften and glorify the violence to the people who watch. The reality, like war itself, is far different. Those who get close to the NFL battlefield are left in awe of its ferocity and speed, the sheer sound of it, as memorable as giant waves crashing repeatedly on the shore. Andy Russell, the Steelers great, broke into the league as a third-team linebacker in 1963. In his first game, the starter, John Reger, collapsed after a brutal hit and swallowed his tongue. Reger went into convulsions on the field, like a man having a seizure. The team doctor searched frantically for a tool to pry open Reger's jaw. Unable to find one, he chipped out his front teeth with a pair of scissors. Blood sprayed everywhere— onto the grass, the doctor, Reger's white jersey. He left the stadium in an ambulance. A few plays later, the second-string linebacker sustained an ankle injury that also put him out of the game. Thus began Russell's 12-year career.

Now, for the first time in its history, the NFL needed a new image, one that instead of glorifying the violence deflected attention from the fact that it was driving men mad. The stakes were obvious. The NFL's success depended not only on the buy-in of millions of fans for whom injuries were an acceptable and even attractive part of the entertainment but also on the parents who submitted their kids to the Darwinian system that led to the glory, however distant, of the NFL. Maroon, in his burst of candor after examining Omalu's slides, had summed it up perfectly: "If only 10 percent of mothers in America begin to conceive of football as a dangerous game, that is the end of football." Or as the *Times* blog had asked, "Is Tackle Football Too Dangerous for Kids to Play?"

And so it came to pass that the NFL found itself reaching out to a new constituency: mommy bloggers.

In the summer of 2012, Lorraine Esposito, a New York life and fitness coach, mother of two teenagers, and author of a blog that was published on WorkingMother.com, received an e-mail from Clare Graff of the NFL's Corporate Communications Department:

"As the mother of a little boy and someone who combs the headlines every day, I see all the stories about concussions in youth sports, as I'm sure you do as well," Graff wrote. "Through working at the NFL, I've been lucky enough to interact with some of the country's most respected neurologists, and I've learned a lot about concussions—what causes them, how to spot the symptoms, and how to treat and prevent them.

"We're inviting parenting/health writers and bloggers to the NFL offices in August, around the time kids head back to school and back to sports. We want to hear what concerns you and your readers about youth sports and injuries, what keeps you up at night, and share some resources with you that may be helpful on the topic."

Esposito was thrilled to be invited to the "Youth Health & Safety Luncheon" at the NFL's offices in New York. She was joined by about 50 people like her, mostly influential women who might be concerned about the continuing bad news about football and brain damage. The group was given a tour of NFL headquarters and introduced to the team that oversaw officials. The luncheon featured the commissioner; Scott Hallenbeck, the executive director of USA Football; Holly Robinson Peete, the wife of former NFL player Rodney Peete "and a football mom"; Elizabeth Pieroth, a neuropsychologist and head injury consultant to the Chicago Bears; and Kelly Sarmiento, a health communications specialist for the Centers for Disease Control and Prevention.

Goodell spoke to the group about the need to change the culture of football. It wasn't totally clear to Esposito what that meant, but she found Goodell solicitous, a good listener.

"To his credit, he really wanted to know," Esposito said. "I asked him to help me define what this cultural change really is. We started talking about the training and equipment. I said, 'That's not what I mean. What's the culture you're talking about?' He said: 'That is a great question, but I don't have an answer for you.'"

Still, Esposito came away convinced that the NFL was committed to creating a healthier and safer sport.

Similar events followed. Amanda Rodriguez, who blogs under the name Dumb Mom, said she learned about some "myths that people should know about. . . . I think that my perception of concussions has changed dramatically. One, I feel like football gets a pretty bad rap as the most dangerous sport. I didn't realize that kids were being concussed in other sports, especially soccer. We learned about that at the NFL. And most concussions don't happen in a sport. Kids get concussed riding their bikes."

After one session, a mommy blogger tweeted: "Football and sports are SO good for kids. Don't let the worry keep your kids from playing sports."

Another, quoting Pieroth, the neuropsychologist who works with the Bears, tweeted: "'We need to balance the hysteria of #concussions with the benefits of sports participation,' says Dr. Pieroth #nflhealthsafety."

For years, the PR machine had disseminated the message that concussions were a nonissue. Now the NFL was pouring its resources into the message that health and safety were *the* issue. All the symbolism of the previous era began to fall away. The image of two helmets crashing together and exploding that preceded *Monday Night Football* for over two decades was quietly discontinued by ESPN at the request of the NFL. ESPN already had ended its popular Monday Night Countdown segment "Jacked Up!" after the first cases of CTE surfaced in 2006. CBS no longer ran "the Pounder Index," another pregame segment, sponsored by McDonald's, in which the biggest hits of the previous week were assessed on a 10-point scale. In January 2011, the league pressured Toyota to pull a commercial that featured a helmet-to-helmet collision between two youth players. Under the direction of Paul Hicks, a veteran of the powerhouse Ogilvy Public Relations, the league crafted a new message that stressed the "evolution" of the sport. The primary vehicle was an interactive website, NFLevolution.com, that highlighted changes in rules and equipment through the decades and a TV commercial directed by Peter Berg, creator of the series *Friday Night Lights*. The commercial showed a kick return that starts in Canton, Ohio, in 1906 with a runner trailing a flying wedge—a blocking technique later banned because of its destructiveness. The return progresses upfield through time, the rules and equipment changing, and ends with Devin Hester, the Bears return man, scoring a touchdown after breaking a recently prohibited horse-collar tackle. Ravens linebacker Ray Lewis delivers the voice-over: "Here's to making the next century safer and more exciting. Forever forward. Forever football."

This was the new era of the NFL. The game had come a long way. It wasn't that long ago that a defensive lineman could sheath his forearm in plaster and bash an offensive lineman in the head. Leg whipping was once legal, as was clotheslining and the crack-back block, which ripped apart the knee ligaments of an untold number of linebackers. But the game continued to evolve.

The commercial, which premiered during the 2012 Super Bowl, featured a number of recognizable greats: Hall of Famer Ollie Matson, who played 14 seasons in the 1950s and 1960s; Rick Upchurch, an electrifying Broncos kick returner in the 1970s and 1980s; and Mel Gray, the great Cardinals wide receiver in the 1970s and early 1980s.

As the commercial continued to run, Matt Crossman, a writer for *The Sporting News,* pointed out that Rick Upchurch and Mel Gray were among the thousands of players suing the NFL, along with Ollie Matson's family. Matson had died in 2011 after years of struggling with dementia. In the end he couldn't speak. His family donated his brain to BU, where Ann McKee diagnosed him with one of the most severe cases of CTE on record.

17

BUZZARDS

On the afternoon of May 2, 2012, Omalu was hunched over a microscope when his phone started blowing up. He ignored it, but when the calls kept coming, he looked down at the number and answered. It was Bailes calling from Chicago, his voice urgent.

"What is this? Is everything okay?" Omalu said.

"Haven't you heard?" said Bailes. "Junior Seau just killed himself."

"Who's Junior Seau?" Omalu replied, predictably.

Bailes told Omalu to get on the Internet. Omalu started reading and absorbed the gist of what had happened that morning in Oceanside, California. Seau, 43, one of the finest linebackers in NFL history, had been found dead of a self-inflicted gunshot wound at his beachfront home.

The implications were obvious. Throughout the country, Seau's suicide provoked shock and profound sadness in a generation of football fans for whom he embodied the cathartic ecstasy of the sport. Seau was an icon in San Diego, a man whose love of life had seemed as real and unflagging as the sun. But to CTE researchers, Seau's death carried a different meaning. He had played in the NFL for 20 years, one of just two defensive players—the other was Redskins cornerback Darrell Green—to make it through two full decades. He had made 1,524 tackles, fourth on the unofficial all-time list. He was a certain Hall of Famer. Like Duerson, Seau had shot himself in the chest; his brain was pristine and intact. As concern about the health effects of football spread, attracting more and more prominent scientists, Seau in death was instantly transformed into a rare and valuable research commodity, his brain the most coveted specimen to come along since the connection between football and brain damage became known.

Omalu, shunned by the NFL and overshadowed by the BU Group, immediately grasped the significance, personal and scientific, even if moments earlier he hadn't known who Junior Seau was.

"What do you need me to do?" he said.

"We need to secure this brain," said Bailes.

Others, of course, had the same idea, including the NFL.

Even the people closest to Seau said they were shocked. His suicide was like peeking behind the facade of the most beautiful building in the world and finding a desert. For decades, there was a fairy-tale quality to Seau's life, except that it was demonstrably real. Raised in a violent ghetto of Oceanside, 40 miles up the coast from San Diego, the son of immigrants from American Samoa who steeped their children in their transplanted culture, Seau had become one of the most talented and beloved players in NFL history.

The NFL had never seen anything like him. He was like a new species, a 6-foot-3, 260-pound floating linebacker who ran the 40-yard dash in 4.61 seconds, bench-pressed 500 pounds, and had a 38-inch vertical leap. In college, Seau had played outside linebacker, with his hand in the dirt, but the Chargers moved him inside, and the effect was devastating. He was mentored by Gary Plummer—Plummer played right inside linebacker, Seau left—who had just turned 30 and was blown away by what his new teammate could do.

Seau sometimes would line up 12 yards deep, "and he'd just fucking blitz!" said Plummer. "He wasn't supposed to and, you know, *bam*. He really changed the game. He was a freelancer, and he had such amazing physical tools he could get away with it. A guy like me, no way, they're going to cut me tomorrow."

San Diego fell in love with Seau during his 13 seasons with the Chargers. Part of it was his improvisational talent and his hometown roots, but in large measure his appeal stemmed from an ability to make people feel better about themselves. Seau was loud, playful, and flirtatious, a giant kid who greeted friends and strangers by yelling, *"Buddeeeee!"* Close friends and family called him June or Junebug. A lifelong surfer, he carried himself with a relaxed confidence, as if he had absorbed the soul of the sea. Seau seemed to know exactly where he came from and what he wanted to give back to the world. He started a charity, the Junior Seau Foundation, to help underprivileged kids in San Diego. During a luncheon for the foundation in the late 1990s, he met a motherly and sweet-natured consultant for the United Way named Bette Hoffman and asked her to help out. Hoffman already had more work than she could handle but couldn't resist. "Junior's personality was bigger than life," she said. "He was so charismatic and so fun and so intriguing. I was used to working with nonprofits; I'd never worked with a football player. But you know, I realized that he had such a compassion for wanting to help the people in San Diego. When he walked into a room, he didn't have to say a word; you knew he was there. He had this amazing capacity when he was talking to someone; people truly believed that he or she was the most important person in the world."

Seau was soon calling Hoffman "Mom" and relying on her to help run his affairs. Together, they built one of the most successful athletic foundations in the country. They also opened a restaurant, Seau's, in Mission Valley that thrived on his good name. From his humble beginnings, Seau had become an engaged and focused community leader. "I would show him budgets for every event and for overall projections, and he was just so sharp with those," said Hoffman. "He would know exactly what we needed to do, how we needed to get there and implement it." Seau served as auctioneer at the Seau Foundation's annual fund-raisers. Before the event, he would memorize the floor plan to know where all the heavy hitters would be sitting and then use his smile and charisma to cajole them into making bids. "He was like a son to me; I really considered him one of my sons," said Hoffman. "He was just so dear, and he was just so sweet."

Seau had had a son with his childhood sweetheart and two boys and a girl with his wife, Gina, a former Chargers marketing associate whom he met as a rookie. Before they divorced in 2001, Gina watched the cult of Junior grow in San Diego—from the afternoon when he was a rookie and a woman asked for his autograph while they were out buying milk and cookies to "four or five years down the road and we couldn't go sit and have dinner without ten, fifteen, twenty interruptions."

During the final years of Seau's career, there were signs that he was changing. Without warning, one day he exploded at his oldest son, Tyler, to the point where the two had to be separated by Junior's friends. "It never got completely physical, but it was close," Tyler said. "I've never really seen him that angry before." Seau played his last down with New England in 2009. By the time he returned to Oceanside, where he had bought a $3.2 million home in 2005, the people closest to him could tell he wasn't right. He seemed totally unprepared for the transition out of football, which was difficult for all players but especially for one who had played almost continuously since his teens. Seau was 40. He had earned over $50 million. But his world quickly began to collapse, financially and spiritually.

Seau was drinking heavily, according to his friends and family. Hoffman was unable to get him to focus on his restaurants or the foundation, a change she had noticed as far back as 2003, after Seau left the Chargers to play in Miami. Now, when Seau made presentations to potential donors, he rambled and lost his train of thought. He had volcanic eruptions of anger, particularly when he drank. His memory seemed to be fading. One day, his son Jake, a star lacrosse player, had a big game in Torrey Pines. Seau's daughter, Sydney, called repeatedly to remind him to be there, including on the morning of the game. "I text him 20 minutes beforehand and I'm like, 'Where are you? They're warming up,'" she recalled. "And he's like, 'What are you talking about? I thought that's tomorrow.' And I'm like, 'No, I called you this morning. We talked about this. You need to be here. Get here now.'"

As Seau's problems grew worse, he withdrew from his family and close friends, going months without seeing his kids. Hoffman became alarmed by his growing gambling addiction, which cost him hundreds of thousands, if not millions, of dollars. "It just became more and more serious," said Hoffman, who had control of Seau's finances. Seau would call her from Las Vegas, sometimes frantic, asking her to wire huge amounts of money to keep him going.

On October 17, 2010, Seau was arrested on charges that he had assaulted his live-in girlfriend, Mary Nolan. She told officers that Seau had "grabbed her by the arm and shoved her into the wall/dresser in their bedroom." Seau was released on $25,000 bail, Nolan never filed a complaint, and the case was dropped. But Seau was inconsolable. The morning after the incident, a few hours after he left jail, Seau was driving up the coast when he ran his Cadillac Escalade off a cliff. The SUV careened down a 100-foot slope and settled in the sand near the water. When Gina learned about the accident, she grabbed the kids and drove to Scripps Memorial Hospital in La Jolla, where Seau had been taken in an ambulance with, remarkably, minor injuries.

Seau was still in the emergency room when his family arrived. "He just looked so broken, and I mean not just physically," said Gina, who stayed close with her ex-husband. "His eyes: He just looked so sad and so defeated, this big guy that barely fits on the bed."

Seau insisted that he had fallen asleep at the wheel, that the accident wasn't a suicide attempt. At the time, Gina believed him. Still, she told him it was an opportunity to turn his life around.

"You've got another chance in life," she said. "You're very blessed. You lived to see another day. What are you gonna do? You have so much to live for. Our kids are progressing so beautifully. You'd be so proud of them. Get in the game."

"You're right, G," said Seau. "You're right."

But soon he disappeared again; Gina and the kids found out from *TMZ* that Seau was back in Vegas just a few weeks after the incident. In January 2011, Bette Hoffman quit as the head of the Junior Seau Foundation. "I was just done; I'd had so much, you know, trying to protect him and cover for him," she said. "I thought, 'What am I doing?' I mean, I couldn't help him. He wouldn't listen to me."

"Oh, Mom," Seau said when Hoffman told him she was quitting. He called her repeatedly, begging her to change her mind. Instead, Hoffman changed her phone number.

Seau's daughter, Sydney, decided to stage a one-girl intervention. Sydney was a high school senior, a promising volleyball player with wavy brown curls and her father's charisma and megawatt smile. She was every bit a daddy's girl; she worshiped her father and wanted to be around him as much as possible: "He was just a light, that's how I'd describe him," she said. That year, Seau had missed most of Sydney's senior season. She had written an English paper about the void her father had left in her life, and it emboldened her to confront him. "I drove over to his house, and I just told him everything," she said. "How I wasn't gonna take a backseat anymore because I was sick of waiting. It hurt me to have to pull so much. It was just hard because I wanted him to want me more than anything. And my whole life was to make him proud and to make him want to see me.

"He just looked in a straight line and cried and didn't hug me, didn't say a word. He just sat on the couch. And that's what really bothered me. How can I express all of this emotion and you just cry and not even want to console me? Like, that's not normal. He just told me that he had never really, truly felt love. And I was like, 'What does that mean?' But it didn't change. He was still really distant."

Sydney decided to attend USC, her father's alma mater, "because that's his second home and I could share that with him." In March 2012, she, Seau, and Gina drove up to Los Angeles for spring orientation. It was the kind of moment Sydney had yearned for. Her parents had been divorced for 10 years, but they all went to dinner together at the Palm before attending a Lakers game. "He was being such a tease and a flirt, and the waitress came by," said Gina. "She goes, 'Oh, you guys are such a cute family.' I was about to say, 'We're not married.' And he said, 'Meet my future wife. This is Gina.'"

"Dad!" exclaimed Sydney, laughing.

Five weeks later, Seau shot himself in the chest with a .357 Magnum revolver.

Unlike Duerson, Seau hadn't left instructions for what to do with his brain, and so it was never known if he shot himself in the chest to preserve it. His girlfriend, Megan Noderer, found him on a queen-sized bed in an upstairs guest room after returning from the gym that morning. After calling 911, Noderer pulled Seau to the floor in an unsuccessful attempt to administer CPR. When police arrived, the bed was strewn with bloodstained pillows and sheets, a gray stocking cap, and the gun, which lay on its left side with five bullets in the chamber and one spent round near the headboard. Seau's cell phone also was on the bed, the SIM card removed, a fact that was never explained.

Seau was placed on a gurney in a body bag and brought down to the garage. Outside, some 400 people had gathered: neighbors, Chargers fans, news crews, Seau's extended Samoan family. Inside the swelter-ing house, Seau's closest relatives and friends milled around in shock amid his trophies, signed helmets, and game photos. In the late morn-ing, the family decided to open the garage for a spontaneous public viewing. Seau lay on his back, the body bag zipped up to his neck, his head exposed. Hoffman bent over and kissed him. "Good-bye, Junior, I love you," she said. "He just looked like he was asleep on the couch," said Hoffman, sobbing at the memory. "He didn't even look like he was dead. I had to wake him up so many times from a nap, and that's how I said good-bye to him." For nearly an hour, the tearful crowd filed past.

That afternoon, Tyler, Seau's 23-year-old son, was still at the house when his phone rang.

It was Omalu and Bailes, asking for his dad's brain.

If the two doctors were concerned about the unfortunate timing— just a few hours after Seau was carted out of the garage—the feeling was superseded by the urgency they felt. Within a day, Seau's body would be autopsied; without preparation, his brain might be buried with him or destroyed. More immediately, there was also the competition: Omalu and Bailes knew that Nowinski and the BU Group would soon make a big push, if they hadn't already, presumably backed by the NFL. They felt they had to move now.

Bailes, Omalu, and Tyler Seau would remember the call differently. Omalu said: "We introduced ourselves, explained what we were doing, about CTE, that we would like him to grant us consent to examine his father's brain." He described Tyler as "very polite" and receptive during the brief call.

But Tyler said he immediately felt pressured by Omalu. "He was very pushy, and he really wanted me to make a decision that night. He pretty much said that we have to do it now because if it's not done the right way, we could lose a lot of the tissue and things like that." Tyler already was under unthinkable pressure; with his father's death, he had become responsible for a host of family decisions. Quiet and thoughtful, four inches shorter and 40 pounds lighter than his dad, Tyler had played linebacker at Palomar Community College in San Diego and Delta State University, a Division II school in Cleveland, Mississippi. Now he was working in Seau's restaurant.

During the call with Omalu and Bailes, Tyler agreed to donate his father's brain to their group.

Omalu initiated the paperwork that would allow him to harvest Seau's brain. He faxed a consent form to Tyler, who initially indicated that he was prepared to sign. At 8:38 that night, Tyler wrote in an e-mail to Omalu: "my guy is on his way here right now so I can sign it and fax it back to you." An hour later he wrote again, asking Omalu to contact David Chao, the San Diego Chargers' doctor, to "cross our Ts and dot our Is before proceeding."

Junior Seau and Chao were close. Tyler said Chao had continued as his dad's personal physician after Seau left the Chargers. Tyler was growing wary about his decision, and he felt Chao was the logical person to help him sort out what to do. But Chao had his own issues. The day after Seau shot himself, the orthopedic surgeon appeared before the Medical Board of California to respond to allegations that he committed acts of "dishonesty or corruption" by failing to report a 2006 drunk driving conviction on an application to evaluate workers' compensation cases. Later that year, the board moved to revoke Chao's medical license over three separate malpractice claims. (DeMaurice Smith, executive director of the NFL Players Association, would take the unusual step of calling for Chao to be replaced as the Chargers' doctor. A panel of independent physicians created under the league's collective bargaining agreement ultimately exonerated Chao. Soon after, Chao resigned his position with the Chargers, citing health and family reasons.)

Now, at Tyler's request, Chao became the point person for what would happen to Seau's brain. The night of Seau's death, Chao called Omalu and berated him, according to Omalu. "That was one of the most arrogant phone calls I've ever been involved with in my life," said Omalu. "This guy was yelling, was extremely arrogant, pretty much questioning who I was." After the contentious call, Omalu e-mailed his credentials and samples of his research to Chao. He was convinced he still had "verbal consent" from Tyler to take Seau's brain. He booked a flight from San Francisco to San Diego to do just that.

By then, at least a half dozen prominent researchers were making a play for Seau's brain. The deputy medical examiner, Craig Nelson, returned from Seau's home to find a sheaf of messages stacked up at the office. "It felt sometimes to me like buzzards were circling," Nelson said. "I have a scientific mind and a medical background, but when someone has just died, things are very fresh. Imagine that your parent dies and then hours later somebody is calling you and saying, 'Hey, would you consider donating this for research?' It can sit a little odd, and when it's such an unexpected death, it makes it harder."

Nelson's buzzards included a Nobel laureate brain researcher, Stanley Prusiner, director of the Institute for Neurodegenerative Diseases at the University of California, San Francisco. Prusiner, a 70-year-old scientist with a cloud of white hair, won the 1997 Nobel Prize in Physiology or Medicine for his discovery of prions, a class of infectious proteins behind brain disorders such as mad cow disease and Creutzfeldt-Jakob disease. Prusiner's specific interest in CTE wasn't clear, but he launched a tag-team effort with Omalu to bid for Seau's brain. Within hours of Seau's death, Prusiner placed calls to the medical examiner's office to try to arrange a meeting with Seau's family. He had his assistant call and e-mail Tyler Seau.

Omalu and Prusiner egged each other on. "Please it is vital you get to the Seau family," Omalu wrote Prusiner in an e-mail the day after Seau's suicide. "I think they will give you/us the brain if you directly speak to them and play the nobel price [sic] card :)"

Prusiner responded by e-mail 12 minutes later that he was planning to fly to San Diego to meet with the Seau family.

But BU was launching its own offensive. At 5:55 A.M. (2:55 California time), the morning after Seau killed himself, popular *Sports Illustrated* football writer Peter King issued a supportive tweet for the BU Group to his more than 1 million followers: "Dedicated researchers in Boston studying deceased players' brains for evidence of trauma attempting to obtain Junior Seau's. Hope they do." King thought the tweet was harmless, but it quickly morphed into a national news story that was picked up by NFL.com, ESPN.com, and other websites. Seau's family was outraged by what they perceived as more tactless pressure. Nowinski and others scrambled to contain the damage. They urged King to "retract" the tweet and apologize to Seau's family. Nowinski later claimed that King had based the tweet on his own assumption that BU would chase after Seau's brain. But King said, in fact, he had confirmed BU's interest. King refused to apologize or make a retraction. "I empathize with them and know how badly they wanted to see Seau's brain," he said. "I was sorry it put them in an awkward situation, because I believe in what they do."

He issued a vague follow-up at 11:13 A.M.: "To clarify researchers seeking Seau's brain: Info not from them. They seek to examine all ex-players who played contact sports. Every one."

When Gina heard about the requests that were pouring in for her ex-husband's brain, she was horrified. "It was the most foreign thing I'd ever heard of, quite honestly," she said. "And the fact that I had to have a conversation with the coroner and ask, 'If we decide to donate it, how do you take it out? And what do you do with it?' And here we are about to have a funeral service. This is an open casket. It was crazy. It was really bizarre."

Not long after the Twitter contretemps, Omalu touched down in San Diego. He was carrying a special "brain briefcase." Nelson, the deputy medical examiner, believed Omalu had permission from Seau's family to take the brain and thus had invited him to participate in the autopsy. Omalu's plan was to remove Seau's brain and fly it back to San Francisco, where he would divvy it up with Prusiner. Omalu headed straight from the airport to the medical examiner's office, a hulking three-story building on the north side of town. Nelson told Omalu he couldn't take any tissue without written consent from Seau's family. That hadn't materialized, and so Nelson asked Joe Davis, the office chaplain, to call Tyler Seau and have him fax it over. Omalu spent much of the morning chatting with Davis, recounting his battles with the NFL and talking about his faith. Omalu then joined Nelson in the autopsy suite, a cool, windowless room with fluorescent lighting and a dozen workstations equipped with gleaming stainless steel tables, oscillating saws, and plastic cutting boards. The office lent Omalu scrubs and a clear plastic visor.

Soot and the imprint of the gun's muzzle were still visible on Seau's chest. He had no alcohol or drugs in his system except for zolpidem, the insomnia medication whose trade name is Ambien, and naproxen, an anti-inflammatory. Nelson made a Y-shaped incision and removed most of Seau's vital organs. Omalu removed the brain and the spinal cord. He sliced Seau's brain with a long knife and placed half in a small tub filled with formalin. The rest he froze under protocols prescribed by Prusiner.

As the autopsy was wrapping up, Davis, the chaplain, received a call back from Tyler. He wasn't calling to sign over his dad's brain. He was in a rage, screaming about Omalu.

"I talked to the NFL," Tyler told Davis. The league, he said, had informed him that Omalu's "research was bad and his ethics are bad."

"He is not to be in the same fucking room as my dad!" he told the chaplain. "He's not to fucking touch my dad! He's not to have anything to do with my dad!"

Davis tried to calm him down.

"Nothing's going to happen without your permission; just rest your heart in that," he said. "But let me ask you, why the U-turn? I mean, you talked to him last night, and the only reason he's here is because you told him to go ahead and buy a plane ticket and come here. So just help me understand why the U-turn."

Tyler repeated that he had talked to "the NFL," without specifying whom, and repeated that he was told Omalu was unethical and his research was flawed. At one point, Tyler mentioned having received advice from Chao. Davis reassured Tyler that nothing would happen without his permission. "But you got to understand," Davis added, "the NFL may very well not want him to do the research because he's the guy that's proving the post-concussion syndrome. You need to think about that." Tyler merely reiterated that he wanted Omalu out.

Davis hung up and went to the autopsy room. He entered with a troubled look on his face.

"Houston, we have a problem," he announced.

It was too late, of course, to keep Omalu away from Seau's brain; he already had dissected it. Nelson felt he was on solid legal ground: He had every right as deputy medical examiner to bring consultants into the autopsy room. But he wanted to protect Seau's family, not insult them. At that moment, Omalu said, he was "persona non grata." He felt like it was a replay of the persecution of his science and his reputation over the previous six years. "It reminded me of the way Casson, Pellman, and Viano dismissed me, actually calling me a fraud as well," he said. "It's the same pattern. To summarize it: a systematic effort to marginalize me, delegitimize me, and dismiss me. To pretty much make me null and void, an outsider not to be trusted."

"Why do I deserve to be treated the way I'm being treated?" Omalu asked, growing emotional. "For doing good work? Isn't that what America is about: doing good work, enhancing the lives of others?"

Omalu returned to San Francisco, depressed, his brain briefcase empty. "My poor wife, who's seen me go through this over and over and over, she cried, you know?" he said. "After that I just said, 'You know what? This is it for me. I think I've done my part.' The Junior Seau case made me regret ever getting involved in CTE."

Prusiner, oblivious to the debacle that had taken place 400 miles to the south, sent Omalu a celebratory e-mail, attaching an article from ESPN.com, which had learned that Omalu had participated in Seau's autopsy. "Your trip to San Diego was really important," the Nobel laureate wrote. "Please see the wonderful attached write-up about you, the CTE identifier. I shall call Tyler and David Chao tomorrow and create a time to meet them in SD."

The chances of that happening were exactly nil. The world again had changed. Omalu and Bailes, Nowinski and Cantu—all of the Dissenters—had succeeded in toppling the NFL's established order. It was an astonishing achievement. Casson and Viano and the MTBI committee were gone. Pellman seemed to be in internal exile, still with the league but unseen. But there was a new order. Those men had been replaced by other men with their own views about what was best for the NFL. Omalu was never part of that world, but now BU, too, was about to be elbowed aside by the league regardless of the framed commitment hung up on the wall back in Boston.

As he appealed to the Seau family through Chao, Nowinski emphasized BU's status as the official brain bank of the NFL. But at the same time Nowinski was trying to close the sale, the NFL was working to direct Seau's brain *away* from BU. At the center of the league's effort were the members of the new concussion committee. Behind the scenes, they had their own strategy to secure Seau's brain. They hadn't succeeded with Duerson's brain a year earlier, but this time they were prepared. To execute their plan, they summoned the same power, resources, and reach that until recently had been used to deny the very existence of brain damage in football players.

The point man was Kevin Guskiewicz, once one of the original Dissenters but now a powerful member of the reconstituted committee. Guskiewicz was one of the critics the NFL had recruited after disbanding the old MTBI committee. Now he found himself working against his former allies, including Bailes, his cofounder of the Center for the Study of Retired Athletes. Guskiewicz and Chao had a mutual friend, a former trainer at UNC, and Guskiewicz advised Chao to send Seau's brain not to Omalu and Bailes or the BU Group but to the NIH, where the head of research for the NFL's new concussion committee, Russ Lonser, worked as chief of surgical neurology. That is, Lonser worked for both the NIH *and* the NFL.

Guskiewicz had never forgotten his revulsion when Omalu put up photos of Webster's corpse three years earlier at the Palm Beach meeting of the Players Association. Guskiewicz said he told Chao that "within the circles that I hang out within the scientific community," Omalu was known for "sensationalizing at times" and for "showing slides of the deceased person—their brain—and that sort of thing." Chao relayed the message to Seau's family: Omalu was bad news. But Guskiewicz wasn't done. He told Chao about his concerns that BU had its own agenda, that McKee was fanning the hysteria about football and brain damage by overstating the prevalence of CTE.

Guskiewicz, like his colleagues on the NFL's new committee, thought donating the brain to the NIH was a tidy solution to a messy situation. The brain race had gotten out of hand. Guskiewicz had an uncle in Latrobe who died of pneumonia in his early forties; the ordeal was traumatic enough without the presence of strangers clamoring for his organs. "All this knocking on doors, the calls, I just can't imagine going through it," Guskiewicz said. "It puts a black mark on the entire neuroscience community because some of us, I think, are perhaps guilty by association. So I think that's concerning."

Two months after Seau's death, after the intervention of three members of the NFL's concussion committee and the team doctor for the San Diego Chargers, his brain was shipped to the NIH.

Two months after that, the NFL donated $30 million to the NIH for concussion research, the largest philanthropic gift in the league's history.

The NFL said there were no strings attached to the donation, a pledge identical to the one the league had made to BU three years earlier.

On one level, it made perfect sense. The chase for Junior Seau's brain had turned into a macabre spectacle, adding to his family's anguish. The NIH could apportion his brain tissue to any independent scientist, not just those whose reputations would be enhanced by the diagnosis. As Gina Seau said, "I didn't care about what people and doctors were competing for. I just cared about a high level of scientific study, doing it properly without bias. I cared about us getting to the bottom of what was really happening without anything to prove. We just wanted the truth."

But of course there was another side to it. In Wheeling, West Virginia, Bob Fitzsimmons watched the battle over Seau's brain with knowing bemusement. The former coach of Team Webster, the man who beat the NFL in court for $1.8 million, Fitzsimmons had followed the league's tortured struggle to get a handle on the concussion crisis for two decades. He wondered how much had really changed. Mike Webster had gone mad and died. Junior Seau had gone mad and died. How many more players were out there? The league had embraced BU's researchers and given them money. When the NFL didn't like the message, it cast BU aside and picked another partner and shelled out more money. Despite numerous offers, Fitzsimmons had decided not to take cases against the NFL in order to focus on the science. But he couldn't help but see a pattern.

"I guess the National Institutes of Health is now involved. I guess they somehow got drafted by the NFL," said Fitzsimmons, still in the firehouse-office where Mike Webster once slept in the basement. "They had an early draft, I think, and they drafted the NIH and paid them a pretty good salary, too, from what I hear."

On the day Seau shot himself, Gary Plummer got a call from a former teammate.

"Please, bro, tell me that there's more to it than just the concussions, tell me that, please," said Steve Young.

The Hall of Fame quarterback was in a panic. For years, Young had been telling himself that he wasn't Mike Webster, that he wasn't even Merril Hoge or Al Toon. He was the Vanilla Guy. He'd had his concussions, but that wasn't what had driven him out of the game. And now people assumed that Junior Seau had shot himself because of concussions. Young wanted to know it wasn't true, had to know it wasn't true.

Plummer knew both men well. Young had none of Seau's problems: the money, the gambling, the drinking, the estrangement from his kids. To be around Steve Young for any length of time was to see how incredibly normal his life was, his conversations interrupted by calls and texts from his wife, wondering why he hadn't completed an errand, or messages from friends making sure he knew it was his day to carpool the kids.

"Steve, you don't have relationship issues like this, you don't have debts and people calling in markers, you're not an alcoholic," Plummer told Young. "I really don't think that in a million years that's going to be an issue for you."

Plummer told Young he thought concussions had been "somewhere in the neighborhood of 10 or 20 percent" of Seau's problems.

Young sounded relieved. "You're right, I know you're right," he said. "Bro, I can't thank you enough."

But of course Seau had had CTE. That was certain. The NIH had distributed unidentified tissue from three different brains to three independent neuropathologists. One of those brains belonged to Seau, another to a person who had had Alzheimer's disease, and the third to a person with no history of traumatic brain injury or neurodegenerative disease. All three neuropathologists concluded that tissue taken from Seau's brain showed definitive signs of CTE. So did two NIH researchers, for a total of five confirmations. The telltale neurofibrillary tangles of tau protein that Omalu first spotted in Webster were found "within multiple regions of Mr. Seau's brain," the NIH reported. Officials refused to speculate on the cause of Seau's brain damage. But his family was told by Lonser he had gotten the disease from "a lot of head-to-head collisions over the course of 20 years of playing in the NFL," said Gina. "And that it gradually, you know, developed the deterioration of his brain and his ability to think logically." Lonser, though, did not express that in any of his public comments.

The discovery that Seau had had brain damage provided no solace to his children; in some ways it made them feel worse. "It didn't take any of the pain away; I feel it almost brought more," said Tyler Seau. "Mainly, because I feel bad that I didn't try harder. And just the pain that he was going through for how many years?" In the weeks leading up to the diagnosis, Jake Seau thought that when it finally came, "it'd answer a lot of questions. And, really, it just gave me more. You know, that's just one question answered that we kind of already knew the answer to. But then there's hundreds more."

Jake Seau had played both football and lacrosse his freshman and sophomore years at The Bishop's School in La Jolla. He was 6-feet-2 and nearly 200 pounds. In football, he played running back and strong safety. In lacrosse, he was a midfielder. By his sophomore year, he had received recruiting letters for both sports. Jake had a growing sense that football was his father's game but probably not his. He didn't have the same passion for it as his dad. Seau never put any pressure on Jake, just told him to keep his options open. Each year, as Jake's love for lacrosse grew, he debated whether to play football. Each year, at the last minute, he would give in and suit up.

But no more. Jake had made a verbal commitment to play lacrosse at Duke, a powerhouse in the sport. Football made him think of his father, and so he no longer watched many games. "I still love football," he said. "I grew up with it; I've always been around it. I love the game." But in the most personal and profound way, he was faced with the same uncomfortable questions that the rest of the country was now confronting. With so many alternatives, how can we let our children, our loved ones, ourselves, play a game that may destroy the essence of who we are? How can we enjoy it as entertainment? When his junior year came around, Jake thought about his father and himself. He thought about his family. And this time he didn't suit up.

"To realize this is the sport that he loved and possibly could have killed him, I just can't play it any longer," Jake Seau said.

SCARS OF THE GLADIATORS

In 1971, a Boston respiratory specialist named Gary Huber was approached by the tobacco industry with a proposal. The companies wanted to give him money to research the connection between smoking and lung disease. It had been almost 20 years since Ernst Wynder had induced cancer in mice by painting them with tar drawn from cigarettes. Huber, who worked at Boston City Hospital's Harvard Medical Unit, had seen one smoker after another come in with emphysema, bronchitis, and lung cancer, but there was little he could do for them. Big Tobacco said it wanted to help.

"We mistrusted them and initially we said no," Huber told PBS's *Frontline* 24 years later, but the industry was persistent. The executives told Huber he'd have total autonomy. Finally he agreed. "This was an industry who made a product that caused disease, and if we were going to do anything about it, I thought we had to work with that industry," said Huber, whose story is recounted in Dan Zegart's *Civil Warriors* and Robert Proctor's *Golden Holocaust: Origins of the Cigarette Catastrophe and the Case for Abolition,* among other places.

Harvard accepted $2.8 million from Big Tobacco, at the time the largest health-related grant the industry had given to a university. Over the next eight years, the grant grew to $7 million. The Harvard Project, started in 1972, produced 27 books and 54 peer-reviewed scientific papers.

The tobacco industry had selected Gary Huber for a reason: He believed the link between cigarettes and disease was unproven. His research had shown that most animals have an "adaptive tolerance" to toxic oxygen and only a few get sick. He had noted that although many people smoked, relatively few seemed to die. Which traits, he wondered, put some people at greater risk?

Big Tobacco's chief lawyer, David Hardy, wined and dined Huber, flying him to Washington to meet with senators, foreign dignitaries, and cabinet members. Hardy offered soothing reassurances about Huber's independence even as he subtly tried to edit his work. Over time, Huber became a "sycophant" of the industry he was studying, Zegart wrote in *Civil Warriors,* believing the support from Big Tobacco would continue no matter where his research led.

Then, in 1977, Huber found that rats exposed to cigarette smoke for six months developed emphysema. When he prepared to announce his findings at a conference in Las Vegas, the tobacco industry sent a lawyer to try to "lessen Huber's inclination to interpret the results as evidence of direct cause and effect." The effort failed. Shortly afterward, Huber discovered that supposedly safer low-tar cigarettes were potentially more dangerous because their smokers puffed more frequently and held the smoke in their lungs twice as long.

When the Harvard Project's grant expired in 1980, Huber begged for more money. Big Tobacco cut him off.

"You just got too close to things you weren't supposed to get into, Gary," a tobacco executive told him.

But Huber continued to work with the industry. Exiled from Harvard with the elimination of his funding, he moved to the University of Kentucky to work at the Tobacco and Health Research Institute despite warnings that Big Tobacco was setting him up. A tobacco lawyer sat on the institute's board. Its signature study involved smoking monkeys that were not allowed to inhale fully, making them unusually healthy smoking monkeys. In Lexington, Huber found himself accused of the manipulation of scientific results, administrative incompetence, and even sexual harassment. Within a year, he'd been fired. He moved on to the University of Texas, where he changed his specialty to nutrition.

When attorneys suing Big Tobacco caught up with Huber in 1997, they showed him internal industry documents to persuade him to testify against his former friends. One memo said programs such as the Harvard Project had been targeted not for their "scientific goals, but rather for . . . public relations, political relations, position for litigation." Huber was stunned to learn that R.J. Reynolds had done the work he was most proud of—producing emphysema in rabbits—10 years before he had.

He broke down in tears, realizing he had wasted 15 years of his life.

"I don't want people to think that I was bought," said Kevin Guskiewicz.

He was sitting in an alehouse in Chapel Hill, North Carolina, sipping his favorite porter, making the case that he was still independent after having joined the NFL's reconstituted concussion committee.

Guskiewicz was an original Dissenter, a respected scientist who had made his name establishing the connection between football and long-term mental illness. He wrote in 2005: "Our findings suggest that the onset of dementia-related syndromes may be initiated by repetitive cerebral concussions in professional football players." Two years later, in another paper that would define his career, he theorized that repeat concussions associated with football led to "biochemical changes" and "neuronal loss"—that is, brain damage.

But now Guskiewicz seemed to be singing a different tune. It was nearly impossible to distinguish his views from those of the NFL. It wasn't just Guskiewicz's attacks on Omalu and McKee or the way he had used the NFL's power to divert Junior Seau's brain to the league's researcher of choice, the NIH.

Guskiewicz no longer seemed to agree even with himself.

"The vast majority of the neuroscience community does not believe that research has established a causal relationship linking repetitive head trauma in football and CTE; I include myself in that," he said after McKee released a study confirming 28 new cases of brain damage in dead football players. This occurred in December 2012. The BU Group now had 50 confirmed cases of former football players with CTE, 33 of whom had played in the NFL. By then, McKee was convinced that "most NFL players are going to get this. It's just a matter of degree."

Guskiewicz said that blaming football for the devastating disease that had spread through the brains of former players such as Mike Webster, John Mackey, Ollie Matson, Dave Duerson, and Junior Seau, among so many others, was like a track team blaming Nike for a rash of ankle injuries simply because the athletes wore that brand of shoe. The same criticism, of course, could have been leveled at Guskiewicz's own game-changing work. In fact, it was—by the NFL.

Guskiewicz had joined the concussion committee in 2010 because he had become convinced that Goodell represented change and was committed to player safety. He thought he could use the NFL's power and resources for the greater good. The league put him in charge of equipment and rules—he literally could change the rules of pro football!—and Guskiewicz immediately went to work. It had long been known that the kickoff was the most dangerous play in football, essentially a 22-car pileup. Guskiewicz persuaded the owners to move up kickoffs to the 35-yard line, ensuring more touchbacks and fewer collisions. Sure enough, concussions on kickoffs dropped 43 percent, according to the league.

Guskiewicz wasn't paid to serve the NFL. His day job was still at the University of North Carolina, where, after he received the MacArthur genius grant, his meteoric rise continued. Long after his start as an ankle-taping apprentice for the Pittsburgh Steelers, Guskiewicz, still exuding a self-effacing boyishness, now chaired the university's department of exercise and sports science. He ran the Center for the Study of Retired Athletes, which he cofounded with Bailes, and the Matthew Gfeller Sport-Related Traumatic Brain Injury Research Center, named after a North Carolina high school player who died from a collision on the field.

But the NFL gave Guskiewicz everything he needed to fulfill his duties for the league. When he needed "big dollars," he said, he would seek out Jeff Pash, the NFL's number two executive, and say, "Jeff, we need to buy six new systems, and it's going to cost $250,000 to install; can you authorize the purchase? And Jeff then does that." The NFL insisted that its new concussion committee—like its old concussion committee—was totally independent, yet the league monitored interviews and filtered communication with the media. Guskiewicz and his colleagues reported directly to Goodell, who came to North Carolina in March 2013 to lecture on football and safety.

People noticed Guskiewicz's transformation. Matt Chaney, a concussion blogger highly critical of the league, satirized him as "Gus Genius" and wrote that he "epitomizes the wily football-funded researcher, morphing from game critic to advocate committee member. The NFL specializes in buying off such pliable 'experts.' Kevin Guskiewicz is no genius; he's just become another football insider of unearned credit and privilege." The blogger Irv Muchnick started calling Guskiewicz "Dr. No Jr."

The most bizarre aspect of Guskiewicz's new role was that he found himself working with Elliot Pellman, his former scientific nemesis, who continued as the NFL's medical director and even attended committee meetings. How Pellman survived baffled even Guskiewicz. "It's a question that many of us have asked," he said. "I mean, I really don't know." Another league-affiliated doctor, half joking, said he assumed Pellman "has incriminating photos hidden somewhere." Pellman, of course, was a walking repository of information about the NFL's concussion policies; the most obvious explanation was the lawyers wanted to keep him close. Guskiewicz said he didn't mind as long as Pellman stayed as far away from him as possible. He said his only interaction with the NFL's medical director was to send him his receipts to get reimbursed for his travel expenses.

Guskiewicz said the former head of the Mild Traumatic Brain Injury Committee was adept at processing his breakfast receipts.

"He does it really well," Guskiewicz insisted. "I have to tell you, if only the university could reimburse me as quickly as he does; it's usually within minutes and the check's in the mail. But I know, it's comical."

There was something poignant about Guskiewicz's ongoing research. He was trying to make a violent game safe. His latest work involved helmet sensors that measured the magnitude and frequency of blows. One of Guskiewicz's sons was playing high school football. On Friday nights, on a glowing field like thousands all over the country—the field where his son played—Guskiewicz watched his sensors pick up one collision after another, play after play after play.

Guskiewicz loved football. He had loved it ever since he had ridden his bike to watch his heroes, men such as Mike Webster and Terry Bradshaw and Mean Joe Greene, from the hill overlooking the Steelers' training camp in Latrobe. The game was part of him, part of his

American story. That's the thing about football, why it's different from cigarettes and coal dust and not wearing your seat belt and a whole range of other things that have been proved bad for us. We love football. Americans by the millions are complicit in making the sport what it has become, for better or worse. The outcome of the NFL's concussion crisis will affect the country. But it will be determined not by the "enemies" or "opponents" of football but by those in love with the sport: the players, the fans, the advertisers, the book writers, the moms and dads and kids. Even the scientists.

Guskiewicz didn't believe his views had changed. He thought the pendulum had swung too far since his studies, before we really know how many people get brain damage from playing football, or how exactly that occurs, or what the true risks are. McKee, for all the publicity surrounding her work, for the many brains she'd examined, had not established "a cause and effect relationship" between football and neurodegenerative disease, Guskiewicz said. Her insistence that she had, and the insistence of others, such as Omalu, Cantu, and even Bailes, had created an unwarranted backlash against the NFL, he thought. "Some of them are beating their fists on the table a little harder than others to say, I'm convinced this exists," Guskiewicz said. "I mean, if it existed to the extent that some people have said, we would have an epidemic on our hands. And I don't think that we have an epidemic."

The Center for the Study of Retired Athletes had evaluated more than 400 NFL players. "I hope that I look as good as three-quarters of them when I'm 55 or 60," said Guskiewicz. "So it's not happening to everybody. There is certainly a quarter of them that need some help, and we've got to figure out how we intervene. But as I've said, three-quarters of them look really pretty good. And I don't think we have a bias. I think we're seeing the typical player walk through our door."

By 2013, the NFL was spending tens of millions of dollars—spread among leading physicians and institutions throughout the country—to become the main sponsor of research that holds the potential of its own undoing. Nearly every prominent scientific group involved in that work—Boston University, the National Institutes of Health, the University of North Carolina—has benefited from the NFL's riches. Does that mean that all the science is tainted or that Kevin Guskiewicz was bought? No. Does it make the research independent and credible? Time will tell.

But once again, the NFL was in control of the science of concussions.

I t wasn't just Guskiewicz. As the league moved into this murky next phase, it was often hard to tell where people stood and whether anything had changed.

Merril Hoge, who retired from the NFL in 1994, the Season of the Concussion, because he couldn't remember his daughter's name and briefly went blind, claimed that football was no more dangerous than riding a bike, an assertion the NFL made repeatedly. Hoge was a board member of USA Football, an organization endowed by the league and identified as the "official youth football development partner of the NFL." He espoused the league's message of teaching proper tackling to take the head out of the game, a concept many players thought impossible and almost laughable.

Hoge used his role as an NFL analyst on ESPN to criticize those who would question the dangers of football. When former quarterback Kurt Warner, who led the Rams to victory in Super Bowl XXXIV and won two MVP awards during a 12-year career, said he would prefer that his sons not play football, remarks similar to those made by former greats such as Bradshaw and Carson, Hoge publicly attacked Warner as "irresponsible" and "uneducated."

Some people seemed to be lining up on both sides of the debate. Cantu, another original Dissenter, now was serving as a senior adviser to the NFL concussion committee. At the same time, he dispensed paid advice to the lawyers suing the league during a February 2012 strategy session in Philadelphia. When the NFL found out about his appearance, league officials sent a warning letter to the lawyers to stay away from Cantu because he worked for them. After discovering Cantu's conflicting roles, the lawyers for the players decided he was tainted as an expert witness and backed away.

The lawsuits, including the first one filed by Jason Luckasevic and his colleagues, had been consolidated into one "mass tort" involving nearly 6,000 former players or their families. That included Bubby Brister, whose long-ago concussion with the Steelers led to the creation of ImPACT and neuropsychological testing in the NFL. It also included the relatives of Junior Seau. Twelve days after the NIH announced that Seau's brain was riddled with CTE, his family sued the NFL. The Seaus alleged that the league "deliberately ignored and actively concealed" the risks of chronic brain damage "from the players, including the late Junior Seau."

By the time the two sides appeared in court in April 2013 for a hearing on the NFL's motion to dismiss the case, Luckasevic and the others had given way to David Frederick, a Washington superlawyer who once clerked for Supreme Court Justice Byron "Whizzer" White, the former star halfback. The NFL was represented by Paul Clement, a former U.S. solicitor general. Both men had argued numerous cases before the Supreme Court. It didn't escape notice that the NFL's chief outside counsel, Covington & Burling, was a veteran of the tobacco wars, one of two law firms—the other was Shook, Hardy & Bacon—that served as "guiding strategists" for Big Tobacco. Before taking over as commissioner, Tagliabue worked as the NFL's lawyer for the powerhouse firm, but it's not known whether he played a role in the tobacco strategy. After retiring as commissioner, he returned to Covington & Burling, where he serves as a senior counsel as part of the firm's Strategic Risk and Crisis Management Team.

For decades, Covington & Burling's lawyers directed litigation, public relations, and opposition research against those who warned against the dangers of smoking. The firm served as the first legal counsel for the Tobacco Institute, which produced industry-friendly research. It helped draft a more lenient liability law, coordinated denials about the dangers of secondhand smoke, and subsidized tobacco-friendly scientific witnesses who were referred to as "whitecoats." In 1987, after the surgeon general concluded that secondhand smoke caused cancer and respiratory disease, Covington & Burling partner John Rupp famously told a group of tobacco executives they were "in deep shit."

Now, in the looming brain wars, the NFL's insurers were warning that the league could face $2.5 billion in damages if it lost its battle with the players. After a federal judge ordered the two sides to mediation, a settlement was announced just one week before the start of the 2013 season. The league agreed to pay $765 million, plus legal fees that were expected to run another $200 million. It was seen by many as a victory for the NFL. There would be no public vetting of what the league knew and when it knew it. No Paul Tagliabue testifying in open court about why on earth he had appointed a rheumatologist to lead a concussion committee. No Dr. No. And that $765 million? It was widely regarded as chump change. As Kevin Mawae, the former president of the NFLPA, tweeted: "NFL concussion lawsuit net outcome? Big loss for the players now and the future! Estimated NFL revenue by 2025 = $27 BILLION.

It had been three years since the NFL's chief spokesman had said it was "quite obvious" that football-related concussions "can lead to long-term problems." No one from the league had uttered a word about that since.

In December 2012, Goodell gave a lecture at the Harvard School of Public Health. He was introduced by the dean, Julio Frenk, who noted that the dangers of secondhand smoke were first identified at Harvard. For 37 minutes, Goodell hit on the NFL's new talking points: Safety is its number one priority; concussions are not confined to football; the league has made rule changes to reduce concussions and is promoting "independent and transparent medical research."

The commissioner emphasized the need to rely on "science and facts, not speculation." He cited a recent study by the National Institute for Occupational Safety and Health (NIOSH) debunking the myth that NFL players had shorter life spans than the general population. He did not, however, note another NIOSH study suggesting that NFL players were four times more likely to develop Alzheimer's or Lou Gehrig's disease.

As he ended his day at Harvard, Goodell took a few questions from the media before being whisked away.

"Is the league's position clear that football has the potential to cause long-term brain damage?" he was asked.

The commissioner hit replay: "What we are doing is making sure that we do everything to make sure that the game is safe. Those conclusions have to be drawn by the medical community."

Seven months later, as training camps prepared to open for the 2013 season, incoming rookies attended a three-day symposium staged by the NFL. On the second day, Cleveland Browns team doctor Mark Schickendantz gave a presentation about health and safety. In a 2011 incident that drew national attention, Schickendantz, an orthopedic surgeon, was among the medical professionals who cleared quarterback Colt McCoy to return to action without receiving a sideline concussion test, despite taking a brutal helmet-to-helmet hit from Steelers linebacker James Harrison. Now, Schickendantz was educating the 2013 rookie class about the dangers of concussions. According to a story in the *Washington Post,* he said, "It's never an insignificant injury. . . . Don't hide it." He discussed the league's new assessment protocols, including the addition of independent neurologists on the sideline.

But as he wrapped up his presentation, Schickendantz told the young players, "Right now, we're learning a little bit more about long-term brain damage." And he added, "No direct cause and effect has been established yet."

Jim Otto wears a silver-and-black sleeve with the Oakland Raiders' logo over his prosthetic right leg.

Otto played center for the Raiders for 15 years. When he first arrived in the San Francisco Bay Area in 1960, he was still carrying around the leather football helmet he had worn at the University of Miami, which couldn't find a plastic one big enough to fit over his size 8 head. Back then, Otto was just 205 pounds and had been passed over in all 20 rounds of the NFL draft. Only the Raiders, the eighth and final team cobbled together to form the American Football League, the newly created rival of the NFL, gave him a shot.

By the time Otto retired, in 1974, the two leagues had merged and the modern NFL had been born. Otto had established himself as one of the finest offensive linemen in the history of the game. "Double O"— his nickname and his number—was the ultimate Raider, at one point starting 210 straight games. He came to see himself as a descendant of the Roman gladiators and "proudly wore the scars of a gladiator." When his helmet cut a gash in the bridge of his nose, he let the blood trickle down his face and smeared it on his jersey. Off the field, Otto was a pleasant-looking man with a crooked smile and a shock of blond hair that he grew longer with the times. On the field he was terrifying: He seemed to age 10 years just cramming the helmet onto his head. Wayne Walker, the Detroit linebacker, said peering through Otto's face mask

was "like looking at a gargoyle." Otto got his bell rung so often playing center, his legs churning like pistons as he drove his head into his
opponent, that his teammates chanted *ding, ding, ding* when he stag-
gered back to the huddle. By the time he was 28, Otto's teammates were
calling him "Pops," partly out of deference to his seniority as an original
Raider and partly because of the quickening destruction of his body. He
titled his autobiography, written with *Oakland Tribune* columnist Dave
Newhouse, *Jim Otto: The Pain of Glory.*

Otto's retirement ushered in an era he referred to as his "middle-
aged horror show."

He got his first artificial knee two years out of the game. His shoul-
ders were replaced. Doctors fused and re-fused the vertebrae in his back.
His knees caused him a kind of perpetual torment: The replacements
wore out or failed to take; horrible infections developed. By the mid-
1990s, Otto's right knee had been replaced six times, his left knee twice.

In 2007, doctors concluded that Otto's right knee would probably
end up killing him. They decided to remove his leg below the thigh. On
the first attempt, they failed to catch all of the infection and decided
to amputate further, taking off another chunk of his thigh. Otto spent
most of the year in a Salt Lake City hospital. The pain was unbear-
able: He cried and begged for stronger medication, which made him
delusional. He saw people dancing outside his window. One night he
woke up and became aware he was standing naked in the hallway on his
remaining leg. Another time he fell between the toilet and the wall and
screamed in vain for help. Doctors strapped him to his bed, and moni-
tors were assigned to his room. His wife, Sally, brought a plaque that
said "Miracles Happen," and Otto believes that's what saved him. The
plaque now hangs in the bedroom of their sprawling ranch-style house
in Auburn, California, on the way to Lake Tahoe from San Francisco.

At 75, Otto is still blessed with an ornery resilience. "If I had a leg,
I'd still be out kicking ass," he said one afternoon. He experienced "tremendous" headaches that felt like someone had hit him with a bat. "I
had a spike go through here just a minute ago," he said at one point. Like
dozens of other players, he was getting treatment for his brain injuries
at the Amen Clinic in Southern California, which he thought helped.
People had approached him about joining the lawsuit, but he refused. As

he wrote in *Jim Otto: The Pain of Glory*: "I'm not a wimp-out. Nobody told me I had to play every week. So I'm not going to sue my former team like other retired players. I'm simply not made that way."

"I take responsibility for everything that happened to my body," he said, falling into a chair in his den one afternoon. When Otto first began in professional football, he made $300 a game. One of his first Raiders paychecks bounced. The NFL, he said wistfully, is "the greatest success story ever in sports. I mean, I would have played for a pat on the back and a bottle of Budweiser after the game and a sandwich, you know? The only thing I'm regretting is that nobody in the NFL has even recognized the fact that I've lost my leg. Nobody has even called me. Someone could have said, 'Boy, Jim, I'm sorry that happened to you.' "

Otto grew up in Wausau, Wisconsin. His father ran deliveries for a meat company and operated the Tidee Didee Diaper Service with Otto's uncle. Otto had viewed football as a means of recognition for a poor boy—"little Jimmy Otto really cleaned somebody's clock"—an escape from the harsh northern Wisconsin winters and the life he foresaw for himself as a welder.

When Otto was established in the NFL, he made a trip back home to rural Wisconsin. One day a high school player came up and introduced himself. He told Otto that he was from a little town near Rhinelander, about an hour north of Wausau. He said he wanted to be just like him. The boy was small for a lineman, stocky and blond. He could have been Otto's little brother. The boy asked Otto for some tips and told him that he, too, planned to play in the NFL someday.

"Great, I'll be looking for you," Otto said.

Now, several years later, in one of his final games as a Raider, two of Otto's linemates, Gene Upshaw and Art Shell, started razzing him.

"Mr. Otto! Oh, Mr. Otto, there's somebody looking for you!" they said.

Upshaw and Shell pointed over to the opposing sideline. A player was trying to get Otto's attention. It was the same boy, now dressed in black and gold.

"Mr. Otto! Mr. Otto!" yelled Mike Webster. "I made it!"

AFTERWORD

Seven weeks before the publication of this book, in the fall of 2013, we received a call from Chris Buckle, the investigations editor at ESPN.com, and Dwayne Bray, who oversees the unit that produces investigative pieces for the network's hard-hitting television program *Outside the Lines*. Chris and Dwayne are our close friends, as well as our editors, so it came as something of a surprise, if not mild shock, when Dwayne informed us that he would be reading a statement over the phone and that neither he nor Chris would be able to take questions.

In the previous 18 months, *League of Denial*, which began as an idea to write a book chronicling the history of the NFL's concussion crisis, had morphed into something more ambitious. *Frontline*, the award-winning PBS investigative series, had signed on to produce a documentary based on the book. ESPN joined as a partner in the project. The result was an extraordinary amount of journalistic firepower trained on the NFL. The ESPN-*Frontline* partnership would generate nine in-depth stories that appeared on TV and the web, including the macabre, cross-country saga of Junior Seau's brain, which appears in greater detail in Chapter 17, and the disclosure that the NFL had been handing out millions of dollars for crippling brain injuries even as the league was denying that football causes brain damage, as revealed in Chapter 9.

The partnership also produced several kumbaya moments celebrating the power of journalism. One took place in a ballroom at the Beverly Hilton hotel that August as PBS, along with the other networks, previewed its fall season. On the same stage where Lady Edith and Lady Mary discussed the plot twists of *Downton Abbey*, we joined a panel to talk about football and the human brain, along with Dwayne, Hall of Fame New York Giants linebacker Harry Carson, and Mike Kirk, who produced and directed the documentary. The highlight was the unveiling of the film's trailer, which set two minutes of NFL violence to a soundtrack of Rihanna singing hauntingly:

Feel it coming in the air
Hear the screams from everywhere
I'm addicted to the thrill
It's a dangerous love affair

The trailer concluded with Ann McKee, the neuropathologist, stating, "I'm really wondering where this stops. I'm really wondering if every single football player doesn't have this."

When the session ended, we all patted ourselves on the back and looked ahead to the simultaneous launch of the book and the film. In hindsight, it seems hopelessly naïve not to have anticipated that the Hollywood-style unveiling of a film titled *League of Denial* might draw the ire of the people who run the $10 billion corporation to which the title referred. And that those people might direct their ire at the network that was, awkwardly, one of the corporation's main business partners, a coproducer of the offending film, and our employer.

The call from Dwayne and Chris came 19 days later. Both were obviously crushed. The statement that Dwayne was compelled to read informed us that ESPN had dropped its partnership with *Frontline*, including the removal of the network's logo from the film. The stated reason was that ESPN had no editorial control over the final product.

The *New York Times* soon presented a parallel narrative: ESPN's withdrawal had come one week after a contentious lunch that included NFL commissioner Roger Goodell and ESPN president John Skipper, according to people with knowledge of the meeting. "The meeting was combative, the people said, with league officials conveying their irritation with the direction of the documentary," the *Times* reported. ESPN's ombudsman, respected former *Times* sportswriter Robert Lipsyte, reported that Skipper made the decision after consulting with lawyers at Disney, ESPN's parent company.

Inside our unit at ESPN, some of us took to calling the event The Implosion. Within minutes of the network's announcement that it was ending the partnership, a *Frontline* editor painstakingly scrubbed all ESPN branding from previous stories and publicity posts related to *League of Denial* and the partnership. Within days of the call from Dwayne and Chris, we flew from San Francisco to Bristol, Connecticut, ESPN's headquarters, to meet with our editors. As astonishment and then anger swept through the investigative unit, one of our colleagues asked, "Are you guys gonna resign?"

But it was never that clear-cut. For nearly two years ESPN had supported, funded, and published the material that ultimately went into *League of Denial*. With nearly every story, the NFL had pushed back—at us, at our bosses, at our bosses' bosses. No one had changed a word. Now the impression was that ESPN had caved to pressure from the league. And yet, despite the public announcement and the firestorm, the partnership lived on in the book and the film, both utterly unchanged.

If the NFL's strategy was to derail *League of Denial*, it was obvious by the time the book and the documentary were released that it had backfired: The publicity drew even more attention to the project, especially the film, which drew ratings 47 percent higher than the average *Frontline* program. ESPN ran two separate nine-minute excerpts from the documentary on *Outside the Lines*, a 5,000-word excerpt from the book was published in *ESPN The Magazine* and on ESPN.com, and our faces were basically plastered all over the network during a series of interviews.

There's a lesson in here somewhere. As the Internet continues to transform journalism, killing newspapers, magazines, and other once-lucrative print products, the most expensive forms of reporting—investigative, explanatory, foreign—are falling by the wayside. To sustain that work in some form means it has to be subsidized—by billionaire philanthropists, by the U.S. government, by Viewers Like You. For its vast ocean of sports content—talk shows, draft previews, injury reports, and, of course, the thousands of games—ESPN also has developed perhaps the largest investigative reporting unit in the country. The unit could not survive on its own. In effect, it is subsidized—irony of ironies—by the riches of the National Football League.

Between 2010 and 2012, Pop Warner, the nation's largest youth football program, saw an exodus of 23,612 players. The 9.5 percent drop in participation is believed to be the largest in the organization's 85-year history.

Pop Warner's medical director was none other than Julian Bailes, the former Pittsburgh Steelers neurosurgeon, who still kept a woodpecker skull on his desk as a reminder of the stakes. It was clear to Bailes what was going on: Joe Maroon's long-ago warning to Bennet Omalu—*If only 10 percent of mothers in America begin to conceive of football as a dangerous game, that is the end of football*—was becoming a reality. Bailes, whose 10-year-old son Clint played Pop Warner in suburban Chicago, was certain that concerns about head injuries were "the number one cause" for the drop.

The trend, of course, did not escape the attention of the NFL. Fortunately, the league had an answer: The head would simply be removed from the sport.

The NFL would accomplish this feat through a $1.5 million initiative the league called Heads Up. The five-part tackling technique taught young players to keep their heads up and lead with their shoulders. "You have to be tough to play football, but no one has a tough brain," explained Stanley Herring, a Seattle Seahawks doctor and a member of the NFL's reconfigured concussion committee, in a promotional video for the program. "And so the right thing to do is take the head out of the game."

The NFL spread the gospel of Heads Up through USA Football, the league's youth arm. NFL teams hosted dozens of seminars for coaches and parents. NFL players and coaches touted the program online and in commercials. The league recruited 100 former players as Heads Up "ambassadors" to youth leagues in every state. Goodell was front and center, promoting Heads Up and its slogan, "For a Better, Safer Game." During the 2013 season, the NFL and the Chicago Bears hosted a Moms Football Safety Clinic at the Bears facility in Lake Forest, Illinois. Some 200 mothers were trained in Heads Up tackling. The clinic was held just one week after an HBO *Real Sports*/Marist Poll revealed that one third of adults said they were "less likely" to let their kids play football because of concerns over head injuries.

Goodell described the challenges faced by parents as nothing new: "My mom went through the same thing. I played nine years. I wouldn't give up a single day of that. Moms were always rightfully concerned about their children, but there's never been a safer time to play football." The commissioner called Heads Up a program the NFL "created this year to teach kids how to better tackle." His wife, Jane Skinner, a former

Fox News anchor, also weighed in, telling the assembled mothers, "I was talking with one of my favorite neurosurgeon friends today . . . and he said he had a message for all of you tonight. He said, 'I can tell you, your kids are more likely to get injured on their bike going to sports practice than they are on the sports field.'"

There was no scientific evidence to support the assertion that Heads Up reduced the potential for concussions. Nor was there evidence that the head could somehow be removed from play.

To Nate Jackson the whole thing was preposterous. Jackson had spent six injury-plagued seasons with the Denver Broncos, primarily as a special teams player. Upon retiring, he penned a memoir called *Slow Getting Up: A Story of NFL Survival from the Bottom of the Pile.* Jackson described Heads Up's tackling techniques as "laughable"—an unrealistic approach for players moving at high speeds and colliding from different angles. This, he said, would be true at all levels, and anybody who ever played should understand that.

Jackson called Heads Up "a product that the NFL is selling" to "create the illusion that the game is safe or can be made safe. It's rather shameless. I think it's sad. I think it's indicative of what the league's motives are: profit, profit, profit."

Asked what he would say to parents who had been told their children's heads were going to be taken out of harm's way, Jackson replied, "I would say, 'You're being lied to.'"

In April 2014 the NFL gave USA Football $45 million to support Heads Up and other youth programs. In its first year, Heads Up was adopted by more than 2,700 youth leagues. With the grant, USA Football would have the funds to pursue its goal of reaching 10,000 youth football leagues across the country.

When the $765 million concussion settlement was announced on the eve of the 2013 season, its proponents argued that it was the quickest way to help aging former players, many of whom urgently needed the money. The players might be dead before they ever saw a dime if they held out for a better deal, the argument went.

But as the season—and another offseason—passed, it became clear that it would probably be years before the NFL was forced to pay anything. It didn't take long for players and lawyers to start doing the math, and one immediate question was whether there was enough money in the deal to cover all the neurologically crippled NFL retirees out there.

Hundreds were scraping by on workers' compensation or disability benefits, as well as the relatively meager allocations of the 88 Plan. In theory, all those players or their relatives would be eligible for the maximum benefits outlined in the settlement: $3 million for dementia, $4 million for CTE, $5 million for ALS. The dollars added up quickly. At least 251 former players had been diagnosed with dementia or ALS, according to the league and the players union. Combined with the 59 confirmed CTE cases, it appeared that retired players and their relatives could collect more than a billion dollars, vastly exceeding the settlement amount.

"I'm trying to figure out how the math works," said Brent Boyd, the outspoken former Vikings lineman.

The NFL and the colead counsel for the players, Chris Seeger, promised there was plenty of money to go around. Seeger said a team of actuaries and economists had done the projections and guaranteed everything would be fine. But Seeger was unable to convince the federal judge overseeing the case, Anita Brody. She rejected the first attempt to get the settlement approved because she, too, wasn't sure there was enough money. "I am primarily concerned that not all retired NFL football players who ultimately received a qualifying diagnosis or their related claimants will be paid," she wrote in denying the request to approve the settlement.

Brody asked the NFL and Seeger to produce the actuarial data that was key to the deal. Seeger promised he would make it public. But nine months after the settlement was announced, still only a select few had seen it; many, in fact, wondered if the NFL was trying to keep the actuarial data from getting out for as long as it could, for the data no doubt included the league's own estimates about how many of its players would come down with the same disease that had turned Mike Webster and many others into raging and delusional madmen.

That was one more thing about the settlement: Iron Mike, the man who started it all, didn't qualify. The negotiators set a cutoff date of

2006, arguing that the statute of limitations in most states prevented wrongful death claims going back any further. Any player who died earlier was ineligible; their relatives couldn't collect a penny. It was the last indignity to the Webster family, whose battles with the NFL had now lasted nearly as long as Webster's Hall of Fame career. Pam Webster couldn't believe it; when she heard the news, she cried.

And then she and Sunny Jani, Webster's former caretaker and the man who rescued him from a bus station, along with rest of Team Webster, sued the NFL, again.

By the spring of 2014, Ann McKee was still very much in the game. The NFL had kept McKee from studying Junior Seau's brain and had reneged on its deal to direct the brains of dead football players to BU, but that hadn't stopped the flow of cases. So much had changed for McKee in the seven years since she had become the face of CTE research, but the one constant was that she kept finding florid disease in the brains of dead football players. In the fall of 2012, during one of our first interviews with McKee, she said she'd examined the brains of 34 ex-NFL players and found CTE in 33 of them. Now, less than two years later, the number had nearly doubled—McKee, tragically, was 59 for 62.

McKee was receiving funding through the NFL's $30 million donation to the NIH, though that was perhaps not by the league's design. Of that money, $12 million had been steered toward CTE studies; one component was to confirm McKee's earlier work. McKee thought it was repetitive but necessary, "a huge opportunity" not only to validate her work but also to extend its reach. She recognized, of course, that given the NFL's involvement—it wasn't so long ago she had called the league's researchers "delusional"—there were political undercurrents to the funding.

"Let me just say that I never forget about the politics," she said.

For all its resistance, the NFL also was very much in the game. In one year alone the league announced that it would donate at least $50 million to science, much of it focused on the kind of concussion-related studies it once ridiculed. The NFL had emerged as perhaps the leading force in the country, if not the world, in the study of traumatic brain injury. For years scientists had to beg for money to study the brain; now an industry with $10 billion in annual revenue was handing out checks liberally. To some it was a reflection of the NFL's reinvigorated effort to protect its players—Goodell repeatedly called this the league's top priority. But to many who knew the history, the NFL's strategy was troubling.

"The reality is you can't put this in the hands of the NFL to govern," said Michael Oriard, the former Chiefs offensive lineman who became an English professor at Oregon State and an NFL historian. "Even with the best possible intentions, the corporate NFL has its needs and interests. You don't let the tobacco industry regulate what's safe in terms of smoking."

For five years Goodell had been repeating his mantra—"We're going to let the medical people decide"—when asked about the connection between football and brain damage. But none of the NFL-funded research seemed designed to help the medical people decide. The research tended to focus on the general population and not those most directly impacted by the NFL's product: football players. Nor did the research begin to answer the most fundamental question, the one on the minds of parents, fans, and an increasing number of players: What is the actual risk of playing America's most popular sport?

Even the $30 million grant to the NIH came with strings attached. No one questioned the NIH's independence. And yet, the NFL could tell the NIH how it *didn't* want its money spent. And by partnering with NIH, the league had picked an organization prohibited from targeting a specific group for study. In other words, the NFL had given $30 million to an agency that wasn't allowed to study football players exclusively.

This point provoked a battle between the owners and the players union over how the league would spend its vast resources. When the two sides signed a new collective bargaining agreement in 2011, they agreed to donate $100 million to medical research. But from the beginning, the owners and the players were divided on how the money should be allocated. The league proposed giving all $100 million to NIH. But this was a nonstarter for the union—the football players wanted the research to be focused on football players.

Some researchers believed the NFL was trying to avoid certain results. One, Eric Nauman, a professor of biomedical engineering at Purdue, had made progress showing how "sub-concussive hits"—the kind that occur at the line of scrimmage on every down—degrade the brain over time. But Nauman couldn't get funding from the league.

"I get the sense that there's some influence over what they'd like to find or what they wouldn't like to find," Nauman said. "The NFL, they're not necessarily in the business of the public good, they're in *their* business. So I can understand why they might not be pushing some of the research."

Perhaps most telling was the research that wasn't being conducted. The one piece of information most relevant to football's future was the percentage of players expected to get brain damage. There were some ominous numbers out there (none more than McKee's 59 out of 62). But McKee admitted her figures were skewed; all the players had been symptomatic before they died. She knew that nothing could be said definitively until players—healthy and diseased—could be tracked over the lengths of their careers and beyond. That kind of longitudinal study would cost tens of millions of dollars; $100 million might do the trick.

The league knew this. The players knew this. The scientists knew this. And yet, as of this writing, there was no such study in the pipeline.

ACKNOWLEDGMENTS

Mental illness has the perverse effect of silently transforming the very identity of the people it afflicts. This book wouldn't have been possible without the help of dozens of NFL families—players, wives, parents, children—who agreed to share their painful stories with us. To them we extend our heartfelt thanks. We are especially grateful to Team Webster— Pam Webster, Colin Webster, Garrett Webster, Brooke Webster, Sunny Jani, Bob Fitzsimmons, Charles Kelly, and Jim Vodvarka—who spent countless hours recounting the life and death of Mike Webster, recognizing that, even more than his Hall of Fame career, Webby's greatest legacy may be to advance the search for the truth about football and brain damage. A special thanks to Julian Bailes for sparking the idea for this book.

We are especially grateful to our wise and courageous editors, Dwayne Bray and Chris Buckle, our colleagues at *Outside the Lines* and ESPN.com's Enterprise/Investigative unit, and others throughout the empire. Particular thanks to Greg Amante, John Barr, Willie Weinbaum, Dave Lubbers, Arty Berko, T. J. Quinn, Vince Doria, Jena Janovy, Patrick Stiegman, Rob King, Don Skwar, Tim Hays, Bob Ley, David Brofsky, Steve Vecchione, and, yes, even Carolyn Hong. Special thanks to Greg Garber, Craig Lazarus, and Christine Caddick, who described the origins of their early reporting and provided critical material; and to Peter Keating, who did the same. Chad Millman plied us with contacts from his fine book (written with Shawn Coyne): *The Ones Who Hit the Hardest: The Steelers, The Cowboys, The '70s, and the Fight for America's Soul.* Rayna Banks gathered enormous amounts of archival material that proved critical, as did Simon Baumgart, Jenna Shulman, and Lindsay Rovegno. Chris Mortensen graciously emptied his bulging electronic Rolodex for us, a gift that kept on giving. Shaun Assael kindly dug out some of his old reporting and provided material and insights.

Phil Bennett, the outgoing managing editor of *Frontline* and former managing editor at the *Washington Post,* turned our modest project into something vastly more ambitious: not only a book but also a two-part documentary film and a yearlong reporting partnership, with stories published simultaneously by ESPN and *Frontline*. Phil also read drafts of the manuscript and made improvements in every chapter, a kind of editing magic he generously has performed on Steve's copy for nearly 20 years. We also are immeasurably grateful to Sabrina Shankman, whose reporting for the film and the book thoroughly enriched both. Thanks also to *Frontline*'s Michael Kirk, Jim Gilmore, Mike Wiser, Lauren Ezell, Colette Neirouz Hanna, Raney Aronson, David Fanning, Pam Johnston, Patrice Taddonio, Tom Jennings, Travis Fox, and Caitlin McNally.

Alan Schwarz blew open the concussion story with three years of relentless reporting in the *New York Times*. Alan embraced our book from the beginning and shared some of his previously unpublished research, along with his own backstory. Julie Tate constructed a database of all the plaintiffs in the growing lawsuit against the NFL, excavated useful documents, and, in the end, held us accountable. Kevin Fixler and Jordan Conn provided dogged research on a variety of topics, including the history of the helmet and the marketing of NFL violence. David Maraniss gave us one huge research tip early on that made our lives considerably easier. The esteemed photographer Brad Mangin somehow managed to make us look presentable, and he also provided two superb shots for the insert. We are thankful to all.

Matt Chaney's indispensable listserv, which he fills with biting commentary and the latest articles on concussions, repeatedly alerted us to material we hadn't seen. We're also grateful to Irv Muchnick (Concussioninc .net), Dustin Fink (TheConcussionBlog.com), and the lawyer Paul Anderson (NFLConcussionLitigation.com), who also enhanced our understanding of the issue. Chuck Finder helped us navigate the concussion research community in Pittsburgh; his *Steelers Encyclopedia* also proved invaluable. Many thanks to Tim Gay for translating the physics of football. Thanks also to Marcy Thorne and her colleagues at "A Better Type."

We are grateful to Mauro DiPreta, editor in chief at Crown Archetype, for his passion for this project and his unwavering support. Also from Crown/Random House, thanks to Tammy Blake, Ellen Folan, Carisa Hays, Min Lee, Lisa Buch, Elizabeth Rendfleisch, Mark Birkey, Meredith McGinnis, and Christina Foxley; and to Deborah Bull for helping us nail down all the photos. Maury Gostfrand was exceedingly patient and steadfast in helping us navigate our relationship with *Frontline*. Scott Waxman was bullish on this book from the moment we first discussed it, and we have benefited from his magic touch.

We are blessed with incredibly supportive families who endured more than their share of tedious updates on "the book."

Mark: Unending thanks to my wife, Nicole, and my kids, Max and Ella. I will never be able to fully express how lucky I am to be living amongst such a loving, supportive, smart, and funny family. Also, I'm grateful to all my in-laws and nephews and nieces—Sylvie, Oliver, Amelie, Isae, Doug, Duncan, Ariel, Luanne, Kyan, and Jocelyne. Thanks to Glenn Schwarz and Ron Kroichick, who endured book talk for months on end during our regular "mayo" lunches and never wavered in their interest and support. Thanks to my dear friend Michael Heenan, who ushered me through my internal challenges with a remarkable sense of understanding. Thanks to Lance Williams, who taught me so much about reporting and whose friendship I cherish. Thanks to T. J. Quinn, who understands it all. And thanks to my hermano, an extraordinary journalist, for this incredible journey; the ride has been wild yet fulfilling, and I'm so grateful we took it together.

Steve: Thanks to my wife, Maureen, and my son, Will—my family, my everything—for filling my days with love, happiness, support, and understanding. Thanks also to my wonderful new in-laws: Bob and Doreen Fan, Elliot Fan and Elaine Grace Chu, and Coby and Jenna. Thanks to our amazing lifelong friends Bud Geracie and Donna Kato, residents of the Budonna Wing, who introduced us to a new world of joy and contentment. Thanks to Karl Vick, whose friendship spans oceans. In loving memory, thanks to Anthony Shadid, Green Bay Packers fanatic, who lost his life reporting in Syria last year but continues to inspire journalists around the world, including and especially me. Thanks to my coauthor, my amazing brother, for bringing me along for this ride and all the others.

To our accomplished and wonderful mother, Ellen Gilbert, our hero and inspiration, thanks for supporting us—again—like all the other messes we've gotten ourselves into.

SOURCE NOTES

This book was built on a foundation of more than 200 interviews conducted in 2012 and the first half of 2013. The interviews took place throughout the United States; one or both authors made six separate reporting trips to Pittsburgh, the epicenter of the NFL's concussion crisis. Among the principal characters who agreed to participate, most were interviewed on more than one occasion.

We also benefited greatly from thousands of documents, including previously unpublished medical records, NFL memorandums, letters, and personal e-mails that were provided to us by various sources. We also reviewed court records, congressional testimony, medical journals, and a large body of research on the NFL and concussions that preceded our work, in some cases by several years.

A handful of journalists provided critical early reporting that raised awareness of this issue and highlighted the struggles of retired NFL players facing mental disabilities. They include Alan Schwarz, whose reporting for the *New York Times* forced the NFL and the medical community to confront the urgency of the concussion crisis; Jeanne Marie Laskas, whose stories in *GQ* provided the first documentation of the league's efforts to stifle Bennet Omalu; Greg Garber, whose ESPN stories foreshadowed the crisis by nearly two decades; Michael Farber, whose 1994 piece in *Sports Illustrated* was similarly prescient; and Peter Keating, whose stories for *ESPN The Magazine* and ESPN.com revealed how Elliot Pellman's Mild Traumatic Brain Injury Committee understated the seriousness of concussions.

Those journalists all made our work easier; in addition to his insights and earlier reporting, Schwarz generously provided audio recordings of previously unpublished interviews with Pellman and Ira Casson. We are deeply grateful.

We made numerous requests to interview the NFL officials who figure prominently in this story, including Commissioner Roger Goodell; his predecessor, Paul Tagliabue; and the previous leaders of the Mild Traumatic Brain Injury Committee. The NFL, still embroiled in a lawsuit involving thousands of its former players, denied those requests and declined to cooperate.

PROLOGUE

Behold the mighty woodpecker: Numerous articles have been written about the Chinese woodpecker study. See "Why Don't Woodpeckers Get Concussions?" *Toronto Star,* Oct. 27, 2011. **Displayed a woodpecker skull:** Julian Bailes interview, 2012. **During a closed-door meeting:** Multiple sources, including Bailes, provided details about the NFL's concussion conference. **The body of Mike Webster:** Information about Webster's physical condition at the time of his death is from interviews with his family and doctors and his medical records. **Hall of Fame:** From video of Webster's induction on July 26, 1997. **An arsenal of weapons:** Colin Webster interview, 2012. **Addicted to Ritalin:** Jim Vodvarka interview, 2012. **"Oh, probably about 25,000 times":** "Webster Still Feeling Bumps on Road to Hall," *Capital Times* (Madison, WI), July 11, 1997. **Thousands of letters:** Webster's family, doctors, friends, and attorney provided copies of his personal correspondence. **As Webster lay dead:** Bennet Omalu interview, 2012. **A media empire:** Walt Disney Company, 2012 Annual Report. **The network pays the NFL:** "ESPN Extends Deal with N.F.L. for $15 Billion," *New York Times,* Sept. 8, 2011. **ESPN's bet:** Barry Blyn interview, 2012. **"Ultimate reality show":** Mike Florio, Pro Football Talk blog, Dec. 26, 2010. **"Contact ballet":** Michael Oriard, *Reading Football,* p. 2. **A football-loving physicist:** Timothy Gay, *Football Physics,* pp. 29–30. **"Journal of No NFL Concussions":** Kevin Guskiewicz interview, 2012. **"Frequent repetitive blows":** David C. Viano et al., "Concussion in Professional Football: Comparison with Boxing Head Impacts—Part 10," *Neurosurgery,* Dec. 2005. **Which concluded it was false:** FTC letter, April 24, 2013. **Nearly 6,000 retired players:** NFLConcussionLitigation.com. **Riding a bike:** "Researchers Discover 28 New Cases of Brain Damage in Deceased Football Players," ESPN.com, Dec. 3, 2012. **Abolishing tackle football:** "Preventing Sports Concussions among Children," *New York Times,* Oct. 6, 2012. **We asked her:** Ann McKee interview, 2012. **An estimated $40 billion:** ESPN was estimated to be worth nearly half the value of Disney, its parent company. See "Why ESPN Is Worth $40 Billion as the World's Most Valuable Media Property," Forbes.com, Nov. 9, 2012. **"You mean that guy":** The account of Webster's autopsy and Omalu's methodology was drawn from interviews with Omalu, Webster's medical records, and a viewing of an autopsy conducted by Omalu in French Camp, CA.

CHAPTER 1

Opening day of training camp: "Jack Lambert: 'I'll Play Somewhere,'" *Pittsburgh Press,* July 16, 1974. **The Nutcracker:** Details about the Nutcracker derived from several sources, including "OU's Gift to Football," *The Oklahoman,* Aug. 22, 2010; David Maraniss, *When Pride Still Mattered,* p. 219; "Belichick Pines for Oklahoma," *Boston Herald,* July 29, 2006. **Noll turned it into a public spectacle:** Interviews with Jon Kolb, Stan Savran, and Art Rooney Jr., 2012. **"You think I'm mean":** "A Living Legend Called Mean Smilin' Jack," *Sports Illustrated,* July 12, 1976. **Lambert's legend:** Art Rooney Jr., *Ruanaidh,* p. 337; "Rowser Trade for 2 Choices," *Pittsburgh Press,* Jan. 30, 1974; "Jack Lambert: 'I'll Play Somewhere,'" *Pittsburgh Press,* July 16, 1974. **Webster, in contrast, was small and slow:** Art Rooney Jr., *Ruanaidh,* pp. 341–343; Rooney Jr. interview, 2012. **It was a clear day:** www.almanac.com/weather and www.wunderground.com/history. **There was the whistle and then the explosion:** "Jack Lambert: 'I'll Play Somewhere,'" *Pittsburgh Press,* July 16, 1974; interviews with Robin Cole, Dan Radokovich, and Kolb, 2012. **Rarely has the urge to escape:** Kolb interview, 2012. **West Virginia clinical psychologist:** Mike Webster's medical records. **Webster childhood:**

Interviews with Bill Webster, Pam Webster, Garrett Webster, Reid Webster, and Billy Makris, 2012; Webster's medical records; court records; "Blood and Guts," ESPN.com, Jan. 25, 2005. **There was a kind of desperation in the way he prepared:** Makris interview, 2012. **The University of Wisconsin:** Interviews with Reid Webster, Bill Webster, Pam Webster, Greg Apkarian, 2012. **Her upbringing was everything Webster's was not:** Pam Webster interview, 2012. **The greatest single draft:** Art Rooney Jr., *Ruanaidh,* pp. 343–346; "Steelers Haul in 1974 among Best Ever," ESPN.com, April 21, 2003. **Webster was the biggest long shot:** Art Rooney Jr., *Ruanaidh,* pp. 342–343. **"I'm gonna go home and get bigger":** Ralph Berlin interview, 2012. **The Red Bull Inn:** Interviews with Jon Kolb and Colin Webster, 2012; "Reflections in Iron," StartingStrength.com, 2011. **Brought his training home with him:** Interviews with Pam Webster, Colin Webster, and Garrett Webster, 2012. **Pushing a sled:** Chuck Finder, *The Steelers Encyclopedia,* p. 147. **Webster's training regimen included anabolic steroids:** Webster's medical records. **Rocky Bleier . . . Steve Courson, later admitted using steroids:** "I Used Steroids, Bleier Says," *Pittsburgh Post-Gazette,* May 15, 1985. **Webster stopped at nothing:** Interviews with Colin Webster, Pam Webster, and Garrett Webster, 2012; "Reflections in Iron," Starting Strength.com, 2011. **The strongest man in the game:** "Big Night," *ESPN The Magazine,* July 21, 2003; "The Strongest Man in Football," CBS video, 1980. **Webster appeared in every game:** ProFootballReference.com. **Webster was slightly goofy:** Interviews with Charles Kelly and Tunch Illkin, 2012. **Pittsburgh was being depopulated:** http://www.census.gov. **An estimated 30,000 steelworkers were laid off:** Robert W. Bednarzik and Joseph Szalanski, "An Examination of the Work History of Pittsburgh Steelworkers," Institute for Labor Study, 2012. **Webster built the stable family life:** Interviews with Pam Webster, Colin Webster, Garrett Webster, and Brooke Webster, 2012. **Sometimes overruled Bradshaw in the huddle:** Interviews with Bleier and Savran, 2012. **One of Webster's greatest assets:** Interviews with Harry Carson, Fred Smerlas, and Gerry Sullivan, 2012. **Training camp:** Interviews with several former Steelers players and coaches, including Kolb, Radokovich, Cole, and Gerry Mullins, 2012. **It was not recorded:** Webster's Steelers medical records. **Webster rarely acknowledged:** Interviews with family members and former teammates and coaches, 2012. **Admitted to the hospital:** Bob Stage interview, 2012. **Webster never missed a snap:** ProFootballReference.com. **When the streak finally ended:** "Turk Has Unenviable Task of Replacing Webster," *Pittsburgh Press,* Sept. 3, 1986. **His name was Merril Hoge:** Hoge interview, 2012. **The Steelers effectively cut Webster:** "Webster among Free Agents Who Jump Ship," *The Sporting News,* April 10, 1989. **He was devastated:** Interviews with Pam Webster, Colin Webster, Garrett Webster, and Sunny Jani, 2012. **Took a job in Kansas City:** Interviews with Tim Grunhard, Bob Moore, and Marty Schottenheimer, 2012. **As for Webster, he was done:** Interviews with Pam Webster, Colin Webster, and Garrett Webster, 2012. **On a medical form:** Webster's medical records. **A 3,000-square-foot home:** Pam Webster interview, 2012.

CHAPTER 2

Noll had a question: Joe Maroon interview, 2012. **A Renaissance man:** "Teacher, Scientist, Innovator, Coach," *Sports Illustrated,* Aug. 23, 2007. **In one series of early experiments:** T. A. Gennarelli et al. "Acceleration Induced Head Injury in the Monkey," *Acta Neuropathologica Supplement,* 1981. **Oddly shaped sphere of Jell-O:** Joe Maroon, Ann McKee interviews, 2012; Mitch Berger interview, 2013, et al. **"Nobody thought":** Jeff Barth interview, 2012. **A front-page article:** "Silent Epidemic," *Wall Street Journal,* Nov. 24, 1982. **The results were startling:** Jeffrey T. Barth, *Mild Head Injury,* 1989. **Novel "secrets":** Joseph Maroon, *The Longevity Factor.* **When Maroon sold:** "Pittsburgh Medical Center Buys Properties Partly Owned by Staff Surgeon," *Pittsburgh Post-Gazette,* Sept. 15, 1999. **Personal experience with concussions:** Mark Lovell interview, 2012. **One of the first guinea pigs:** Much of Merrill Hoge's concussion history was drawn from Merrill Hoge interview, 2012, interviews with Maroon and Lovell, and Hoge's subsequent lawsuit against Bears team physician John Munsell. See *Hoge v. Munsell,* No. 98 WL 0996 (Ill. Lake County Ct, July 5, 2000). **He told a reporter:** "Injury Will Keep Hoge Out," *Chicago Tribune,* Oct. 4, 1994. **Hoge's baseline scores:** Henry "Tim" Bream III, "Postconcussion Syndrome: A Case Study," *Human Kinetics,* 1996. **"Fuck Ass Shit Test":** Lovell interview, 2012. **Neurosurgeon was shaken:** Maroon interview, 2012.

CHAPTER 3

Turned into a nightmare: This account of Webster's unraveling is from interviews with Pam Webster, Colin Webster, Garrett Webster, Bob Stage, and Billy Makris, 2012. **Webster returned to Kansas City:** Interviews with Grunhard, Moore, and Schottenheimer, 2012. **Sunny Jani was his given name:** This section on Webster's relationship with Sunny Jani is based on interviews with Jani, 2012. **Sleeping in his car:** Mike Webster Feature, ESPN, Feb. 2010; "Man on the Moon," ESPN .com, Jan. 26, 2005. **Living out of his truck:** Interviews with Garrett Webster and Jani, 2012. **Mike's life was coming apart:** Pam Webster interview, 2012; court records. **His health continued to get worse:** Webster's medical records. **Super Glue to stanch the bleeding:** Pam Webster and Garrett Webster interviews, 2012. **Offices of Dr. Stanley Marks:** Webster's medical records. **At the Amtrak station:** Joe Gordon interview, 2012; "Man on the Moon," ESPN.com, Jan. 26, 2005. **Gordon was a Pittsburgh native:** "Joe Gordon, Former Steelers Director of Communications," *Pittsburgh Sports Daily Bulletin,* Aug. 5, 2012. **Gordon decked an Oakland TV reporter:** "Steelers vs. Ravens Latest in a Long Line of Football Feuds," *Pittsburgh Post-Gazette,* Jan. 16, 2009. **Gordon also was impressed by Webster's generosity:** Gordon interview, 2012. **The train station:** The details of Gordon's encounter with Webster at the Pittsburgh Amtrak station and Webster's extended stay at the downtown Hilton are from Gordon interview, 2012, and "Man on the Moon," ESPN.com, Jan. 26, 2005. **ESPN aired a story:** Mike Webster feature, ESPN, July

1996. **The fallen hero:** "Webster's Induction Comes Amid Chaos," *Houston Chronicle,* July 26, 1997; "Humbled Hero; Webster Fights to Overcome Despair," *Atlanta Journal-Constitution,* July 25, 1997; "A Life Off-Center," *Pittsburgh Post-Gazette,* July 24, 1997; "A Man of Steel Crumbles," *St. Petersburg Times,* July 24, 1997; "From Super Bowls to Sleeping in Bus Stations," Associated Press, July 20, 1997. **A business opportunity:** Interviews with Garrett Webster, Colin Webster, and Jani, 2012. **Webster asked Bob Stage:** Stage interview, 2012. **A check for $175,000:** Interviews with Garrett Webster and Jani, 2012. **Webster repeatedly rebuffed offers:** Interviews with family, friends, and former players, 2012. **The ceremony:** Details derived from video of the Hall of Fame ceremony. **Bradshaw rarely had set foot in Pittsburgh:** "Bradshaw: It's Great to Be Home," *Pittsburgh Post-Gazette,* Oct. 20, 2002. **At Bradshaw's own induction:** "Bradshaw Delivers Sermon That Revives Steelers Memories," *Pittsburgh Press,* Aug. 6, 1989. **Ritalin was one of his best friends:** Interviews with Dr. James Vodvarka, Dr. Charles Kelly, Garrett Webster, and Jani, 2012; Webster's medical records. **Bob Stage cringed:** Stage interview, 2012. **"I expected more":** "A Bittersweet Day in Canton," *Pittsburgh Post-Gazette,* July 27, 1997. **Webster's festering enmity:** Interviews with Colin Webster, Garrett Webster, Pam Webster, and Jani, 2012.

CHAPTER 4

The conference: "Concussion from the Inside: The Athlete's Perspective," *Sports-Related Concussion,* 1999. **"Somebody somewhere isn't bleeding":** "A Steeler Turns Anger into Commodity," *New York Times,* Oct. 24, 1993. **Sitting in the audience:** Micky Collins interview, 2012. **Sexy paper:** Michael W. Collins et al., "Relationship between Concussion and Neuropsychological Performance in College Football Players," *Journal of the American Medical Association,* 1999. **A rising star:** Maroon interview, 2012. **The son of a Louisiana Supreme Court justice:** Julian Bailes interview, 2012. **"May be anticipated":** "Chronic Traumatic Brain Injury," *Sports-Related Concussion,* 1999. **Collins told:** "Tests Offer Key to Concussions," *Detroit News,* Sept. 8, 1999. **Slapped the turf:** "Steelers Are Betting the Ranch on Lloyd," *Pittsburgh Post-Gazette,* June 1, 1997. **"A cannonball hitting me":** Associated Press, Nov. 27, 1992. **"A process of remembering":** "Post-Concussion Syndrome," *NFL Gameday,* Oct. 23, 1994. **One of the smartest players in the league:** "From Football to Finance," *Capital Times* (Madison, WI), Nov. 24, 1995. **Weeping softly:** "With Sadness in His Eyes, Toon Bids Farewell," *New York Times,* Nov. 28, 1992. **Penalty box:** "NFL May Consider Using a Penalty Box," *New York Times,* Nov. 29, 1994. **Lacerating his tongue:** Associated Press, Oct. 23, 1994. **Three questions:** "Aikman Left Woozy by Sixth Concussion," *Dallas Morning News,* Oct. 24, 1994. **The prototypical new player:** For more information on how Lawrence Taylor transformed the NFL, see the classic first chapter of Michael Lewis's book *The Blind Side* (electronic). **The physical consequences:** Tim Gay interview, 2012. **Football players got bigger:** Timothy Gay, *Football Physics,* 2004. **When it came time to edit:** Greg Garber, e-mail. **"A disgrace":** "Playing the Hits Is NFL's Disgrace," *Plain*

Dealer (Cleveland, OH), Oct. 26, 1994. **"A tragedy"**: "The NFL Is Asking for a Tragedy," *New York Times,* Nov. 27, 1994. **"Hey, they do occur"**: "Suiting Up with a Concussion Is a Dangerous Game," *Times Union* (Albany, NY), Jan. 31, 1995. **Maroon did his own calculations:** "The Breaks of the Game," *Baltimore Sun,* Dec. 28, 1994. **Tagliabue appeared:** "Tagla-Boo," *Sports Illustrated* (Scorecard), Dec. 26, 1994. **A staggering bet:** "Fox Network Outbids CBS for Rights to Pro Football," *New York Times,* Dec. 18, 1993. **Steinberg was astonished:** Leigh Steinberg interview, 2012. **The immediate consequences:** "Aikman Recalls Little of NFC Title Game," *Dallas Morning News,* Jan. 25, 1994. **Sometimes vomiting:** Steinberg interview, 2012. **A year later:** "Looking at Concussions, and the Repercussions," *New York Times,* Feb. 18, 1995. **Plummer's view:** Gary Plummer interview, 2013. **28 team doctors:** "NFL Medical Standards, Practices Are Different Than Almost Anywhere Else," *Washington Post,* March 16, 2013. **10 or 20 deep:** Ben Lynch interview, 2012. **"Straddling a line"**: "Players Schooled on Concussions," *Orange County Register,* Feb. 18, 1995.

CHAPTER 5

Living with his oldest son, Colin: Colin Webster interview, 2012. **Dad was in trouble in Philadelphia:** Colin Webster interview, 2012. **Webster's mental or physical deterioration:** Details of Webster's deteriorating physicial condition are from interviews with Colin Webster, Garrett Webster, and Jani, 2012; Webster's medical records; and "A Steeler's Melting Point," ESPN.com's five-part series on Webster, Jan. 24–28, 2005. **Courson was concerned:** Vodvarka interview, 2012. **Vodvarka had grown up:** Details of Vodvarka's biography and his first meeting with Webster are from Vodvarka interview, 2012. **People hanging around Webster:** Interviews with Colin Webster, Garrett Webster, and Jani, 2012. **The Bert Bell/Pete Rozelle NFL Player Retirement Plan:** Plan documents. **Viewed the plan with contempt:** There are numerous accounts detailing the frustrations of former players with the NFL retirement plan. The Senate Committee on Commerce, Science, & Transportation held hearings on the subject on Sept. 18, 2007. **Deserved disability benefits:** Vodvarka interview, 2012. **Neither of them slept:** Bob Fitzsimmons interview, 2012. **When Mike and Sunny first went to meet him:** Jani interview, 2012. **The man to turn to:** Fitzsimmons interview, 2012; Fitzsimmons biography at www.fitzsimmons firm.com. **He sent him first to see Fred Krieg:** Fitzsimmons interview, 2012; Webster medical records. **Fitzsimmons also sent Webster:** Kelly interview, 2012; Webster's medical records. **Fitzsimmons turned finally to a forensic psychiatrist:** Webster's medical records. **Webster came to believe it was his destiny:** Interviews with Colin Webster, Garrett Webster, Jani, Fitzsimmons, Vodvarka, and Kelly, 2012. **Webster raged:** Interviews with Garrett Webster, Colin Webster, and Jani, 2012. **An array of firearms:** Colin Webster interview, 2012. **Legal pads and notebooks:** Nearly every person close to Webster who was interviewed provided copies of personal correspondence. **Fingers were so mangled:** Interviews with Garrett Webster and Jani, 2012. **Fitzsimmons cleared out a storage room:** Interviews with

Garrett Webster, Fitzsimmons, and Jani, 2012. **His bitterness was palpable:** Letters provided by Fitzsimmons. **Threatened to become the first player to quit the Hall:** Interviews with Colin Webster, Garrett Webster, and Jani, 2012. **Super Bowl rings into yet another money-raising scheme:** Jani interview, 2012. **Sunny called Fitzsimmons in a panic:** Interviews with Garrett Webster, Jani, and Fitzsimmons, 2012. **Acutely aware of what was happening to him:** Kelly interview, 2012. **"Mr. Webster, you're under arrest":** Details of the arrest and the events surrounding it are from court records; interviews with Colin Webster, Garrett Webster, Jani, Vodvarka, and Fitzsimmons; and "Ex-Steeler Webster Faces Forged Prescription Charge," *Pittsburgh Post-Gazette,* Feb. 26, 1999. **Drug use was out of control:** Vodvarka interview, 2012. **Helped get him out of the charges:** Fitzsimmons interview, 2012; court records. **Cut Webster off:** Vodvarka interview, 2012. **Fitzsimmons scrambled together a press conference:** Details of the run-up to the press conference and the event are from interviews with Colin Webster, Fitzsimmons, Vodvarka, and Jani, 2012; and "Hall of Fame Center Says He Has Brain Injury from Football," Associated Press, March 10, 1999. **Jail might be the best option:** Vodvarka interview, 2012. **A mini-debate:** "Opinions of Webster's Ailments and Treatment Vary," *Pittsburgh Post-Gazette,* March 15, 1999. **Four doctors weren't enough:** Court documents and Webster's disability case records. **Their paranoia:** Jani interview, 2012. **The NFL's handpicked neurologist:** Details of the meeting are derived from 2012 interviews with Dr. Edward Westbrook and Jani as well as Webster's disability case records. **Edward Westbrook was not in denial:** Westbrook interview, 2012. **The retirement board granted:** Webster's disability case records. **Thousands of former players were suing:** NFLConcussionLitigation.com. **"Proverbial smoking gun":** Fitzsimmons interview, 2012. **A hollow victory:** Webster's disability case records. **He couldn't get over the injustice:** Vodvarka interview, 2012, and 1999 letter. **No alternative except to sue:** Fitzsimmons interview, 2012. **IRS garnished most of the payments:** Court documents and Webster disability case records. **Pissing into [oven]:** Colin Webster interview, 2012. **Like high school buddies:** Garrett Webster and Jani interviews, 2012. **His incoherent letters:** Provided by Bob Fitzsimmons. **The two men had once been close:** Stage interview, 2012. **Chest pains and trouble breathing:** Details of the Webster's death are from interviews with Garrett Webster, Jani, Fitzsimmons, and Vodvarka, 2012. **The Steelers paid for the funeral:** Interviews with Jani and Gordon, 2012. **Who's Who of Steelers greats:** "200 Offer Final Tribute to Steelers' Webster," *Pittsburgh Post-Gazette,* Sept. 28, 2002. **He watched with disgust:** Colin Webster interview, 2012. **Why just Mike?:** Pam Webster interview, 2012. **Phone rang at Bob Fitzsimmons's office:** Interviews with Bennet Omalu and Fitzsimmons, 2012.

CHAPTER 6

"The flippancy": Steve Young interview, 2013. **The great-great-great-grandson:** Adam Lazarus, *Best of Rivals,* p. 37. **The Brett Favre part:** Young interview, 2013. **Young was merely frustrated:** Young interview, 2013. **Hid behind offensive line-**

men: Leigh Steinberg interview, 2013. **"A pinata":** "Swarm Puts Hurt on Young," *San Francisco Chronicle,* Sept. 20, 1999. **"It's basically got to stop":** "Offensive Line Feels the Heat," *San Francisco Chronicle,* Sept. 20, 1999. **Invited her family:** Young interview. **"The emperor":** "Young Should Quit While He Still Can," *Hartford Courant,* Oct. 17, 1999. **Still too dangerous:** Associated Press, Oct. 14, 1999. **"Risk factor":** "Young Could Play, but Says He Won't," *Los Angeles Times,* June 13, 2000. **More steeped in Steelers lore:** Kevin Guskiewicz interview, 2012. **The data had suggested to him:** Julian Bailes interview, 2012. **A 10-page survey:** *Health Survey of Retired NFL Players,* Center for the Study of Retired Athletes, Chapel Hill, NC. **The survey highlighted:** "What Football Tells Us about Everyday Fitness," *Los Angeles Times,* June 2, 2003. **More ominous:** Kevin Guskiewicz, "Recurrent Concussion and Late-Life Cognitive Impairment," *Neurosurgery,* Oct. 2005. **College football players:** Kevin Guskiewicz, "The NCAA Concussion Study," *JAMA,* 2003. **Three times more likely:** Kevin Guskiewicz, "Risk of Depression in Retired Professional Football Players," *Medicine & Science in Sports & Exercise,* 2007. **His complaint:** *Hoge v. Munsell,* No. 98 WL 0996 (Ill. Lake County Ct, July 5, 2000). **Trivial matters set him off:** Merril Hoge interview, 2012. **Bears' doctor:** Munsell deposition, Nov. 19, 1997. **Hoge described:** Hoge testimony, July 14, 2000. **The crux:** Munsell deposition. **"Save a lot of time":** Hoge testimony. **The jury awarded:** "Hoge Wins Lawsuit against Doctor," *Chicago Tribune,* July 22, 2000. **Fogel suddenly found himself:** Robert Fogel interview, 2012. **The letter:** Letter from William J. Rogers, Munsell attorney, to Fogel, March 30, 2000.

CHAPTER 7

Pellman had called: Mark Lovell interview, 2012. **Nearly half:** NFL Subcommittee on Mild Traumatic Brain Injury, Status Report, Nov. 1996. **Reflecting years later:** Henry Feuer interview, 2013. **He had not produced:** PubMed, the database of biomedical literature maintained by the National Library of Medicine and the National Institutes of Health, does not list Pellman as an author of any previous concussion or brain research. **Most complete professional biography:** "Medical Adviser for Baseball Lists Exaggerated Credentials," *New York Times,* March 30, 2005. **"I don't know who any neuropsychologists are":** "Doctor Yes," *ESPN The Magazine,* Oct. 28, 2006. **Barr was struck:** William Barr interview, 2012. **"Occupational risk":** "The Worst Case," *Sports Illustrated,* Dec. 19, 1994. **The same year:** "Injuries in NFL to Big-Name Players Heighten Awareness," *Times-Picayune* (New Orleans, LA), Nov. 14, 1999. **During a 1999 playoff game:** Kyle Brady interview with John Barr, 2013. **Liked Pellman immensely:** Kevin Mawae interview with John Barr, 2013. **"Red Brick Broadway":** Kevin Mawae interview with John Barr, 2013. **"Comical":** Kevin Guskiewicz interview, 2012. **Pellman offered one explanation:** "Background on the National Football League's Research on Concussion in Professional Football," *Neurosurgery,* Oct. 2003. **"That's my understanding":** Mark Lovell interview, 2012. **In a statement to ESPN:** Paul Tagliabue e-mail to ESPN, Aug. 13, 2013. **NFL definition of a concussion:** MTBI Status Report. **"Willing test subjects":**

Chris Withnall, confidential memo to Riddell Inc., "A New Performance Index for Mild Traumatic Brain Injury (MTBI)," Nov. 15, 2000. **Lovell thought he'd probably be ousted:** Lovell interview, 2012. **$12,000 in seed money:** MTBI Status Report. **"Strongly recommend":** Memorandum, Paul Tagliabue, June 10, 1998. **Mitchell's responsibilities:** Dorothy Mitchell biography, Brune & Richard LLP. **"Worked tirelessly":** "Concussion in Professional Football," *Neurosurgery,* Oct. 2003. **Expert witness:** Details of the aborted McShane project and the dispute over his testimony are from John McShane interview, 2013, and documents forwarded to Munsell's attorneys by the NFL. Court transcripts indicate Hoge's attorney was unaware that Mitchell, as head of the NFL's counsel for policy and litigation, provided the documents. "Frankly, I don't know how they obtained these records," Hoge's attorney, Robert Fogel, told the court. **A number of early NFL concussion projects:** MTBI Status Report. **Wearing their hair long:** Beau Riffenburgh, "History of Pro Football Equipment," *Official NFL Encyclopedia.* **"Head harnesses":** John J. Miller, *The Big Scrum,* p. 180. **A Chicago company:** Riddell Sports Inc., company history. **"The Humper":** For the definitive story of Hardy Brown, see Jim Dent, *Twelve Mighty Orphans: The Inspiring True Story of the Mighty Mites Who Ruled Texas Football.* Brown learned to play football in a Fort Worth orphanage after witnessing his bootlegger father murdered with a shotgun. "You see these westerns with guys who have niches [*sic*] on their belt for the guys they killed? Hardy Brown had niches in his belt for all the jockstraps he got," Rams quarterback Norm Van Brocklin told NFL Films. **"Elliot waltzing":** Bob Cantu interview, 2012. **"A fantasy":** Mark Lovell interview, 2012. **"Incredible stuff":** "Troy Vincent: Another Case Study in Concussions," *Philadelphia Daily News,* Dec. 24, 1999. **The committee examined:** Elliot J. Pellman et al., "Concussion in Professional Football," *Neurosurgery,* Oct. 2003. **Apuzzo:** Apuzzo's biography is available at keckmedicalcenterofusc.org/doctor/bio/view/72257. **Clearly was thrilled:** "USC Neurosurgeon Is a Giant on the Field and Off," *USC News,* Feb. 9, 2001. **"Really enjoyed the association":** Cantu interview, 2012. **"King of Concussions":** During a conference on CTE in the fall of 2012 at the Cleveland Clinic's Lou Ruvo Center for Brain Health in Las Vegas, a researcher introducing Cantu said: "He truly is the king of concussions, and it's really a pleasure to invite him up to the podium." **Cantu had grown up:** Bob Cantu interview, 2012. **"Recommendations from rat data?":** Linda Carroll and David Rosner, *The Concussion Crisis,* p. 250 (electronic). **A bland guest editorial:** Paul Tagliabue, "Tackling Concussions in Sports," *Neurosurgery,* Oct. 2003. **More effusive and colorful:** Michael L. J. Apuzzo, "Galen 2003: Critical Analysis of Brain Injury in Sport," *Neurosurgery,* Oct. 2003. **Another study:** Elliot J. Pellman et al., "Concussion in Professional Football, Part 2," *Neurosurgery,* Dec. 2003. **The reaction was positive:** *Neurosurgery,* Dec. 2003 (comments). **NFL Paper Number 3:** Elliot J. Pellman et al., "Concussion in Professional Football, Part 3," *Neurosurgery,* Jan. 2004. **Response . . . was guarded:** *Neurosurgery,* Jan. 2004 (comments). **Yet another NFL study:** Elliot J. Pellman et al., "Concussion in Professional Football, Part 4," *Neurosurgery,* Oct. 2004. **They were rejecting:** Julian Bailes and Kevin Guskiewicz interviews, 2012. **Cantu . . . had misgivings:** Cantu interview, 2012. **Stilted language**

of science: Elliot J. Pellman et al., "Concussion in Professional Football, Part 4," *Neurosurgery,* Oct. 2004 (comments).

CHAPTER 8

Roughly 17,500 deaths: Details on the Allegheny County coroner's policies and the circumstances in which the coroner took Webster's body into custody are from Chief Deputy Medical Examiner Joe Dominick interview, 2012. **Who happened to be working that day:** Omalu interview, 2012; Omalu's CV. **Unlikely character:** This section is from several interviews with Bennet Omalu, 2012; interviews with Fr. Carmen D'Amico, Julian Bailes, Cyril Wecht, and Bob Fitzsimmons; and Bennet Omalu, *Play Hard, Die Young: Football Dementia, Depression, and Death.* **At the coroner's office:** Omalu interview, 2012. **Cyril Wecht, a Pittsburgh legend:** Wecht interview, 2012; www.cyrilwecht.com; "Cyril H. Wecht: Up Close and Personal," *Pittsburgh Post-Gazette Magazine,* Oct. 24, 1999. **Bennet Ifeakandu Onyemalukwube:** This account of Omalu's childhood and immigration to the United States is derived from Omalu interviews, 2012; Omalu, *Play Hard, Die Young: Football Dementia, Depression, and Death*; and Omalu's CV. **The conflict claimed at least 1 million lives:** "Nigeria: Biafra War 30 Years On," Associated Press, Jan. 14, 2000. **"An asinine, pseudoscientific sham":** "40 Years on, Arlen Specter and Cyril Wecht Still Don't Agree on How JFK Died," *Pittsburgh Post-Gazette,* Nov. 16, 2003. **A one-year fellowship:** Omalu's CV. **"Bennet, you remind me of myself":** Omalu interview, 2012. **"Junior Wecht":** Omalu interview, 2012. **"A saying in Arabic":** Dr. Abdulrezak Shakir interview, 2012. **Private medical consultations:** Omalu interview, 2012. **Omalu placed the 3½-pound brain:** Details of how Webster's brain was removed and prepared for study are from 2012 interviews with Ron Hamilton, Ann McKee, and Omalu; Webster autopsy report. **Omalu forgot about it:** Omalu interview, 2012. **St. Benedict the Moor:** www.stbtmchurch.org. **Away from work:** D'Amico interview, 2012. **Slides of Webster's brain:** Omalu interview, 2012. **The buildup of tau:** This brief explanation of the tau protein, how it's detected, and how it destroys brain cells is from 2012 interviews with Dr. Dan Perl, Omalu, Hamilton, and McKee. **Omalu knew from his training:** Interviews with Omalu and Hamilton, 2012. **A landmark paper:** Dr. Harrison Martland, "Punch Drunk," *JAMA,* 1928. **"Slug-nutty":** "Too Many Punches, Too Little Concern," *Sports Illustrated,* April 11, 1983. **A British neuropathologist:** JA Corsellis et al., "The Aftermath of Boxing," *Psychological Medicine,* 1973. **Omalu's working theory:** Omalu interview, 2012. **Omalu was ready to seek a second opinion:** This account of how Omalu confirmed that Webster had CTE and assembled the research paper detailing the findings is drawn from 2012 interviews with Steve DeKosky, Omalu, and Hamilton. **A representative from the NFL Hall of Fame:** Steve DeKosky interview, 2012. **The paper was completed:** Early drafts provided by Omalu; Omalu et al., "Chronic Traumatic Encephalopathy in a National Football League Player," *Neurosurgery,* July 2005. **Omalu first submitted:** Omalu and Hamilton e-mails. **"The official journal of the NFL committee on MTBI":**

Omalu e-mail to Hamilton and DeKosky. **How naive they had been:** Interviews with Omalu, Hamilton, and DeKosky, 2012.

CHAPTER 9

Paper Number 5: Elliot J. Pellman et al., "Concussion in Professional Football, Part 5," *Neurosurgery,* Nov. 2004. **A number of conclusions:** Elliot J. Pellman et al., "Concussion in Professional Football, Part 5," *Neurosurgery,* Nov. 2004. **Confidential documents:** The NFL produced the documents on Oct. 28, 2004, in response to discovery requests for "all other benefit claims for TBD (total and permanent disability) in which the Plan participant has asserted that: (1) the claim is based on mental disability, and (2) the mental disability was alleged to have resulted from repetitive trauma to the head or brain from League football activities." The NFL listed 11 such claims (besides Webster's) and produced incomplete case histories for several. The players' names were blacked out. It is impossible to tell from the documents the total number of players who received benefits from the NFL on the basis of claims of mental disability related to football. **One was Gerry Sullivan:** Sullivan's case history shows that he was awarded benefits for both mental and orthopedic disabilities. An independent psychiatrist determined that Sullivan was totally and permanently disabled "due to cognitive impairment and behavioral disinhibition." A neurologist brought in by the NFL disagreed. The retirement board granted benefits on the basis of the reports of the psychiatrist and an orthopedist. **The appellate court:** *Jani v. Bert Bell/Pete Rozelle NFL Player Retirement Plan,* Fourth Circuit Court of Appeals, unpublished opinion, Dec. 13, 2006. **So far as to declare:** David C. Viano et al., "Concussion in Professional Football, Part 10," *Neurosurgery,* Dec. 2005. **"Virtually worthless":** "Study of Ex-NFL Players Ties Concussion to Depression Risk," *New York Times,* May 31, 2007. **Numerous studies:** J. S. Delaney et al., "Concussion during the 1997 Canadian Football League Season," *Clinical Journal of Sports Medicine,* 2000; J. S. Delaney et al., "Concussions among University Football and Soccer Players," *Clinical Journal of Sports Medicine,* 2002. **At his alma mater:** Guskiewicz brought up the NFL midway through his commencement speech to emphasize the need for "perseverance, surrounding yourself with good people, and carefully making decisions." He said: "In 2005 and 2007, I published (along with a group of 5 colleagues) two research papers that have defined my career as a neuroscientist. The findings of my research outlined in these papers appeared to be incriminating toward arguably one of the most popular and profitable industries in America—professional football, yes—the NFL. Our four-year study identified a high probability of developing later life cognitive impairment and depression once a player had sustained 3 or more concussions during their NFL career. It was the last thing the NFL wanted to hear, and the league's own medical committee immediately began dismissing our findings and trying to hire other doctors and scientists to 'put out the fire.' The NFL was in damage control mode. Its committee members began pointing fingers at our research and even initiated its own study. This was 'industry-funded research' at its best. Members of the league's committee even suggested that we were out to ruin the game of football. It was a difficult time for our group, because we knew our research was solid, and we refused to be intimidated and just walk away. The irony of this is that my 3 boys were playing Pop Warner Football at the time, and if I wanted to paint this ugly picture of the game—would I really allow my own children to participate in the sport? All along, we had claimed that our goal was to identify risk factors for concussion and long-term effects to help improve the game and to help preserve the sport of football." **Protector of the league:** Bob Cantu interview, 2012. **Conclusions of NFL Paper Number 6:** Elliot J. Pellman et al., "Concussion in Professional Football, Part 6," *Neurosurgery,* Dec. 2004. **The response:** Elliot J. Pellman et al., "Concussion in Professional Football, Part 6," *Neurosurgery,* Dec. 2004 (comments). **A lark:** Bill Barr interview, 2012. **Coauthored a chapter:** Mark R. Lovell and William Barr, "American Professional Football," *Traumatic Brain Injury in Sports,* pp. 209–219. **Madison Square Garden:** Barr interview, 2012. **He was incredulous:** Barr interview, 2012. **Pellman later denied:** "Doctor Yes," *ESPN The Magazine,* Oct. 28, 2006. **Barr began to contact:** Barr e-mail correspondence with Rick Naugle, Chris Randolph, and John Woodward. **This was false:** "Doctor Yes," *ESPN The Magazine,* Oct. 28, 2006. **Lovell denied:** Mark Lovell interview. **Maroon seemed taken aback:** Pellman et al., "Concussion in Professional Football, Part 6," *Neurosurgery,* Dec. 2004 (comments). **A letter to his dean:** Letter from Barr to Richard I. Levin, Vice Dean for Education, Faculty and Academic Affairs, NYU School of Medicine, April 29, 2005. **Five papers in as many months:** "Concussion in Professional Football," Parts 4–8, ran monthly between Oct. 2004 and Feb. 2005 in *Neurosurgery.* Committee members told the authors that the NFL project evolved into a series of 16 papers but that no specific number was originally planned. **Concussions were so minor:** Elliot J. Pellman et al., "Concussion in Professional Football, Part 7," *Neurosurgery,* Jan. 2007. **"Concussion prone":** Elliot J. Pellman et al., "Concussion in Professional Football, Part 12," *Neurosurgery,* Feb. 2006. **For $500,000:** "NFL Helmet Manufacturer Warned on Concussion Risk," *Frontline,* May 1, 2013. This article, written by Sabrina Shankman, was part of a reporting partnership between *Frontline* and ESPN's *Outside the Lines.* The original article can be found at pbs.org/wgbh/pages/front line/sports/concussion-watch/nfl-helmet-manufacturer-warned-on-concussion -risk; and espn.go.com/espn/otl/story/_/id/9228260/report-warned-riddell-no -helmet-prevent-concussions-nfl-helmet-maker-marketed-one-such-anyway/. **A confidential report:** Report from Chris Withnall, senior engineer, Biokinetics, prepared for Riddell Inc., Nov. 15, 2000. **"Full stop":** *Frontline,* May 1, 2013. **Riddell provided the helmets:** Mark Lovell interview, 2012. **Collins, who led the study:** Micky Collins et al., "Examining Concussion Rates and Return to Play in High School Football Players Wearing Newer Helmet Technology: A Three-Year Prospective Cohort Study," *Neurosurgery,* Feb. 2006. **A blistering commentary:** Micky Collins et al., "Examining Concussion Rates and Return to Play in High School Football Players Wearing Newer Helmet Technology: A Three-Year Prospective Cohort Study," *Neurosurgery,* Feb. 2006 (comments).

CHAPTER 10

Apuzzo continued to rubber-stamp: Cantu, the section editor, said other peer reviewers were recruited to evaluate the papers after he and Guskiewicz refused; the publication of the NFL concussion series continued until just before the MTBI committee was disbanded. **Agreed to publish Omalu's paper:** Omalu e-mails. **Support Cantu's theory:** Cantu interview, 2012. **The torturous review process:** Omalu e-mails and interview, 2012. **An original version:** Omalu and Hamilton e-mails. **The paper was published:** Bennet I. Omalu et al., "Chronic Traumatic Encephalopathy in a National Football League Player," *Neurosurgery,* July 2005. **Donald Marion:** Omalu interview, 2012; Hamilton e-mails; Donald Marion interview, 2012. **Omalu wrote to his colleagues:** Omalu e-mail to DeKosky and Hamilton. **The NFL's letter:** Ira R. Casson, Elliot J. Pellman, and David C. Viano, "Correspondence," *Neurosurgery,* May 2006. **A shot of Johnnie Walker Red:** Omalu interview, 2012; Omalu, *Play Hard, Die Young: Football Dementia, Depression, and Death.* **He did some quick research:** Omalu interview, 2012; Omalu, *Play Hard, Die Young: Football Dementia, Depression, and Death.* **Omalu e-mailed:** Hamilton e-mails. **Hamilton wasn't at all amused:** Hamilton interview, 2012, and e-mails. **The men exchanged e-mails:** Hamilton e-mails. **Dug further into the history:** Omalu, Hamilton, and DeKosky interviews, 2012. **He had discovered another case of CTE:** Omalu, Hamilton, DeKosky, and Wecht interviews; Hamilton e-mails. **Terry Long killed himself:** Long autopsy report. **Long was like Webster:** Long biography from ProFootball Reference.com; Bailes interview, 2012; "Long, Terrence L," *TribLive,* obituaries; and "Long Carries His Weight with Steelers," *Pittsburgh Press,* Aug. 6, 1985. **Tested positive for steroids:** "Long's Road Back," *Pittsburgh Post-Gazette,* Dec. 4, 1991. **Dramatic downward spiral:** Omalu, *Play Hard, Die Young: Football Dementia, Depression, and Death*; "Final Days Were Troubled for Former Steeler," *Pittsburgh Post-Gazette,* June 10, 2005. **"Ground Zero":** "Heads Up," *Pittsburgh Post-Gazette,* Sept. 7, 2000. Upon launching the UPMC concussion program, Micky Collins told Chuck Finder: "What we really want to do is make Pittsburgh ground zero." **The autopsy:** Dr. Abdulrezak Shakir interview, 2012; Long autopsy; Omalu interview, 2012. **Omalu repeated the process:** Bennet I. Omalu et al., "Chronic Traumatic Encephalopathy in a National Football League Player: Part II," *Neurosurgery,* Nov. 2006. **Omalu sent the slides to Hamilton:** Omalu and Hamilton interviews, 2012; Hamilton e-mails. **He went straight to the media:** "Wecht: Long Died from Brain Injury; Had Head Trauma from NFL Days," *Pittsburgh Post-Gazette,* Sept. 14, 2005. **The NFL responded swiftly:** "Surgeon Disputes Findings; Disagrees with Wecht That Football Killed Long," *Pittsburgh Post-Gazette,* Sept. 15, 2005. **Wecht called Omalu at home:** Omalu and Wecht interviews, 2012. **A 1987 letter written by Maroon:** "Cause of Death Sparks Debate," *Pittsburgh Post-Gazette,* Sept. 16, 2005. **Even more confusing:** "Suicide Ruling in Long's Death Hasn't Ended Controversy," *Pittsburgh Post-Gazette,* Jan. 26, 2006. **Finishing touches:** Hamilton e-mails. **Omalu, Hamilton, and DeKosky wrote:** Bennet I. Omalu et al., "Correspondence," *Neurosurgery,* May 2006. **Published the Long study six months later:** Bennet I. Omalu et al.,

"Chronic Traumatic Encephalopathy in a National Football League Player: Part II," *Neurosurgery,* Nov. 2006. **The phone rang at Omalu's desk:** Omalu and Bailes interviews, 2012; Omalu, *Play Hard, Die Young: Football Dementia, Depression, and Death,* 2008. **Bailes told Omalu:** Bailes and Omalu interviews, 2012. **One of Cantu's former patients:** Chris Nowinski and Omalu interviews, 2012; Omalu, *Play Hard, Die Young: Football Dementia, Depression, and Death.* **A new breed of Dissenter:** Nowinski biography from Nowinski interview, 2012; Christopher Nowinski, *Head Games: Football's Concussion Crisis.* **Killer Kowalski's Pro Wrestling School:** www .killerkowalskis.com. **"A dynamic individual":** Cantu interview, 2012. **Nowinski was checking SI.com:** Nowinski interview, 2012. **Andre Waters:** Biography from ProFootballReference.com; "Pro Football's Necessary Headaches to NFL Players," *Philadelphia Inquirer,* Oct. 30, 1994. **Nowinski played a hunch:** Nowinski interview, 2012. **While trying to get his book published:** Nowinski and Alan Schwarz interviews, 2012. **Primarily a baseball writer:** Schwarz interview, 2012; Alan Schwarz, *The Numbers Game: Baseball's Lifelong Fascination with Statistics,* 2005. **The story on the Waters results:** This account of the background on how the Andre Waters story developed is drawn from 2012 interviews with Schwarz, Nowinski, and Omalu. **Waters had brain damage:** "Expert Ties Ex-Players' Brain Damage to Football," *New York Times,* Jan. 18, 2007. **When Bailes contacted Omalu:** Bailes and Omalu interviews, 2012. **Omalu and Maroon had struck a truce:** Omalu and Maroon interviews, 2012; Hamilton e-mails. **Gathered in Hamilton's office:** This account of the meeting is drawn from 2012 interviews with Omalu, Bailes, Hamilton, DeKosky, and Maroon.

CHAPTER 11

Profoundly affected: Harry Carson interview, 2012. **"Dick in the dirt":** Harry Carson, *Captain for Life,* p. 209 (electronic). **No player had hit him harder:** Harry Carson, *Captain for Life,* p. 184 (electronic). He confessed: Carson interview, 2012. **He went back:** "Two Authors of N.F.L. Study on Concussions Dispute Finding," *New York Times,* June 10, 2007. **Riddell developed PowerPoint presentations:** A history of the controversial Revolution helmet study, Riddell's marketing strategy, and the relationship between Riddell and ImPACT is summarized in a partial opinion issued in Riddell's lawsuit against Schutt. The court established a series of "undisputed facts," which included the findings that Riddell provided salary support for Collins and Lovell; ImPACT agreed not to sell concussion software at "any places in conflict with Riddell"; ImPACT agreed to pay Riddell for any sale "completed through a Riddell initiated contact"; and data compiled in 2002 and 2003, the first two years of the three-year study, produced "nearly identical concussion rates" in Year 1 and a difference that was "not statistically significant" in Year 2. The opinion granted Riddell summary judgment to toss out Schutt's claims that Riddell falsely advertised the concussion-reducing properties of the Revolution helmet. Schutt "has failed to identify literally false statements or show that it has been harmed by plaintiff statements," Judge Barbara B. Crabb wrote. See *Riddell,*

Inc. v. Schutt Sports, Inc. **The two pieces ran:** " 'I don't want anyone to end up like me'; Plagued by postconcussion syndrome and battling an amphetamine addiction, former Patriots linebacker Ted Johnson is a shell of his former self," *Boston Globe,* Feb. 2, 2007; and "Dark Days Follow Hard-Hitting Career in N.F.L.," *New York Times,* Feb. 2, 2007. The main difference in the two pieces was MacMullan's revealing interview with Belichick. The Patriots' coach declined comment to the *Times.* **"88 Plan":** "Wives United by Husbands' Post-N.F.L. Trauma," *New York Times,* March 14, 2007. **"Many elderly people":** *New York Times,* March 14, 2007. **1982 study:** Ira R. Casson et al., "Neurological and CT Evaluation of Knocked Out Boxers," *Journal of Neurology, Neurosurgery, and Psychiatry,* 1982. **Sports Illustrated brought in Casson:** Robert Boyle and Wilmer Ames, "Too Many Punches, Too Little Concern," *Sports Illustrated,* April 11, 1983. **In a 2010 article:** Ira R. Casson, "Do the 'Facts' Really Support an Association between NFL Players' Concussions, Dementia and Depression?" *Neurology Today,* June 3, 2010. **Goldberg said he walked away thinking:** Bernard Goldberg interview, 2013. **Inherited a nightmare:** Bob Stern interview, 2013. **After taking office:** Don Van Natta Jr., "His Game, His Rules," *ESPN The Magazine,* March 5, 2013. **"Why did they ask you?":** Julian Bailes interview, 2012. **The daylong meeting:** Unless otherwise noted, this account of the NFL's tumultuous 2007 concussion summit comes primarily from interviews with Mark Lovell, Micky Collins, Julian Bailes, Kevin Guskiewicz, Bob Cantu, and Bill Barr. The timeline is drawn from a written agenda issued by the league to the participants. **"You're looking for an answer":** This quote is from an interview *Times* reporter Alan Schwarz conducted with Pellman and Casson. A recording of the interview was provided by Schwarz. **Goodell also weighed in:** "NFL Personnel Discuss Concussion Management," *St. Petersburg Times* (FL), June 20, 2007. **A bit heated:** Schwarz interview with Pellman.

CHAPTER 12

Omalu wanted to travel to Florida: Details of Florida trip from 2012 interviews with Omalu and Nowinski as well as their respective books. **A two-page document:** Document was provided by Nowinski. **Tossed around names:** Omalu and Nowinski interviews, 2012; Omalu e-mails. **"He can be trusted":** Omalu e-mails. **Omalu brought in his own champion:** The account of how SLI was formed is drawn from interviews with Omalu, Nowinski, Bailes, and Fitzsimmons, and Omalu e-mails. **Resurrected his own concussion summits:** Leigh Steinberg, Nowinski, Omalu, and Bailes interviews, 2012; 2007 National Concussion Summit pamphlet. **"Ticking time bomb":** "Steinberg Labels Concussions 'Time Bomb,' " Associated Press, April 20, 2007. **More disturbing story to tell:** Omalu, Nowinski, Bailes, Lovell, and Guskiewicz interviews, 2012; Omalu PowerPoint presentation. **Sights on the brain of another player:** Bailes and Nowinski interviews, 2012; Omalu e-mails. **Steelers offensive lineman:** Strzelczyk biography from ProFootballReference.com; "What Drove Justin Strzelczyk to His Death?" *Pittsburgh Post-Gazette,* Oct. 21, 2004. **He remembered Strzelczyk:** Bailes interview, 2012. **Schwarz had another**

story: "Lineman, Dead at 36, Exposes Brain Injuries," *New York Times,* June 15, 2007. **The NFL needed a new strategy:** Peter Davies interview, 2012, and e-mails. **Bailes continued to be shaken:** Colleen Bailes and Julian Bailes, interview, 2012. **Casson set out to find an independent expert:** Davies interview, 2012. **A leader in Alzheimer's research:** www.einstein.yu.edu; DeKosky interview, 2012. **Met with the committee at the NFL's headquarters:** Davies interview, 2012. **West Virginia University:** Details of the meeting and the events that followed are from 2012 interviews with Davies, Omalu, Bailes, and Maroon; Omalu and Davies e-mails; the PowerPoint presentation Davies prepared for the NFL; and "Game Brain," *GQ,* Oct. 2009. **"What are you going to do about this?":** This account of Jason Luckasevic's friendship with Omalu and the early conversations about the NFL lawsuit are from 2012 interviews with Luckasevic and Omalu. **On September 18, 2007:** Transcripts from "Oversight of the NFL Retirement System," hearing convened by the Senate Committee on Commerce, Science, & Transportation. **His name was Dave Duerson:** Biography from ProFootballReference.com; Duerson testimony; "Dave Duerson: The Ferocious Life and Tragic Death of a Super Bowl Star," *Men's Journal,* May 2011. **A screaming match:** "Dave Duerson Knew Nothing about Concussions and Players' Best Interests," www.concussioninc.net, Feb. 24, 2011. **Charged with assaulting his wife:** "Dave Duerson: The Ferocious Life and Tragic Death of a Super Bowl Star," *Men's Journal,* May 2011.

CHAPTER 13

Chris Benoit: "The Last Days of Chris Benoit," *Maxim,* Nov. 14, 2007; "Steroids Discovered in Probe of Slayings, Suicide," Associated Press, June 27, 2007. **"I knew him well":** Nowinski e-mail to Omalu and others. **Within days of the murders:** Nowinski interview, 2012, and Omalu e-mails. **ESPN crew showed up:** Arty Berko and Omalu interviews, 2012. **Riddled with CTE:** Omalu, Nowinski, Bailes, Cantu, and Fitzsimmons interviews, 2012. **Raise its national profile:** Omalu and Nowinski interviews; Omalu e-mails; "Why Did Wrestler Kill Wife, Son, Self," *Larry King Live* transcripts, Sept. 6, 2007. **Larry could take only one brain researcher:** Omalu, Nowinski, Bailes, and Fitzsimmons interviews, 2012. **The ESPN piece:** "Brain Chasers," ESPN, *Outside the Lines,* July 28, 2007. **Almost from the beginning:** Omalu and Nowinski interviews, 2012. **SLI began to split apart:** This account of the split is drawn from 2012 interviews with Nowinski, Omalu, Bailes, Cantu, and Fitzsimmons. **"Our Story":** www.sportslegacy.org. **Nowinski had made the connection:** Nowinski and Stern interviews, 2012. **Her name was Ann McKee:** Details of McKee's biography were drawn from interviews with Ann McKee, Chuck McKee, Nowinski, Cantu, and Stern, 2012; "The Woman Who Would Save Football," *Grantland,* Aug. 17, 2012; and www.bu.edu. **Appleton:** "A Place to Place," *Sports Illustrated,* Aug. 11, 1986. **During her Alzheimer's studies:** Ann McKee interview, 2012. **Nowinski got McKee her first brain:** McKee and Nowinski interviews, 2012. **John Grimsley:** Biography derived from ProFootballReference.com; "Former Oiler Grimsley Found Shot to Death," *Houston Chronicle,* Feb. 6, 2008; "Ex-Oilers

Shocked by Loss of Teammate Grimsley," *Houston Chronicle,* Feb. 6, 2008; "Football-Related Head Injuries Affect Players' Loved Ones," *Houston Chronicle,* Oct. 25, 2008. **Two days later, Nowinski called:** Nowinski and McKee interviews, 2012. **She was excited:** McKee interview, 2012. **Her first call:** Ann McKee and Chuck McKee interviews, 2012. **Schwarz broke the story:** "12 Athletes Leaving Brains to Concussion Study," *New York Times,* Sept. 23, 2008. **Omalu was in Lodi:** Omalu interview, 2012. **A Shakespearean drama:** Details surrounding case against Wecht and Omalu's involvement derived from 2012 interviews with both men as well as Shakir and Dominick; "Timeline: The Investigation and Trial of Cyril H. Wecht," *Pittsburgh Post-Gazette,* Jan. 27, 2008. **Brain Injury Research Institute:** Interviews with Omalu, Bailes, Fitzsimmons, and Garrett Webster, 2012. **Another former NFL player died young:** Tom McHale biography from Lisa McHale interview, 2012; ProFootballReference.com; "Ex-Buccaneer Tom McHale Found Dead at 45," *Tampa Bay Times,* Sept. 25, 2008; "Major Breakthrough in Concussion Crisis," *Boston Globe,* Jan. 27, 2009. **The Omalu Group got to McHale's family first:** Omalu e-mails; Nowinski and Omalu interviews, 2012. **Nowinski called Omalu:** Details of the Omalu Group's agreement with Nowinski and subsequent contact with McHale's family are derived from Omalu's e-mails. **Trying to contact Omalu:** Nowinski interview, 2012. **Go public with the results:** Nowinski and Lisa McHale interviews, 2012. **The press conference:** Details derived from Nowinski, McKee, and Lisa McHale interviews, 2012; "Major Breakthrough in Concussion Crisis," *Boston Globe,* Jan. 27, 2009; "Sixth NFL Player's Brain Is Found to Have Brain Damage," *New York Times,* Jan. 28, 2009; BU-CSTE press release. **Learned of BU's announcement on TV:** Omalu interview, 2012. **Coming-out party as a spokeswoman:** "Major Breakthrough in Concussion Crisis," *Boston Globe,* Jan. 27, 2009.

CHAPTER 14

It was that kind of call: McKee interview, 2012. **She asked if Nowinski could attend:** McKee and Nowinski interviews, 2012. **Another expert in neurodegenerative disease:** Daniel Perl interview, 2012; www.hjfcp3.org/military-medical-symposium/symposium-files/Daniel%20Perl-%20MD.pdf. **McKee was nervous but excited:** McKee interview, 2012. **NFL headquarters:** This account of McKee's presentation to the MTBI committee is drawn from 2012 interviews with McKee, Perl, Nowinski, Henry Feuer, Colonel Michael Jaffee, and John Mann. **Call her brother:** Ann McKee and Chuck McKee interviews, 2012. **The young Pittsburgh lawyer:** Luckasevic interview, 2012. **The league could fall back on:** Collective Bargaining Agreement, specifically the role of the retirement board. **One such case:** "Seeing Is Believing," *Sports Illustrated,* June 9, 2003; "Orlando Brown, Who Sued the N.F.L. over Errant Flag, Dies at 40," *New York Times,* Sept. 23, 2011. **Line up consultants:** Luckasevic interview, 2012; contract with Nowinski. **Questions lingered:** "Researchers Consulted with Law Firms," ESPN.com, April 6, 2013. **Fearing it could compromise their independence:** Guskiewicz interview, 2012. **A viable case:** Luckasevic interview, 2012. **Goldberg, Persky & White:** www.gpwlaw.com.

Time to fish around: Luckasevic interview, 2012. **Houston-based firm:** "Vioxx Jury Awards $253 Million in Damages," *Houston Chronicle,* Aug. 20, 2005. **Lanier's lawyers ultimately pulled out:** Luckasevic interview, 2012. **A big win:** "Former Dolphins Receiver O.J. McDuffie Wins $11.5 Million in Malpractice Lawsuit," *Sun-Sentinel* (Fort Lauderdale), May 5, 2010. **Tierney was right:** Luckasevic interview, 2012. **A big gun in Los Angeles:** Tom Girardi interview, 2012; www.girardikeese.com; "Erin Brockovich: The Real Story," *Salon,* April 14, 2000. **NFL Paper Number 16:** Anders Hamburger et al., "Concussion in Professional Football, Part 16," *Neurosurgery,* June 2009. **Another confounding story:** "Dementia Risk Seen in N.F.L. Players Study," *New York Times,* Sept. 29, 2009. **Announced that it would hold hearings:** "Congress to Hold Hearing on N.F.L. Head Injuries," *New York Times,* Oct. 2, 2009. **Democratic committee staffers:** Details of the setup for the hearing and the NFL's reactions are derived primarily from a 2012 interview with Eric Tamarkin, who at the time was counsel to the committee. **"Will's Bill":** Dick Benson testimony. **"Rebel with a cause":** "N.F.L. Players with Head Injuries Find a Voice," *New York Times,* Oct. 28, 2009. **The packed hearing:** Transcripts from written and oral testimony before the committee. **Linda Sanchez:** Biography from www.lindasanchez.house.gov; and "Sanchez Sisters to Make History in the House," womensenews.org, Nov. 19, 2002. **On a shelf in his office at BU:** Nowinski interview, 2012. **400 law firms:** Dan Zegart, *Civil Warriors* (Delacorte Press, 2000), p. 202. **180,000 research papers:** Dan Zegart, *Civil Warriors,* p. 296. **Tobacco fight's version of Omalu:** Dan Zegart, *Civil Warriors,* p. 37. **Started in the morgue:** Ernst Wynder biography: cdc.gov/mmwr/preview/mmwrhtml/mm4843bx.htm. **Among the 62 mice still alive:** Ernst Wynder et al., "Experimental Production of Carcinoma with Cigarette Tar," *Cancer Research,* 1953. **Research group:** Dan Zegart, *Civil Warriors,* p. 37. **"Savage the other side":** Dan Zegart, *Civil Warriors,* p. 38. **"A front":** Victor DeNoble interview, 2012. **A "metaphysical quarrel":** Dan Zegart, *Civil Warriors,* p. 38. **"NFL equals Tobacco":** Stern interview, 2012. **"Graciously" resigned:** "Co-Chairmen of NFL Concussion Panel Resign," Associated Press, Nov. 25, 2009. **Several changes to its concussion policy:** "NFL Changes Return to Play Rules for Concussions," Associated Press, Dec. 3, 2009; "New N.F.L. Rule on Concussions Benches Injured," *New York Times,* Dec. 3, 2009. **The headline that the NFL never wanted to see:** "Is Tackle Football Too Dangerous for Kids to Play?" *New York Times* blog, Nov. 30, 2009. **A guest column:** "Listening to Wisdom from a 10-Year-Old Son about His Head Injury," *New York Times,* Nov. 28, 2009. **A wire report:** "NFL to Ask Its Players to Donate Brains for Study," Associated Press, Dec. 20, 2009. **Schwarz was surprised:** Details of Schwarz's reaction and his call to Aiello derived from 2012 interview with Schwarz. **Nowinski on the phone:** Schwarz and Nowinski interviews, 2012. **The timing of the NFL's announcement:** Nowinski interview, 2012. **The following headline:** "N.F.L. Acknowledges Long-Term Concussion Effects," *New York Times,* Dec. 21, 2009. **Sent a bottle of champagne to BU:** Nowinski interview, 2012.

CHAPTER 15

"Started from zero": Dr. Mitchel Berger interview, 2012. **Head, Neck and Spine Committee:** "NFL Picks Two New Co-Chairs of Concussion Committee," Associated Press, March 18, 2010. **A two-page letter:** The framed letter is posted on the wall at the offices of the BU Center for the Study of Traumatic Encephalopathy, 2012. **A full-fledged member:** Guskiewicz interview, 2012. **Appointing brain surgeons:** "NFL Picks Two New Co-Chairs of Concussion Committee," Associated Press, March 18, 2010. **Ellenbogen:** Dr. Rich Ellenbogen interview, 2012; "Taking Brain Injuries out of Sports," *Seattle Magazine,* Fall/Winter 2012. **Batjer:** Dr. Hunt Batjer interview, 2012. **Batjer and Ellenbogen professed to know very little:** Batjer and Ellenbogen interviews, 2012. **At odds with Ellenbogen's review:** Anders Hamburger et al., "Concussions in Professional Football, Part 16," *Neurosurgery,* Aug. 2007 (comments). **"Like the same old NFL":** "House Panel Criticizes New N.F.L. Doctors," *New York Times,* May 24, 2010; "Panel Criticizes NFL on Safety Research," Associated Press, May 24, 2010. **A man in exile:** Omalu interview, 2012. **BU's researchers literally kept a file:** Stern interview, 2012. **Omalu's exaggerations:** Cantu interview, 2012. **Nowinski was no more charitable:** Transcripts, *Dennis & Callahan Radio Show,* Oct. 14, 2010. **A writer for GQ:** Jeanne Marie Laskas interview, 2012. **Never recognizing the need to filter:** Lovell and Guskiewicz interviews, 2012. **Ban on tackle football:** Cantu interview, 2012; "Preventing Sports Concussions Among Children," *New York Times,* Oct. 7, 2012. **"He got steamrolled":** Collins interview, 2012. **The league's biggest threat:** Bailes interview, 2012. **Omalu's marginalization:** Carson interview, 2012. **On February 17, 2011:** Details of Duerson's death and the scene at the condo from Sunny Isles Beach Police Department Incident/Investigation Report, Feb. 17, 2011; Tregg and Alicia Duerson interviews, 2012; excerpts of texts to Alicia Duerson; excerpts of letter left by Duerson. **Cast a proxy vote:** Mike Webster disability lawsuit court records. **Copy of Sports Illustrated:** "Concussions: The Hits That Are Changing Football," *Sports Illustrated,* Nov. 1, 2010. **A DVD case:** "Trapped: Haitian Nights," *The Movie Database.* **"Football's First Martyr":** "Dave Duerson: Football's First Martyr Can't Die in Vain," *Time,* Feb. 25, 2011. **A star scholar-athlete:** Duerson biography, both rise and fall, derived from Alicia Duerson, Tregg Duerson, and Harold Rice interviews, 2012; "You Have to Accept My Pain: An Interview with Dave Duerson Three Months before His Suicide," *Deadspin,* Feb. 23, 2011; "Dave Duerson: The Ferocious Life and Tragic Death of a Super Bowl Star," *Men's Journal,* May 2011; ProFootballReference.com; bankruptcy records. **Duerson had a radio show:** *Double Time with Double D* radio show, VoiceAmerica, Oct. 21, 2010. **Donating his father's brain:** Details of Duerson family efforts to donate his brain are from 2012 interviews with Tregg Duerson, Alicia Duerson, Kelly Woods, and David Krichavsky. **NFL wasn't nearly as unified:** Berger, Ellenbogen, Batjer, and Guskiewicz interviews, 2012. **BU's rock star:** "The Woman Who Would Save Football," *Grantland,* Aug. 17, 2012. **Conference in Las Vegas:** "Chronic Traumatic Encephalopathy," conference in Las Vegas, Sept. 30–Oct. 1, 2012. **Their most ominous**

assertions: McKee, Cantu, Stern, and Nowinski interviews, 2012. **If CTE was occurring at a deep level:** McKee interview, 2012; Ann C. McKee et al., "The Spectrum of Disease in Chronic Traumatic Encephalopathy," *Brain,* 2012. **One of BU's main critics:** Berger interview, 2012; http://neurosurgery.ucsf.edu/index.php/about_us_faculty_berger.html. **Wasn't a single recorded case:** Ann C. McKee et al., "The Spectrum of Disease in Chronic Traumatic Encephalopathy," *Brain,* 2012. **Self-selecting quality:** McKee, Cantu, Berger, and Ellenbogen interviews, 2012. **"With all due respect":** Cantu interview, 2012. **"The facts are the facts":** Nowinski interview, 2012. **Steer Duerson's brain:** Batjer interview, 2012. **From the new committee's inception:** Ellenbogen, Guskiewicz, and Berger interviews, 2012. **A press conference:** "Duerson's Brain Trauma Diagnosed," *New York Times,* May 2, 2011. **"Drove him to suicide":** McKee interview, 2012. **"I just can't even believe this":** McKee interview, 2012.

CHAPTER 16

Two dozen clients: Ron Feenberg interview, 2011. **A new front:** "Former Pro Athletes Battle against Bill Limiting Workers' Comp," *Sacramento Bee,* April 16, 2013. **A fierce lobbying campaign:** The NFL, with support from the other major sports leagues and 16 California teams, rallied around AB 1309, a bill that would close the loophole. On April 24, 2013, the bill passed out of the California State Assembly's Insurance Committee by a unanimous 11–0 vote and was headed to the full assembly for debate. **Brady and . . . Brees:** "Injured Pro Athletes Deserve Workers' Comp," *San Francisco Chronicle,* June 24, 2013. **Luckasevic had found:** Jason Luckasevic interview, 2012. **One of the first . . . cases:** Jeanne Marie Laskas, "The People V. Football," *GQ,* March 2011. **On July 19, 2011:** See *Vernon Maxwell, et al. v. National Football League, et al.,* Superior Court of the State of California, July 19, 2011. **"We thought maybe":** Tom Girardi interview, 2012. **The next month:** *Charles Ray Easterling and his wife, Mary Ann Easterling; et al. v. National Football League, Inc.,* U.S. District Court for the Eastern District of Pennsylvania, Aug. 17, 2011. Later, the Easterling suit would be described in some accounts as the first brain injury case to be filed against the NFL. It was first to be filed in federal court, where all the cases were later consolidated. **"I won't remember":** "Taking Its Toll," *Outside the Lines,* March 16, 2012. **Painfully familiar:** "Death Isn't the End," *New York Times,* May 4, 2012. **Riddled with CTE:** "Football Player Who Killed Himself Had Brain Disease," *New York Times,* July 27, 2012. **By the time the results were released:** Nathan Fenno and Luke Rosiak of the *Washington Times* compiled the most comprehensive database on the lawsuits, a working online document that allows users to explore the plaintiffs by team, position, and number of seasons played. The database can be found at: washingtontimes.com/footballinjuries/; the website NFLConcussionLitigation.com has maintained the most current information about the lawsuits and the plaintiffs. **50 military service members:** G. Wolf et al., "The Effect of Hyperbaric Oxygen on Symptoms after Mild Traumatic Brain Injury," *Journal of Neurotrauma,* 2012. **Medieval-sounding device:** Julian Bailes interview, 2012.

Pilot study: Gary W. Small et al., "PET Scanning of Brain Tau in Retired National Football League Players: Preliminary Findings," *American Journal of Geriatric Psychiatry,* 2013. **Nearly every NFL team:** The ImPACT website lists many of the company's clients. See ImpactTest.com. **Two heart attacks:** Mark Lovell interview, 2012. **His own research:** Maroon coauthored a study on the use of natural plant extracts to neutralize the chemical reaction that leads to brain disease. See Russell L. Blaylock and Joseph Maroon, "Natural Plant Products and Extracts That Reduce Immunoexcitotoxicity-Associated Neurodegeneration and Promote Repair within the Central Nervous System," *Surgical Neurology International,* 2012. **A letter to the FTC:** Letter from Tom Udall to Federal Trade Commission Chairman Jon Leibowitz, Jan. 4, 2011. **One mouth guard:** Letter from Tom Udall to Federal Trade Commission Chairman Jon Leibowitz, Jan. 4, 2011. **An endorsement:** Letter from Tom Udall to Federal Trade Commission Chairman Jon Leibowitz, Jan. 4, 2011. **"No significant data":** Testimony of Jeffrey S. Kutcher, Senate Commerce Committee, Oct. 19, 2011. **"Don't forget to take your fish oil!":** Peter Davies e-mail correspondence. **FTC ordered:** Letter from Mary K. Engle, the FTC's associate director for advertising practices, to John M. Shanahan, CEO, Newport Nutritionals, Inc., Nov. 7, 2012. **Closed its investigation:** Letter from Engle to John E. Villafranco, representing Riddell Sports Group, Inc., April 24, 2013. **A coffee table book:** *The First 50 Years.* **Their own words:** *The First 50 Years,* pp. 39–83. **"Propaganda organ":** "Steve Sabol, Cinematic Force for N.F.L., Dies at 69," *New York Times,* Sept. 18, 2012. **Origin story:** Michael Oriard, *Brand NFL,* pp. 14–18. **"NFL football is *real*":** Oriard, *Brand NFL,* p. 14. **Swallowed his tongue:** Andy Russell, *A Steeler Odyssey,* p. 15. **Summer of 2012:** E-mail from Clare Graff, NFL Communications, to Lorraine Esposito. **"He really wanted to know":** Lorraine Esposito interview, 2013. **Dumb Mom:** Amanda Rodriguez interview, 2013. **Two helmets crashing:** "N.F.L.'s Policy on Helmet-to-Helmet Hits Makes Highlights Distasteful," *New York Times,* Oct. 21, 2010. **Pull a commercial:** "Unhappy NFL Prods Toyota to Edit TV Ad," Reuters, Jan. 19, 2011. **Pointed out:** On Feb. 4, 2013, Crossman tweeted: "So far I have found three players in the NFL's safety evolution commercial from last night who are suing the league over concussions."

CHAPTER 17

Hunched over a microscope: Bennet Omalu interview, 2012. **Raised in a violent ghetto:** Award-winning sportswriter Jill Lieber Steeg wrote one of the first lengthy profiles on Seau's unlikely rise to NFL stardom for *Sports Illustrated* in 1993. After Seau's suicide, she produced an exhaustive two-part series on the events leading up to his death. See Jill Lieber, "Hard Charger," *Sports Illustrated,* Sept. 6, 1993, and "Junior Seau: Song of Sorrow," *San Diego Union-Tribune,* Oct. 14, 2012. **12 yards deep:** Gary Plummer interview, 2013. **Seau was loud:** The account of Seau's personality changes and the final years of his life is drawn primarily from interviews with members of Seau's family, including three of his four children and Gina Seau, his ex-wife; Bette Hoffman, former director of the Junior Seau Foundation and the executor of his will; and Lieber's *Union-Tribune* articles. **When police arrived:** Junior Seau autopsy report, Aug. 20, 2012. **Placed on a gurney:** The account of the events in Seau's house after his death and Tyler Seau's phone call with Bennet Omalu and Julian Bailes is from interviews with Tyler Seau, Bette Hoffman, Joe Davis, Bennet Omalu, and Julian Bailes. **At 8:38 that night:** E-mail correspondence between Tyler Seau and Bennet Omalu. **Chargers' doctor:** E-mail correspondence between Tyler Seau and Bennet Omalu. **Chao had his own issues:** The Medical Board of California website contains detailed records of the allegations against Chao and issues surrounding his drinking. See: mbc.ca.gov. For additional details of Chao's checkered history, see "The Chargers' Doctor Is a Drunk Quack. Why Haven't They Fired Him?" *Deadspin,* April 24, 2013. On June 13, 2013, Chao stepped down after 17 years as the Chargers' doctor. "I talked to the Chargers about my back problems in March and my desire to spend more time with my newborn twins and young daughter," Chao said in a statement released by the team. **At least a half dozen:** Craig Nelson interview, 2013. **Prusiner placed calls:** Prusiner's interest in obtaining part of Seau's brain is confirmed in e-mails and interviews with Bennet Omalu and Joe Davis. **"I empathize":** Peter King interview, 2013. **Nelson told Omalu:** Nelson interview, 2013. **Soot and the imprint:** Seau autopsy report, Aug. 20, 2012. **"Persona non grata":** Bennet Omalu interview, 2012. **Celebratory e-mail:** E-mail correspondence between Bennet Omalu and Stanley Prusiner. **Nowinski emphasized:** Tyler Seau interview, 2013. **At the center of the league's effort:** The account of the NFL's effort to take control of Seau's brain is drawn from interviews with Tyler Seau, Bette Hoffman, Gina Seau, Kevin Guskiewicz, Rich Ellenbogen, Russell Lonser, and others familiar with the negotiations. **"An early draft":** Bob Fitzsimmons interview, 2013. **Got a call:** Gary Plummer interview, 2013. **That was certain:** "Doctors: Junior Seau's Brain Had CTE," ESPN.com, Jan. 11, 2013. **"I still love football":** Jake Seau interview, 2013.

EPILOGUE

A proposal: The section on Gary Huber's dealings with Big Tobacco is drawn from Dan Zegart, *Civil Warriors,* 2000; and Robert N. Proctor, *Golden Holocaust,* 2011. **50 confirmed cases:** Ann C. McKee et al., "The Spectrum of Disease in Chronic Traumatic Encephalopathy," *Brain,* 2012. **43 percent:** Associated Press, Aug. 7, 2012. **"No genius":** Matt Chaney e-mail to authors, 2013. **Dispensed paid advice:** "Researchers consulted with law firms," ESPN.com, April 6, 2013. **Had given way:** "Concussion Kickoff: Oral Arguments Held in NFL Concussion Litigation," NFLconcussionlitigation.com, April 10, 2013. **"Guiding strategists":** *United States of America v. Philip Morris USA Inc.,* District Court for the District of Columbia Judge Gladys Kessler, Aug. 17, 2006, p. 97. **Directed litigation:** Ibid., p. 68. **"Whitecoats":** Robert Proctor, *Golden Holocaust,* p. 545, and "Proposal for the Organization of the Whitecoat Project," Bates 3990006961/3990006964, at the University of California, San Francisco Legacy Tobacco Documents Library. See http://legacy.library.ucsf.edu/tid/ecr82i00/pdf. **"Deep shit":** Robert

Proctor, *Golden Holocaust,* p. 303, and "Project Down Under: Conference Notes," June 24, 1987, Bates 2021502102-2134 (p. 4). See http://legacy.library.ucsf.edu/tid/njh56b00/pdf. **When he first arrived:** Jim Otto interview, 2012. **Descendant of the Roman gladiators:** Jim Otto with Dave Newhouse, *Jim Otto: The Pain of Glory,* p. 7. **A gash:** Jim Otto with Dave Newhouse, *Jim Otto: The Pain of Glory,* p. viii. **"Looking at a gargoyle":** Jim Otto with Dave Newhouse, *Jim Otto: The Pain of Glory,* p. 143. **"Middle-aged horror show":** Jim Otto with Dave Newhouse, *Jim Otto: The Pain of Glory,* p. 2. **Probably end up killing him:** Otto interview, 2012. **"I'm not a wimp-out":** Jim Otto with Dave Newhouse, *Jim Otto: The Pain of Glory,* p. 6.

BIBLIOGRAPHY

BOOKS

Bailes, Julian E., Mark R. Lovell, and Joseph C. Maroon (eds.). *Sports-Related Concussion.* St. Louis, MO: Quality Medical Publishing, 1999.

Blount, Roy. *About Three Bricks Shy of a Load: A Highly Irregular Lowdown on the Year the Pittsburgh Steelers Were Super but Missed the Bowl.* Boston: Little, Brown, 1974.

Bradshaw, Terry, and David Fisher. *It's Only a Game.* New York: Pocket Books, 2001.

Cantu, Robert C., and Mark Hyman. *Concussions and Our Kids: America's Leading Expert on How to Protect Young Athletes and Keep Sports Safe.* Boston: Houghton Mifflin Harcourt, 2012 (Electronic).

Carroll, Linda, and David Rosner. *The Concussion Crisis: Anatomy of a Silent Epidemic.* New York: Simon & Schuster, 2011 (Electronic).

Carson, Harry. *Captain for Life: My Story as a Hall of Fame Linebacker.* New York: St. Martin's Press, 2011 (Electronic).

Cook, Kevin. *The Last Headbangers: NFL Football in the Rowdy, Reckless '70s, the Era That Created Modern Sports.* New York: W. W. Norton, 2012.

Dent, Jim. *Twelve Mighty Orphans: The Inspiring True Story of the Mighty Mites Who Ruled Texas Football.* New York: Thomas Dunne/St. Martin's, 2007.

Finder, Chuck. *The Steelers Encyclopedia.* Philadelphia: Temple University Press, 2012.

Gay, Timothy J. *Football Physics: The Science of the Game.* Emmaus, PA: Rodale, 2004.

Greenfield, Susan. *The Human Brain: A Guided Tour.* New York: Basic, 1997 (Electronic).

Harris, David. *The League: The Rise and Decline of the NFL.* Toronto: Bantam, 1986.

Hoge, Merril, and Brent Cole. *Find a Way: Three Words That Changed My Life.* New York: Center Street, 2010.

Kramer, Jerry (with Dick Schaap). *Instant Replay: The Green Bay Diary of Jerry Kramer.* New York: New American Library, 1968.

Lazarus, Adam. *Best of Rivals: Joe Montana, Steve Young, and the Inside Story Behind the NFL's Greatest Quarterback Controversy.* Boston: Da Capo Press, 2012.

Levin, Harvey S., Howard M. Eisenberg, and Arthur L. Benton (eds.). *Mild Head Injury.* New York and Oxford: Oxford University Press, 1989.

Lewis, Michael. *The Blind Side: Evolution of a Game.* New York: W. W. Norton, 2006 (Electronic).

Lovell, Mark R., Ruben J. Echemendia, Jeffrey T. Barth, and Michael W. Collins (eds.). *Traumatic Brain Injury in Sports: An International Neuropsychological Perspective.* Lisse, The Netherlands: Swets & Zeitlinger, 2004.

Maroon, Joseph. *The Longevity Factor: How Resveratrol and Red Wine Activate Genes for a Longer and Healthier Life.* New York: Atria Books, 2009.

Millman, Chad, and Shawn Coyne. *The Ones Who Hit the Hardest: The Steelers, the Cowboys, the '70s, and the Fight for America's Soul.* New York: Gotham, 2010 (Electronic).

Muchnick, Irvin. *Duerson.* Berkeley, CA: Concussion Inc., 2011 (Electronic).

Muchnick, Irvin. *UMPC: Concussion Scandal Ground Zero.* Berkeley, CA: Concussion Inc., 2012 (Electronic).

National Football League Properties, Inc. *The First Fifty Years: A Celebration of the National Football League in Its Fiftieth Season.* New York: Simon and Schuster, 1969.

Nowinski, Christopher. *Head Games: Football's Concussion Crisis from the NFL to Youth Leagues.* East Bridgewater, MA: Drummond Publishing Group, 2007.

Omalu, Bennet. *Play Hard, Die Young: Football Dementia, Depression, and Death.* Lodi, CA: Neo-Forenxis, 2008.

Oriard, Michael. *Brand NFL: Making and Selling America's Favorite Sport.* Chapel Hill: University of North Carolina Press, 2007.

Oriard, Michael. *Reading Football: How the Popular Press Created an American Spectacle.* Chapel Hill: University of North Carolina Press, 1993.

Otto, Jim (with Dave Newhouse). *Jim Otto: The Pain of Glory.* Champaign, IL: Sports Publishing Inc., 2000.

Plimpton, George. *Paper Lion.* New York: Harper & Row, 1966.

Proctor, Robert. *Golden Holocaust: Origins of the Cigarette Catastrophe and the Case for Abolition.* Berkeley, CA: University of California, 2011.

Rooney, Art Jr. (with Roy McHugh). *Ruanaidh: The Story of Art Rooney and His Clan.* Pittsburgh, PA: Art Rooney Jr., 2008.

Russell, Andy. *An Odd Steelers Journey.* Champaign, IL: Sports Publishing Inc., 2002.

Solomon, Gary S., Karen M. Johnston, and Mark R. Lovell. *The Heads-Up on Sport Concussion.* Champaign, IL: Human Kinetics, 2006.

Tatum, Jack, and Bill Kushner. *They Call Me Assassin.* New York: Everett House, 1979.

Zegart, Dan. *Civil Warriors: The Legal Siege on the Tobacco Industry.* New York: Delacorte, 2000.

SCIENTIFIC ARTICLES

Barth, Jeffrey T., et al. "Mild Head Injury in Sports: Neuropsychological Sequelae and Recovery of Function." In *Mild Head Injury,* edited by Harvey S. Levin, Howard M. Eisenberg, and Arthur L. Benton, 256–275. New York: Oxford University Press, 1989.

Blaylock, Russell L., and Joseph Maroon. "Immunoexcitotoxicity as a Central Mechanism in Chronic Traumatic Encephalopathy—A Unifying Hypothesis." *Surgical Neurology International* 2 (July 30, 2011): 107.

Casson, Ira R. "Do the 'Facts' Really Support an Association Between NFL Players' Concussions, Dementia and Depression?" *Neurology Today,* June 3, 2010: 6–7.

Casson, Ira R., et al. "Neurological and CT Evaluation of Knocked-Out Boxers." *Journal of Neurology, Neurosurgery and Psychiatry* 45 (1982):170–174.

Casson, Ira R., Elliot J. Pellman, and David C. Viano. "Correspondence." *Neurosurgery* 58 (May 2006): E1003.

Casson, Ira R., Elliot J. Pellman, and David C. Viano. "Correspondence." *Neurosurgery* 59 (Nov. 2006): E1152.

Collins, Michael W., et al. "Relationship Between Concussion and Neuropsychological Performance in College Football Players." *Journal of the American Medical Association* 282 (Sept. 8, 1999): 964–970.

Collins, Micky, et al. "Examining Concussion Rates and Return to Play in High School Football Players Wearing Newer Helmet Technology: A Three-Year Prospective Cohort Study." *Neurosurgery* 58 (Feb. 2006): 275–285.

Corsellis, JA, et al. "The Aftermath of Boxing." *Psychological Medicine* (Aug. 3, 1973): 270–303.

Guskiewicz, Kevin M., et al. "Association Between Recurrent Concussion and Late-Life Cognitive Impairment in Retired Football Players." *Neurosurgery* 57 (Oct. 2005): 719–726.

Guskiewicz, Kevin M., et al. "Cumulative Effects Associated with Recurrent Concussion in Collegiate Football Players." *Journal of the American Medical Association* 290 (Nov. 19, 2003): 2549–2555.

Guskiewicz, Kevin M., et al. "Recurrent Concussion and Risk of Depression in Retired Professional Football Players." *Medicine & Science in Sports & Exercise* 39, no. 6 (2007): 903–909.

Hamberger, Anders, et al. "Concussion in Professional Football: Morphology of Brain Injuries in the NFL Concussion Model—Part 16." *Neurosurgery* 64 (June 2009): 1174–1182.

Hart, John Jr., et al. "Neuroimaging of Cognitive Dysfunction and Depression in Aging Retired National Football League Players." *JAMA Neurology* 70, no. 3 (March 2013): 326–335.

Lehman, Everett J., et al. "Neurodegenerative Causes of Death among Retired National Football League Players." *Neurology* 79 (Nov. 6, 2012): 1–6.

Martland, Harrison S. "Punch Drunk." *The Journal of the American Medical Association,* Vol. 91, 15 (Oct. 13, 1928): 1103–1107.

McCrea, Michael, et al. "Acute Effects and Recovery Time Following Concussion in Collegiate Football Players." *Journal of the American Medical Association* 290 (Nov. 19, 2003): 2556.

McKee, Ann C., et al. "Chronic Traumatic Encephalopathy in Athletes: Progressive Tauopathy Following Repetitive Head Injury." *Journal of Neuropathology and Experimental Neurology* 68 (July 2009): 709–735.

McKee, Ann C., et al. "The Spectrum of Disease in Chronic Traumatic Encephalopathy." *Brain,* Dec. 3, 2012: 1–22.

Omalu, Bennet I. "Chronic Traumatic Encephalopathy (CTE) in a National Football League Player: Case Report and Emerging Medicolegal Practice Questions." *Journal of Forensic Nursing* 6 (2010): 40–46.

Omalu, Bennet I. "Correspondence." *Neurosurgery* 58 (May 2006): E1003.

Omalu, Bennet I. "Emerging Histomorphologic Phenotypes of Chronic Traumatic Encephalopathy in American Athletes." *Journal of Forensic Nursing* 69 (July 2011): 173–183.

Omalu, Bennet I., et al. "Chronic Traumatic Encephalopathy in a National Football League Player." *Neurosurgery* 57 (July 2005): 128–134.

Omalu, Bennet I., et al. "Chronic Traumatic Encephalopathy in a National Football League Player—Part II." *Neurosurgery* 59 (Nov. 2006): 1086–1093.

Omalu, Bennet I., et al. "Chronic Traumatic Encephalopathy in a Professional American Wrestler." *Journal of Forensic Nursing* 6 (2010): 130–136.

Pellman, Elliot J., et al. "Concussion in Professional Football: Reconstruction of Game Impacts and Injuries." *Neurosurgery* 53 (Oct. 2003): 799–814.

Pellman, Elliot J., et al. "Concussion in Professional Football: Location and Direction of Helmet Impacts—Part 2." *Neurosurgery* 53 (Dec. 2003): 1328–1341.

Pellman, Elliot J., et al. "Concussion in Professional Football: Epidemiological Features of Game Injuries and Review of Literature—Part 3." *Neurosurgery* 54 (Jan. 2004): 81–96.

Pellman, Elliot J., et al. "Concussion in Professional Football: Repeat Injuries—Part 4." *Neurosurgery* 55 (Oct. 2004): 860–876.

Pellman, Elliot J., et al. "Concussion in Professional Football: Injuries Involving 7 or More Days Out—Part 5." *Neurosurgery* 55 (Nov. 2004): 1100–1119.

Pellman, Elliot J., et al. "Concussion in Professional Football: Neuropsychological Testing—Part 6." *Neurosurgery* 55 (Dec. 2004): 1290–1305.

Pellman, Elliot J., et al. "Concussion in Professional Football: Players Returning to the Same Game—Part 7." *Neurosurgery* 56 (Jan. 2005): 79–92.

Pellman, Elliot J., et al. "Concussion in Professional Football: Helmet Testing to Assess Impact Performance—Part 11." *Neurosurgery* 58 (Jan. 2006): 78–96.

Pellman, Elliot J., et al. "Concussion in Professional Football: Recovery of NFL and High School Athletes Assessed by Computerized Neuropsychological Testing—Part 12." *Neurosurgery* 58 (Feb. 2006): 263–274.

Small, Gary W., et al. "PET Scanning of Brain Tau in Retired National Football League Players: Preliminary Findings." *American Journal of Geriatric Psychiatry* 21 (Feb. 2013): 138–144.

Viano, David C., and Elliot J. Pellman. "Concussion in Professional Football: Biomechanics of the Striking Player—Part 8." *Neurosurgery* 56 (Feb. 2005): 266–280.

Viano, David C., et al. "Concussion in Professional Football: Brain Responses by Finite Element Analysis—Part 9." *Neurosurgery* 57 (Nov. 2005): 891–916.

Viano, David C., et al. "Concussion in Professional Football: Comparison with Boxing Head Impacts—Part 10." *Neurosurgery* 57 (Dec. 2005): 1154–1172.

Viano, David C., et al. "Concussion in Professional Football: Performance of Newer Helmets in Reconstructed Game Impacts—Part 13." *Neurosurgery* 59 (Sept. 2006): 591–606.

Viano, David C., Ira R. Casson, and Elliot J. Pellman. "Concussion in Professional Football: Biomechanics of the Struck Player—Part 14." *Neurosurgery* 61 (Aug. 2007): 313–328.

Viano, David C., et al. "Concussion in Professional Football: Animal Model of Brain Injury—Part 15." *Neurosurgery* 64 (June 2009): 1162–1173.

Weir, David R., James S. Jackson, and Amanda Sonnega. "Study of Retired NFL Players." *University of Michigan Institute for Social Research,* Sept. 10, 2009: 1–37.

PHOTO INSERT CREDITS

INDEX

Aiello, Greg, 74, 215, 277, 284–85
Aikman, Troy, 71, 76–78, 79, 82, 117, 125, 167, 283
Ali, Muhammad, 71, 216
Allegheny General Hospital, 31, 35, 37, 44, 63, 67
Alzheimer's disease, 158, 192, 235, 255, 259, 267, 268, 277, 312
    see also dementia
Amen Clinics, 310, 351
American Academy of Neurology, 32, 68–69
American Association of Neurological Surgeons, 205, 234
American College of Sports Medicine, 141
American Orthopaedic Society for Sports Medicine, 136
Anapol Schwartz PC, 309
Anderson, Dave, 73
Appleton, Wisc., 255–56
Apuzzo, Michael L. J., 139–40, 172
    at Concussion Summit, 219–21, 226–27
    as Neurosurgery editor, 139, 140, 141–43, 146, 172–73, 180–82, 188, 189, 197, 226, 291
    as NY Giants consultant, 139–40, 220, 227
Arfken, Cynthia, 210–11
Atlanta Falcons, 177
Atwater, Steve, 40

Bailes, Colleen, 235
Bailes, Julian, 67–68, 81, 82, 116, 117, 119, 126, 144, 150, 174,
    203, 207, 233–34, 261, 262–63, 266, 277, 293, 336, 344
    concussion prevention devices developed by, 311–12
    at Concussion Summit, 1–2, 219, 220, 224–25, 272
    Guskiewicz and, 113, 114–15
    long-term brain damage studied by, 67–69, 113, 114, 146, 198, 202
    MTBI papers reviewed by, 146, 175
    Omalu and, 197–98, 205, 234–35
    and Seau's brain autopsy, 324–25, 330
    SLI and, 232, 234, 252–54
Barr, Bill, 128, 140, 175, 207, 312
    Collins's confrontation with, 223–24
    at Concussion Summit, 219, 220, 221
    Lovell attacked by, 221–22, 223
    MTBI papers criticized by, 176–78, 221
    Pellman and, 175–76, 178, 179–80
Barr, John, 129
Barth, Jeff, 33–35, 37, 38, 66, 67, 114, 126, 128, 159
Bartkowski, Steve, 75–76
baseball, 5, 127, 239
Batjer, Hunt, 288–90, 304
Baxter, Fred, 177
Belichick, Bill, 14, 214, 259
Bell, Todd, 299–300
Benoit, Chris, 249, 250
Benson, Dick, 278
Benson, Will, 278
Berbick, Trevor, 216
Berg, Peter, 323
Berger, Mitch, 286, 302–4

Berko, Arty, 250
Berlin, Ralph, 21, 113–14
Bert Bell/Pete Rozelle NFL Player
    Retirement Plan, 86–87, 91,
    272–73, 294
  benefits for long-term brain damage
    granted by, 168–70
  Webster lawsuit against, 101, 105,
    168–70, 192
  and Webster's disability claim,
    98–101, 168
beta-amyloid plaques, 158, 259, 268
Bettman, Gary, 74
Biokinetics, 143, 184
Biologic Effects of Tobacco, The
    (Wynder), 280
Blackledge, Ron, 27
Bleier, Rocky, 22, 25, 40, 96
Blount, Mel, 96, 104
Bonds, Barry, 127
Boston City Hospital, 341
Boston Globe, 213
Boston University School of Medicine,
    253, 254, 255, 257, 264
  see also BU Group
boxers, 216
  Parkinson's disease in, 159
  Punch-Drunk Syndrome in, 89, 90,
    97, 110, 158–59, 161, 190, 191,
    192, 197, 257, 259, 268, 302
Boyd, Brent, 87, 243–45, 280
Bradshaw, Terry, 3, 4, 23, 25, 67, 104,
    347
  at Webster's Hall of Fame induction,
    58–60, 62
Brady, Kyle, 129, 130, 177
Brady, Tom, 307
brain, anatomy of, 32–33
brain damage, long-term, 6, 117–18
  Bailes's and Jordan's research on,
    67–69, 113, 114, 146
  Casson's denial of, 215–18, 219,
    225
  MTBI Committee's denial of,

145–47, 167–68, 170, 174–75,
    198, 210, 234, 239, 269–71
  NFL's acknowledgment of, 284–85,
    290
  NFL's ignoring of evidence on, 2,
    280
  Webster as advocate for issue of,
    94–95
  see also chronic traumatic
    encephalopathy (CTE);
    concussions, sports-related
Brain Injury Association of America,
    102
Brain Injury Research Institute,
    261–62
  see also Omalu Group
Brain-Pad, 315–16, 317
Brain Surgery (Apuzzo), 139
Brees, Drew, 307
Brister, Bubby, 31, 35, 40, 347–48
Brooks, Michael, 70
Brown, et al. v. N.F.L., 273
Brown, Hardy, 135, 364n
Brown, Jerome, 40
Brown, Orlando, 273
Bryant, Waymond, 20
BU Group, 253–54, 330, 343
  brain bank of, 259, 284, 287, 301,
    303, 304, 305
  competition between Omalu group
    and, 261–62, 290–91
  NFL concussion committee's
    disparagement of, 301, 302–3, 304
  NFL's donation to, 283–84, 287, 301
  and Seau's brain autopsy, 332–33,
    335–36
  Super Bowl press conference of,
    263–65
Butkus, Dick, 5

Caddick, Christine, 73
Caito, Fred, 42
California, workers' compensation
    cases in, 306, 307

California Superior Court, 309
Campbell, Earl, 168
Cantu, Bob, 136–37, 140–41, 174, 198, 203, 207, 217, 250–51, 291, 292, 302, 303–4, 347
   concussion guidelines of, 141–42
   at Concussion Summit, 219, 221, 222
   helmet study paper attacked by, 186–87
   Johnson's incipient dementia diagnosis by, 214
   as *Neurosurgery* sports section editor, 140, 142, 143, 146–47, 171–74, 175, 180, 186–87
   NFL donation and, 284, 287
   Nowinski and, 200–201, 254
   on SLI board, 232, 252
Captain for Life (Carson), 208
Carson, Harry, 25, 63–64, 73, 209–10, 347
   on backlash against Omalu, 293
   and Webster's death, 207–9
Casson, Ira, 126, 128, 171, 210, 234, 270–71, 277, 278, 279
   boxing brain damage study of, 70–71, 216
   brain damage evidence denied by, 215–18, 219, 225
   at Concussion Summit, 2, 221, 224
   Goldberg's interview of, 217–18
   Guskiewicz's research attacked by, 217
   McKee's findings attacked by, 268–69, 270
   as MTBI Committee cochair, 215, 235–36, 237, 238, 239, 266, 286
   Omalu's research attacked by, 189–92, 215, 335
   resignation of, 283, 286
CBS, 75, 322–23
Center for the Study of Retired Athletes, 226, 336, 344, 346
Center for the Study of Traumatic Encephalopathy, *see* BU Group

Chaney, Matt, 344
Chao, David, 331, 334, 335–36
Chicago Bears, 20, 41–43, 118–22, 132, 177, 178, 296, 309–10
Chrebet, Wayne, 130
chronic traumatic encephalopathy (CTE), 7–8, 163, 190–91, 194–96, 197, 205, 257, 259, 261–64, 266, 272, 300, 311, 312
   Bailes's Concussion Summit presentation on, 224–25
   SLI Super Bowl press conference on, 263–65
   steroid use and, 238–39
   subconcussive blows as possible cause of, 302
   tau protein buildup in, 224, 225, 236, 267, 268
   see also brain damage, long-term; concussions, sports-related
"Chronic Traumatic Encephalopathy in a National Football League Player" (Omalu et al.), 163–65, 188–92, 202, 215, 257
Chrostowski, Leszek, 201–2
Civil Warriors (Zegart), 281, 341, 342
Cleveland Browns, 168, 177
Cobb, Randall "Tex," 216
Coben, Larry, 309–10
Cohen, Will, 283
Colangelo, Ron, 128
Cole, Robin, 16
collective bargaining agreement (CBA), 272–73
Collins, Michael "Micky," 64–65, 69, 159, 175, 183, 215, 226, 292–93, 313
   Barr confronted by, 223–24
   brain research of, 65–66, 137
   helmet study of, 184–87, 211, 315, 369*n*–370*n*
   ImPACT and, 113, 183
   Lovell as mentor to, 66–67
Colucci, Anthony, 281

concussion, definitions of, 32, 115, 132
concussions, sports-related:
  Barth's research on, 33–35, 37, 38
  depression and, 116, 117
  early dementia and, 116, 144, 145
  fans' growing awareness of, 69–70, 71–72, 125
  guidelines for, 31–32, 35–36, 37–38, 141–43
  Guskiewicz's research on, 114–18
  lack of research on, 32, 78
  Lovell and Maroon's test for, *see* ImPACT; Pittsburgh Steelers Test Battery
  medical entrepreneurs and, 310–14
  NFL's downplaying of, 74–75, 82, 144–45
  1996 conference on, 63–65
  physics of, 138
  seriousness of, as underplayed, 32–33
  Steinberg and, 77–79, 80–82, 110, 125
  see also brain damage, long-term; chronic traumatic encephalopathy (CTE)
Concussion Summit, 1–2, 218–28, 229, 234, 254, 266, 272
Congress, U.S., 7, 87, 216, 242
  see also House of Representatives, U.S.; Senate Commerce Committee
Congress of Neurological Surgeons, 139
Conyers, John, 278–79
Corcoran, John, 199
Corsellis, J. A. N. "Nick," 159, 192
Council for Tobacco Research, 281
Courson, Steve, 22, 23, 85
Crabb, Barbara B., 369*n*–370*n*
Creutzfeldt-Jakob disease, 332
Crossman, Matt, 323
Crowe, Cameron, 76
Culp, Curley, 25

Culverhouse, Gay, 278
Curinga, Lou, 21

D'Alessandro, David, 262
D'Amico, Carmen, 149, 156–57
Davies, Peter, 235–39, 259, 267, 269, 317
Davis, Joe, 333, 334
Deese, Derrick, 108
Defense and Veterans Brain Injury Center, 268
DeKosky, Steve, 161–64, 189, 191–92, 196–98, 205, 209–10, 257, 259
Delsohn, Steve, 251, 310
dementia, 116, 144, 145, 198, 214–15, 232, 233, 243, 308
  see also Alzheimer's disease; brain damage, long-term; chronic traumatic encephalopathy (CTE); Punch-Drunk Syndrome
DeNoble, Victor, 281
Denver Broncos, 70, 110
Dissenters, 174, 180, 181, 187, 198, 203, 207, 218, 219, 254, 287, 335, 343
Dominick, Joe, 148–49, 155
Dotsch, Rollie, 14
Duerson, Alicia, 294, 296–99, 300, 304
Duerson, Dave:
  Alicia assaulted by, 298
  background of, 295–96
  business career of, 297–99
  concussions of, 294–95, 296
  CTE diagnosed in, 7, 304–5
  as desiring to donate brain to research, 295, 300, 304
  mental problems of, 297–98
  NFL concussion policy defended by, 244–45, 294
  on NFL disability board, 294, 299
  as player representative, 244, 296–97
  suicide of, 7, 293–95, 300, 305

Duerson, Tregg, 294, 299, 300–301, 304
Duper, Mark, 308

Easterling, Ray, 310
Ellenbogen, Richard, 288–90, 304, 314
Elway, John, 110
ESPN, 70, 109, 118, 204, 207, 249–50,
    311, 322, 347
  authors' investigation supported by,
    4, 8–9
  market research of, 4–5
  NFL contract of, 4, 8, 73
  SLI story of, 249–50, 251
  Webster story of, 57
Esposito, Lorraine, 321

Facenda, John, 319–20
False Glory: Steelers and Steroids
    (Courson), 22
Federal Trade Commission (FTC), 6,
    315, 317–18
Feenberg, Ron, 306–7
Feuer, Hank, 126, 133, 170–71,
    210–11, 269, 277, 288
Finder, Chuck, 194
First Fifty Years, The (NFL), 318–19
Fitzsimmons, Bob, 261, 262, 337
  in NFL lawsuit, 101, 105, 168–70
  Omalu's call to, 105
  SLI and, 232, 252–54
  Webster's disability case and, 87–92,
    98–101
  Webster's friendship with, 89, 92, 94,
    96, 105
Fogel, Robert, 119, 120, 121, 122
football:
  brain damage caused by, see brain
    damage, long-term; chronic
    traumatic encephalopathy (CTE);
    concussions, sports-related
  Hoge's defense of, 347
  inherent brutality in, 5–6, 39, 134
  U.S. obsession with, 5, 345–46
football, high school and college,

  concussions in, 97, 114, 141, 181,
    183, 185–86, 210, 211, 264, 278
football, Pee Wee and middle school,
    concussions in, 211, 283, 288
Football Physics (Gay), 72
football players, retired, 198
  brains of, as scientific commodities,
    7, 8
  dementia in, 144, 145, 243, 308
  Guskiewicz's surveys and, 115–17
  health insurance problems of, 68
  in negligence lawsuits, 7, 241–42,
    272–76, 307, 308–9, 347–49
  neurological problems of, 68–69
  suicides by, 7, 193–94, 201, 204, 249,
    293–95, 310, 324–25, 329–30
  see also individual players
forensic pathology, 154–55, 160
Fox Network, 75
Framingham Heart Study, 255, 259
Frenk, Julio, 349
Frontline, 184, 341

Garber, Greg, 70, 73, 109, 204
Garcia, Jeff, 110
Gaunt, Sarah E., 99–100
Gay, Tim, 5, 72–73
Giordani, Bruno, 34
Girardi, Tom, 276, 309
Goldberg, Bernard, 217–18
Goldberg, Persky & White, 272,
    274–75
Golden Holocaust (Proctor), 341
Goodell, Charles, 219
Goodell, Roger, 220, 221, 228, 240,
    322, 344, 349
  Casson and Viano resignation to,
    283, 286
  Concussion Summit and, 1, 218–19,
    272
  Judiciary hearing testimony of,
    278–80
Gordon, Joe, 55, 61, 91, 104
Graff, Clare, 321

Gray, Mel, 323
Green, Darrell, 324
Green Bay Packers, 7, 255, 257
Greene, Joe, 14–15
Grimsley, John, 258–59, 285
Grimsley, Virginia, 258, 285
Grossman, Randy, 96
Grunhard, Tim, 28–29, 51
Guskiewicz, Kevin, 137, 159, 174, 175,
    203–4, 207, 227–28, 274, 313, 336
  on backlash against Omalu, 292
  Bailes and, 113, 114–15
  brain damage research of, 114–18,
    130–31, 145, 146, 198, 202
  causal relationship between
    concussions and CTE questioned
    by, 343–44, 346
  at Concussion Summit, 218, 219,
    220, 226, 272
  health surveys of, 115–17
  MacArthur "genius grant" of, 113,
    287, 344
  MTBI papers reviewed by, 146–47,
    171–72, 175, 180–81
  NFL attack on research of, 170–71,
    217, 366n–367n
  on NFL concussion committee,
    287–88, 336, 343–47

Halas, George, 135
Halberstam, David, 74–75, 87
Haley, Dick, 20–21
Hallenbeck, Scott, 321
Hall of Fame Players Association, 162
Ham, Jack, 15
Hamilton, Ronald, 159–62, 163, 164,
    189, 191–92, 194, 196–98, 205,
    234, 259
Hampton, Rodney, 308
Hardy, David, 342
Harris, Franco, 104
Harrison, James, 350
Harvard Brain Tissue Resource Center,
    231

Harvard Project, 341–43
Harvard School of Public Health, 349
Haynes, Mike, 58
HBO, 266, 279
*Head Games: Football's Concussion
    Crisis* (Nowinski), 201, 232, 280
helmet design, 6, 134–36, 315, 317,
    369n–370n
  MTBI Committee and, 134, 136–
    38, 142–43, 184–87, 211–12
  NOCSAE standards for, 143–44
  see also Riddell
Hester, Devin, 323
Hicks, Paul, 323
Himmelhoch, Jonathan, 90, 96, 97
Hoffman, Bette, 326, 327, 328, 330
Hoge, Merril, 27–28, 39–41, 63, 73,
    97, 117, 171, 178, 312
  concussions of, 40–45, 64–65, 71,
    118–22
  concussion test and, 39, 44, 65
  football defended by, 347
  Munsell sued by, 118–22, 125,
    128–29, 132–34
  retirement of, 45, 63, 79, 109, 125,
    189
House of Representatives, U.S.:
  Committee on Government Reform
    of, 127
  Judiciary Committee football
    hearings of, 277–83, 287, 289–90
Hovda, David, 141
Huber, Gary, 341–43
Huff, Sam, 244–45

Ide, Thad, 185
Ilkin, Tunch, 23, 27, 40
ImPACT (Immediate Post-Concussion
    Assessment and Cognitive
    Testing), 38–39, 44, 67–68, 97,
    112–13, 174, 182–83, 194, 215,
    223, 317, 348
  financial success of, 312–13, 314
  helmet study and, 185, 369n–370n

Jaffee, Col. Michael, 268–69, 270

Jani, Sunny, 51–54, 57–58, 85, 88, 94, 95, 103–4

Jerry Maguire (film), 76, 79

Johnson, Billy "White Shoes," 168

Johnson, Keyshawn, 177

Johnson, Ted, 213–14, 218, 259–60, 263

Jolly, Tom, 203

Jones, Barbara, 232

Jordan, Barry, 68–69, 82, 126, 144, 146

Journal of Forensic Nursing, The, 291

Journal of Neurology, Neurosurgery, and Psychiatry, 216

Journal of the American Medical Association (JAMA), 65–66, 69, 164, 175

Joyner, Seth, 40

Junior Seau Foundation, 326, 328

Kansas City Chiefs, 28–29, 50–51

Keating, Peter, 128, 176, 204, 207

Kelly, Charles, 89–90, 94–95, 96, 97, 103

Kelso, Mark, 63

Kent State University, 14, 15

Kentucky, University of, 342

Kim, Duk Koo, 216

Kinetic energy, 72–73

King, Peter, 332–33

Klint, Jim, 109

Kolb, Jon, 14, 16, 21, 23, 26

Krieg, Fred, 89, 96, 97

Kutcher, Jeffrey, 316

Lambert, Jack, 2, 14, 15–16, 20, 67

Lane, Dick "Night Train," 136

Larry King Live, 250–51

Laskas, Jeanne Marie, 291

Lavin, Shelly, 297

Lawrence University, 256, 259

Lewis, Ray, 323

Lewy bodies, 159–60

Livingston, Bill, 73

Lloyd, Greg, 64

Lombardi, Vince, 13, 138

Long, Terry, 193–96, 233

Longevity Factor, The (Maroon), 36, 317

Long Island Jewish Medical Center, 128, 235

Lonser, Russ, 336, 338

Lorenz, Konrad, 319

Lovell, Mark, 35, 36, 37–38, 64, 65, 80, 82, 200, 215, 217, 221–22, 292, 313

    Barr's attack on, 221–22, 223

    brain damage research of, 126, 128, 137, 178, 182

    Collins mentored by, 66–67

    in helmet study, 185, 211, 315, 369n

    in Hoge lawsuit, 119, 125, 132, 178

    ImPACT and, 38–39, 44, 67–68, 97, 112–13, 174, 182–83, 312–13

    on MTBI committee, 125–26, 131, 137, 174–75, 178–79, 185, 313

    MTBI papers coauthored by, 175, 178–79, 182

    as NFL Neuropsychology Program head, 132, 174–75, 176–77, 183

Luckasevic, Jason:

    NFL lawsuit of, 241–42, 272–76, 307, 308–9, 347

    Omalu's friendship with, 240–42, 272, 308–9

Lynch, Ben, 80

MacArthur Foundation, 113, 287, 344

McCoy, Colt, 350

McDuffie, O. J., 275

McHale, Lisa, 261, 262, 263, 264

McHale, Tom, 261–65

McKee, Ann, 7–8, 257, 284, 301–2, 303, 304, 305, 323, 336, 346

    background of, 255–57

    at BU Group Super Bowl press conference, 264–65

McKee, Ann *(continued)*:
    Grimsley's brain autopsied by,
        258–59
    Judiciary Committee testimony of,
        282–83
    McHale's brain autopsied by, 263
    MTBI presentation of, 266–71
    on subconcussive blows as cause of
        CTE, 302
McKee, Chuck, 256, 259, 271
Mackey, John, 214–15, 218
Mackey, Sylvia, 215
McLuhan, Marshall, 318
McMahon, Jim, 106, 309–10
MacMullan, Jackie, 213
McNeill, Fred, 307, 310, 312
McNeill, Gavin, 308
McShane, John, 133–34
Makris, Billy, 18–19
Malanga, Gerard, 211
Mancini, Ray, 216
Mann, John, 267, 269, 270–71
Mansfield, Ray, 21
Mara, Wellington, 58
Marion, Donald, 189
Mariucci, Steve, 108, 109
Marks, Stanley, 55
Maroon, Charles, 36
Maroon, Joe, 31–32, 35, 63, 64, 66–67,
        74, 114, 126, 171, 178, 180, 205,
        224, 235, 316
    concussion testing and, 37–39
    entrepreneurship of, 35–37
    helmet study and, 315, 317
    Hoge and, 43–46, 119
    ImPACT and, 38–39, 44, 67–68, 97,
        113, 182–83, 194, 312, 317
    on implications of Omalu's findings,
        205–6, 314, 321
    Long autopsy results rebutted by,
        195–96
    on MTBI Committee, 215, 236
    Omalu's evidence examined by,
        205–6, 236, 237

    as Steelers' neurological consultant,
        31–32, 35, 37–39, 67
    Webster's CTE diagnosis questioned
        by, 97–98
Marshall, Wilber, 71, 72
Martland, Harrison, 158–59, 191
Massachusetts General Hospital,
        231
Matson, Ollie, 323
Matthew Gfeller Sport-Related
        Traumatic Brain Injury Research
        Center, 344
Mawae, Kevin, 129–30, 349
Michigan, University of, 277
Miller, Chris, 71
Miller, Jeff, 277, 278
Mitchell, Dorothy C., 133
Mix, Ron, 162
Monday Night Football, 4, 322
Montana, Joe, 107
Moon, Warren, 78, 79
Moore, Bob, 50
Morgan, Gerry, 135
Muchnick, Irvin, 245
Mudd, Howard, 318
Mullins, Gerry, 26
Munsell, John, 42, 119
    Hoge's lawsuit against, 118–22,
        125, 128–29, 132–34
Musick, Phil, 15, 16

National Football League (NFL):
    acknowledgment of brain damage
        link by, 284–85, 290
    Alzheimer's study commissioned by,
        276–77
    brain damage evidence ignored by,
        2, 271–72, 273, 276, 280
    brain-injury claims rejected by, 87
    BU Group donation of, 283–84,
        287, 301
    collective bargaining agreement of
        (CBA) of, 272–73
    concussion crisis downplayed by,

74–75, 82, 144–45, 166–68, 174,
197, 322
concussion policy changes of, 283
Concussion Summit of, *see* Concussion Summit
congressional hearings on, 242–44,
277–83, 287, 289–90, 294
disability plan of, *see* Bert Bell/Pete
Rozelle NFL Player Retirement
Plan
88 Plan of, 214–15, 218, 243, 276
ESPN's contract with, 4, 8, 73
Hoge's lawsuit and, 121–22
Luckasevic lawsuit against, 241–42,
272–76, 306–10, 347
mass tort lawsuit against, 7, 100,
347–48
mommy bloggers campaign of,
321–22
neuropsychological testing mandate
of, 215, 276, 350
NIH donation of, 337
1994 "Season of the concussion" in,
71, 201, 347
players' increased size and ability in,
71–72
research spending by, 346–47
safety campaign of, 322–23
Seau's brain autopsy and, 8, 334,
335–36, 343
steroid ban in, 22
three-day symposium staged by,
349–50
tobacco industry compared to, 6–7,
244, 280–83
wealth and power of, 5, 6, 89, 130,
197, 219, 280
National Heart Institute, 255
National Hockey League (NHL), 183
National Institute for Occupational
Safety and Health (NIOSH), 349
National Institutes of Health (NIH),
304
NFL donation to, 337

Seau's brain autopsy and, 336, 337,
343
National Operating Committee on
Standards for Athletic Equipment
(NOCSAE), 143–44
Naugle, Rick, 177–78
Nelson, Craig, 332, 333, 334
Nelson, Steve, 308
Neurology Today, 217
Neurosurgery, 139, 140, 172–73, 226,
291
MTBI papers published in, 142–47,
164, 166–67, 170, 171–72,
174–75, 176, 177, 179, 180–81,
220, 276, 289
Omalu papers published in, 164–65,
188, 189, 197
peer-review process at, 146–47,
171–72, 181–82
Riddell helmet study published in,
185–86
Newhouse, Dave, 351
New York Giants, 6, 130, 139–40, 220,
227
New York Jets, 70, 128, 129–30, 131,
145, 175–76, 180
New York State Athletic Commission, 68
New York Times, 8, 73, 127–28, 176–77,
203, 204, 254, 259, 264, 283, 321
Johnson story in, 213
MTBI stories in, 210–11
NFL brain damage acknowledgment
story in, 284–85
Strzelczyk story in, 234
Waters story in, 204, 207, 210, 229
New York University Medical Center,
175, 180
NFLevolution.com, 323
NFL Films, 319–20
NFL Hall of Fame, 3, 56–62, 83, 162
NFL Head, Neck and Spine Committee (concussion committee),
286–90, 301, 302–3, 304,
335–36, 337, 343–47

NFL Mild Brain Injury Surveillance
    Study, 132, 139, 144
NFL Mild Traumatic Brain Injury
    (MTBI) Committee, 75, 79, 122,
    126, 130, 159, 203–4, 227, 237,
    238, 260, 272, 276, 286
  conclusions published by, 6, 145–47,
    167–68, 170, 171–72, 174–75,
    221, 227
  concussion as defined by, 132
  in demand for retraction of Omalu
    paper, 189–92, 196–98
  Guskiewicz's research attacked by,
    170–71
  helmet design and, 134, 136–38,
    142–43, 184–87, 211–12
  long-term brain damage denied by,
    145–47, 167–68, 170, 174–75,
    198, 210, 234, 239, 269–71
  Lovell and, 125–26
  NFL Neuropsychology Program data
    and, 175, 221
  research studies by, 132, 138–39,
    142–47, 164, 166–67, 171–72,
    174–75, 176–81, 220, 276, 289
NFL Neuropsychology Program,
    174–75, 183, 221
NFL Players Association, 38, 68, 115,
    244, 284, 290, 292, 300
NFL Retired Players Association, 116
Noderer, Megan, 329
Nolan, Mary, 328
Noll, Chuck, 13, 14, 20, 26, 28, 29, 38,
    39, 41, 104, 193, 194, 314
  concussion guidelines questioned by,
    31–32, 35, 36, 38
Noll, Marianne, 104–5
North Carolina, University of (UNC),
    114, 226, 344
  Center for the Study of Retired
    Athletes at, 115, 202, 344, 346
Nowinski, Chris, 201, 202–3, 204,
    207, 213, 233, 249, 254, 257, 260,
    280, 285, 292, 304

  advocacy role of, 198, 201, 229, 230,
    263
  background of, 198–200, 204
  as brain hunter, 201–2, 231, 233–34,
    257–58, 304, 330
  and BU Group Super Bowl press
    conference, 263, 264
  concussions of, 198, 200–201
  Duerson's brain and, 301
  Judiciary Committee testimony of,
    282
  Luckasevic lawsuit and, 274
  McHale brain autopsy and, 262–63
  at McKee's MTBI presentation,
    266–67, 268, 271
  and NFL's donation to BU Group,
    284
  Omalu Group's break with, 252–54,
    291
  Omalu's relationship with, 198,
    201, 202, 229–32, 234, 249–50,
    251–52
  and Seau's brain autopsy, 333,
    335–36
  SLI founded by Omalu and, 230–32,
    234
Numbers Game, The (Schwarz), 203

Oakland Raiders, 5, 350
Omalu, Bennet, 150–51, 156–57, 198,
    205, 207, 234–35, 257, 259, 260,
    290–91, 312, 338
  background of, 9, 153–54
  backlash against, 291–93
  Bailes and, 197–98, 205
  in break with SLI, 252–54
  in call to Fitzsimmons, 105
  in conversations with the dead, 9, 152
  Davies and, 236–37
  as excluded from Concussion
    Summit, 220, 229
  Hamilton as mentor to, 159–60
  intellect of, 149, 150, 162
  Long's CTE diagnosed by, 194–96

Luckasevic's friendship with, 240–42, 272, 308–9

McHale's brain autopsied by, 262, 264

Maroon and, 205–6

NFL's attacks on, 227, 240–41, 259, 272, 292–93, 333, 335

Nowinski's relationship with, 198, 201, 202, 229–30, 249–50, 251–52

personal belief system of, 149–50

personality of, 149, 150, 160, 162, 291–92

Players Association presentation of, 292

in response to MTBI retraction demand, 189–92, 196–98

and Seau's brain autopsy, 324–25, 330–35

SLI founded by Nowinski and, 230–32, 234

at Steinberg seminar, 232–33

Waters's CTE diagnosed by, 203, 213, 291

Webster autopsied by, 4, 5, 9–10, 151–53, 155–56, 157–58, 159, 194, 207

Wecht as mentor to, 154–55, 164, 260

Omalu, John, 153

Omalu Group, 252–54, 261, 264
    competition between BU Group and, 261–62

On Aggression (Lorenz), 319

Oriard, Michael, 5, 320

Otto, Jim, 350–52

Otto, Sally, 351

Pacheco, Mark, 216

Pain of Glory, The (Jim Otto), 351

Parcells, Bill, 129, 145, 208

Parkinson's disease, 159–60

Parrish, Bernie, 244–45, 287

Pash, Jeff, 133, 228, 287, 344

Paterno, Joe, 31

Payton, Connie, 300

Peete, Holly Robinson, 321

Peete, Rodney, 321

Pellman, Elliot, 129–30, 132–33, 145, 226, 266, 276, 345

Barr and, 175–76, 178, 179–80, 221–22

in demand for Omalu paper retraction, 189–92

embellished credentials of, 127–28, 129, 176–77

helmet design project of, 136, 137, 184–87

in Hoge lawsuit, 122, 125, 128–29, 134

as ignorant of brain injury research, 128–29

as lead author on MTBI papers, 142–45, 166–67, 174, 177, 179, 181

Long autopsy results rebutted by, 196

McKee's findings attacked by, 269

as MTBI Committee chairman, 127, 130, 131–32, 137, 142, 144, 174, 181, 204, 270, 286

Omalu attacked by, 227, 335

removed as MTBI Committee chairman, 215

as rheumatologist, 127, 128, 131, 137, 144, 191

Perfetto, Eleanor, 302

Perl, Daniel, 267, 269–70, 271

Perles, George, 14

Perrin, Dave, 114

Peterson, Carl, 50, 93

Pieroth, Elizabeth, 321, 322

Pittsburgh, University of, 34–35
    Medical Center at, see University of Pittsburgh Medical Center

Pittsburgh *Post-Gazette,* 36, 61, 97, 194, 195

Pittsburgh Steelers, 1, 2, 20, 21, 23, 55, 112–14, 130, 193
    concussion testing and, 38–39

Pittsburgh Steelers *(continued):*
full-contact practices of, 26, 41
Maroon as neurological consultant to, 31–32, 35, 37–39, 67
Nutcracker drill of, 13–16
Webster released by, 28
Webster's growing hatred of, 90–91, 104
Pittsburgh Steelers Test Battery, 65, 67–68, 97, 112
see also ImPACT
Plummer, Gary, 79–81, 107, 108, 111, 117, 325, 337–38
Powell, John, 126
Pro Bowl, 24
Proctor, Robert, 341
ProHEALTH Care Associates, 129
Prusiner, Stanley, 332, 333, 334, 335
Punch-Drunk Syndrome (dementia pugilistica), 89, 90, 97, 110, 158–59, 161, 190, 191, 192, 197, 257, 259, 268, 302

Quarry, Jerry, 216

Randolph, Chris, 177–78, 312
Ratzan, Stuart, 275
Reger, John, 320
"Relationship between Concussion and Neuropsychological Performance in College Football Players" (Collins), 65–66
Rice, Harold, 297
Riddell, 135, 184–85, 223
false and misleading claims of, 6, 211–12, 315, 316
FTC investigation of, 315, 317–18
retired players' suit against, 7
Revolution helmet of, 184–86, 187, 211–12, 315, 317, 369*n*–370*n*
UPMC helmet study funded by, 184–86, 316, 317–18
Ritalin, 3, 55, 60, 83, 86, 89, 94, 95–97, 98

Rodriguez, Amanda, 322
Rooney, Art, Jr., 14, 15, 20–21
Rooney, Art, Sr., 61, 114
Rooney, Dan, 38, 55, 61, 91, 104
Rozelle, Pete, 219, 310, 319
Russell, Andy, 15, 320
Russomanno, Herman, 275–76, 309

Sabol, Ed and Steve, 319
Sanchez, Linda, 279–80, 289
San Diego Chargers, 325–26
San Francisco 49ers, 107–8
Sapp, Warren, 107–8
Sarmiento, Kelly, 322
Savran, Stan, 14
Schickendantz, Mark, 349–50
Schottenheimer, Marty, 28–29, 50
Schulten, Katherine, 283
Schutt, 212, 369*n*–370*n*
Schwarz, Alan, 213, 215, 226, 227, 234, 260, 264, 276, 283–84
MTBI stories by, 210–11
Nowinski and, 203, 254
Waters story by, 204, 207, 210
Seau, Gina, 326–27, 328, 333, 337, 338
Seau, Jake, 327, 339
Seau, Junior:
autopsy of, 7, 324–25, 330–35, 343
CTE diagnosed in, 7, 338–39, 348
personality change of, 327–28, 338
suicide of, 7, 324–25, 329–30, 338
Seau, Sydney, 327, 328–29
Seau, Tyler, 7, 327, 330–31, 332, 339
second impact syndrome, 141
Seifert, George, 107
Senate Commerce Committee, 315
NFL retirement system hearing of (2007), 242–44, 277, 294
sports equipment hearings of (2011), 316–17
Shakir, Abdulrazak, 155, 194
Shanahan, Mike, 110
Shankman, Sabrina, 184
Shell, Donnie, 41

Shula, Don, 58–59

Skipper, John, 8

Small, Gary, 312

Smith, Cy, 168

Smith, DeMaurice, 331

Sports Brain Guard, 316–17

Sports Illustrated, 75, 128, 216, 255, 319

Sports Legacy Institute (SLI), 230–32, 234, 250, 259, 274

  brain samples acquired by, 202, 231, 233–34, 249, 257–58

  BU affiliation with, 253, 254–55

  disharmony in, 251–54

  ESPN's piece on, 249–50, 251

  see also BU Group

Stage, Bob, 24, 27, 47–48, 58, 61, 103

Stallworth, John, 20

Stautner, Ernie, 318

Steinberg, Gary, 109

Steinberg, Leigh, 75–77, 118, 207

  concussion crisis seminars of, 78–79, 80–82, 106, 110, 125, 178, 232–33

Stern, Bob, 218–19, 254–55, 283, 284

Stern, David, 74

steroids, 22, 127, 193, 238–39

Stingley, Darryl, 73

Strzelczyk, Justin, 233–34, 295

suicides, 7, 193–94, 201, 202, 204, 249, 293–95, 310, 324–25, 329–30

Sullivan, Gerry, 168–69, 366*n*

Swann, Lynn, 20, 63, 104

Tagliabue, Paul, 62, 79, 87, 125, 132–33, 210, 215, 218–19, 240, 286

  Apuzzo and, 140, 172

  concussion crisis downplayed by, 74–75, 144

  Pellman and, 127, 128, 131

  statement to ESPN, 131

Tamarkin, Eric, 278

Tatum, Jack, 296

tau protein, 157–58, 224, 225, 235, 255, 256–57, 258–59, 265, 267, 268, 312, 338

Taylor, Lawrence, 71–72

Team Webster, 53, 57, 60, 83, 85, 86, 88, 96, 98, 337

Ted Johnson Rule, 215

Testaverde, Vinny, 71, 73

They Call It Pro Football (film), 319–20

They Call Me Assassin (Tatum), 296

Thomas, Derrick, 41

Tierney, Jack, 275–76

Tobacco and Health Research Institute, 342

tobacco industry:

  Harvard Project funded by, 341–43

  link between smoking and cancer denied by, 281–82

  NFL compared to, 6–7, 244, 280–83

Tomczak, Mike, 63

Toon, Al, 70, 73, 117

  concussions of, 70–71, 131

  retirement of, 79, 109, 125, 126, 189

Udall, Tom, 314–16

United States Football League, 107

University of Pittsburgh Medical Center (UPMC), 36, 66, 112–13, 149, 154, 174, 183, 194, 312, 313

  helmet study of, 184–87, 211–12, 315, 316, 317–18

Upchurch, Rick, 323

Upshaw, Gene, 244–45, 297, 299

Viano, Dave, 143–44, 210, 211, 221, 227–28, 266, 335

  in demand for Omalu paper retraction, 189–92

  McKee's findings attacked by, 269, 270

  as MTBI Committee cochair, 215, 227, 286

  resignation of, 283, 286

Virginia, University of, 33, 34

Vodvarka, James, 85–86, 89, 90, 95–96, 97, 100

Waeckerle, Joe, 222

Walker, Wayne, 350

Wallace, Steve, 81

Wall Street Journal, 33, 281

War and Peace in the Global Village (McLuhan), 318

Warner, Kurt, 347

Washington, Joe, 299

Washington Post, 80, 215, 350

Washington State, football safety laws in, 288, 314

Waters, Andre, 210, 229
  CTE in, 203, 204, 213, 291
  suicide of, 201, 204, 295

Webster, Betty, 17–18

Webster, Bill, 17, 19

Webster, Brooke, 24, 83–84

Webster, Colin, 17, 23, 58, 83, 86, 91, 95, 96, 101, 104

Webster, Garrett, 22, 49–50, 54, 102, 103–4, 207, 242–43, 261

Webster, Joey, 17–18

Webster, Mike:
  as advocate for brain-damage issues, 94–95
  autopsy of, 2, 4, 5, 9–10, 151–52, 233
  brain disease diagnosed in, 89–90
  as Chiefs' strength and conditioning coach, 50–51
  childhood of, 17–19
  concussions of, 138
  consecutive-play streak of, 27
  constant pain of, 49
  death of, 104, 148, 207–9, 295
  deep-seated fear as motivator of, 24, 26–27, 28
  disability case of, 87–92, 95, 98–101, 168
  divorce of, 54
  elected to Hall of Fame, 56–58
  erratic behavior of, 3, 10, 29–30, 47, 48–51
  and family history of mental illness, 17

financial problems of, 47, 48–49, 54

in first training camp, 13–16

Fitzsimmons's friendship with, 89, 92, 94, 96, 105

forged prescription arrest of, 95–97, 98

growing hatred of Steelers and NFL expressed by, 90–91, 104

at Hall of Fame induction, 3, 58–62, 83

headaches of, 26

head injuries as unreported by, 26

head used as battering ram by, 25

heart attack as cause of death of, 10, 148

heart disease of, 103–4

intensity of, 19–20, 21

Jani and, 51–54, 57–58, 85, 94, 103–4

Kansas City house of, 29–30, 47, 48

letters of, 91–93, 102–3

mental and physical deterioration of, 3, 53, 54–55, 57, 84, 85–86, 90, 91, 101–3

NFL lawsuit of, 101, 168–70, 192

in 1974 Steelers draft, 20

in Nutcracker drill, 15–16

Otto and, 352

paranoia of, 50, 61, 90–91

pills and supplements taken by, 22–23, 84, 86

as prankster, 23

Pro Bowl appearances by, 24

psychiatric exams of, 89–90

religious beliefs of, 16–17

retirement of, 29, 47

Ritalin addiction of, 3, 55, 60, 83, 86, 89, 94, 95–97

Stage and, 47–48, 61

steroid use by, 22

stun guns owned by, 84–85

Super Bowl rings of, 52, 94

training regimen of, 19, 21–22

at University of Wisconsin, 19–20

unrealistic business plans of, 48, 56, 58, 83
weapons owned by, 3, 84–85, 91
Westbrook's examination of, 98–99
Webster, Mike, brain of:
Alzheimer's brain vs., 158, 161
beta-amyloid plaque in, 158
CTE diagnosed in, 207, 338
DeKosky's examination of, 162–63
Hamilton's examination of, 160–61
normal external appearance of, 10, 152
Omalu's autopsy of, 157–58, 159, 194
Omalu's decision to preserve, 10, 152–53, 155–56
Omalu's paper on, 163–65, 188–92, 202, 215, 257
tau buildup in, 157–58, 235
Webster, Pam, 20, 21, 24, 26, 29, 50, 54, 60, 104–5, 168
Mike's erratic behavior and, 29–30, 47, 48–49
at Webster's Hall of Fame induction, 61
Webster, Reid, 18, 19
Wecht, Cyril, 152–53, 154–55, 160, 164, 194–96, 260
Weiner, Anthony, 290
Wenzel, Ralph, 302
Werley, Jonette, 156
Westbrook, Edward, 98–99, 169
West Chester University, 171
White, Reggie, 40

Widmeyer Communications, 250
Wiley, Clayton, 205
Wilkinson, Bud, 13
Williams, Aeneas, 108
Wilson, Otis, 296
Winning with Integrity (Steinberg), 76
Wisconsin, University of, 19–20
Withnall, Chris, 184
Wolfley, Craig, 22
Woodard, John, 177–78
woodpeckers, brains of, 1, 2
workers' compensation, former players' claims for, 306–7
World Class Expeditions, 258
Worley, Tim, 41–42
Woschitz, Frank, health survey of, 68, 69, 113, 114
Wynder, Ernst, 281, 283, 341

Yates, Tony, 64, 126, 145, 221–22
Young, Barbara Graham, 108, 111
Young, Steve, 79, 171
background of, 106–7
concussions of, 107–12, 167, 283, 337–38
retirement of, 111, 112
Youngblood, Jack, 292
"Youth Health & Safety Luncheon," 321–22

Zackery Lystedt Law, 288, 314
Zamorano, J. R., 71, 77
Zegart, Dan, 281, 341, 342